CANCER OBSTETRICS *AND* GYNECOLOGY

CANCER OBSTETRICS *AND* GYNECOLOGY

Editors

Edward L. Trimble, M.D., M.P.H.
Head of Surgery Section
Cancer Therapy Evaluation Program
National Cancer Institute
Bethesda, Maryland;
Associate Professor
Departments of Gynecology, Obstetrics, and Oncology
Johns Hopkins University School of Medicine
Baltimore, Maryland

Cornelia Liu Trimble, M.D.
Director of Colposcopy Clinics
Department of Gynecology and Obstetrics
Johns Hopkins Hospital
Baltimore, Maryland;
Assistant Professor
Departments of Gynecology, Obstetrics, and Oncology
Johns Hopkins University School of Medicine
Baltimore, Maryland

LIPPINCOTT WILLIAMS & WILKINS
A **Wolters Kluwer** Company
Philadelphia • Baltimore • New York • London
Buenos Aires • Hong Kong • Sydney • Tokyo

Acquisitions Editor: Stuart Freeman
Production Editor: Melanie Bennitt
Manufacturing Manager: Kevin Watt
Cover Designer: Christine Jenny
Compositor: Lippincott Williams & Wilkins Desktop Division
Printer: Edwards Brothers

227 East Washington Square
Philadelphia, PA 19106-3780 USA
LWW.com

Printed in the USA

Library of Congress Cataloging-in-Publication Data
Cancer obstetrics and gynecology / edited by Edward L. Trimble, Cornelia Liu Trimble.
p. cm.
Includes bibliographical references and index.
ISBN 0-7817-1410-9 (alk. paper)
1. Cancer in women. 2. Cancer in women—Complications. 3. Generative organs, Female—Cancer. 4. Generative organs, Female—Cancer—Complications. I. Trimble, Edward L. II. Trimble, Cornelia Liu.
[DNLM: 1. Neoplasms—complications. 2. Neoplasms—psychology. 3. Pregnancy Complications, Neoplastic. 4. Reproduction. 5. Sexuality. WQ 240 C2155 1999]
RC281.W65C356 1999
616.99′465—dc21
DNLM/DLC 99-21823
for Library of Congress CIP

Care has been taken to confirm the accuracy of the information presented and to describe generally accepted practices. However, the authors, editors, and publisher are not responsible for errors or omissions or for any consequences from application of the information in this book and make no warranty, expressed or implied, with respect to the currency, completeness, or accuracy of the contents of the publication. Application of this information in a particular situation remains the professional responsibility of the practitioner.

The authors, editors, and publisher have exerted every effort to ensure that drug selection and dosage set forth in this text are in accordance with current recommendations and practice at the time of publication. However, in view of ongoing research, changes in government regulations, and the constant flow of information relating to drug therapy and drug reactions, the reader is urged to check the package insert for each drug for any change in indications and dosage and for added warnings and precautions. This is particularly important when the recommended agent is a new or infrequently employed drug.

Some drugs and medical devices presented in this publication have Food and Drug Administration (FDA) clearance for limited use in restricted research settings. It is the responsibility of the health care provider to ascertain the FDA status of each drug or device planned for use in their clinical practice.

10 9 8 7 6 5 4 3 2 1

To DL and all those women with cancer in whose care

we have been privileged to participate.

Contents

Contributing Authors

Barbara L. Andersen, Ph.D. *Professor, Departments of Psychology and Gynecology and Obstetrics, Ohio State University, 1885 Neil Avenue, Columbus, Ohio 43210*

Deborah K. Armstrong, M.D. *Active Staff, Department of Oncology, Johns Hopkins Hospital, Baltimore, Maryland; Assistant Professor, Department of Oncology, Johns Hopkins University School of Medicine, 600 North Wolfe Street, Baltimore, Maryland 21287*

Joanna Brell, M.D. *Moll Cancer Center, Fairview Hospital, Physician Suite, 2nd Floor, 18200 Lorain Avenue, Cleveland, Ohio 44111*

Robert E. Bristow, M.D. *Assistant Professor, Department of Gynecology and Obstetrics, Johns Hopkins Hospital and Johns Hopkins University School of Medicine, 600 North Wolfe Street, Houck 248, Baltimore, Maryland 21287*

Anuradha Chakravarthy, M.D. *Assistant Professor, Department of Radiation Oncology, Vanderbilt University Medical Center and Vanderbilt University School of Medicine, 1301 22nd Avenue South, Suite 902, Nashville, Tennessee 37232*

Jennifer Cohen-Kogan, M.D. *Department of General Internal Medicine, Hospital of the University of Pennsylvania, 3100 Spruce Street, 3rd Floor, Silverstein, Suite D, Philadelphia, Pennsylvania 19104*

Linda R. Duska, M.D. *Instructor, Department of Gynecologic Oncology, Massachusetts General Hospital, Gillette Center for Women's Cancer, Cox 120, 100 Blossom Street, Boston, Massachusetts 02114*

Jairo E. Garcia, M.D. *Director of IVF Program, Department of Reproductive Endocrinology, Johns Hopkins Hospital, Baltimore, Maryland; Associate Professor, Department of Reproductive Endocrinology, Johns Hopkins University School of Medicine, 600 North Wolfe Street, Houck 249, Baltimore, Maryland 21287*

Carolyn Johnston, M.D. *Clinical Assistant Professor, Department of Obstetrics and Gynecology, University of Michigan, 1500 East Medical Center Drive, WHL4606, Ann Arbor, Michigan 48109*

Matt Kalaycio, M.D. *Director of Leukemia Program, Department of Hematology and Medical Oncology, Cleveland Clinic Foundation, 9500 Euclid Avenue, Cleveland, Ohio 44195*

Michael E. Lantz, M.D. *Director, Department of Gynecology and Obstetrics, Johns Hopkins Bayview Medical Center, Baltimore, Maryland 21224; Assistant Professor, Department of Gynecology and Obstetrics, Johns Hopkins University School of Medicine, 600 North Wolfe Street, Baltimore, Maryland 21287*

James F. Lilja, M.D. *Fellow, Department of Obstetrics and Gynecology, University of Michigan, 1500 East Medical Center Drive, WHL4602, Ann Arbor, Michigan 48109*

J. Rebecca Liu, M.D. *Fellow, Department of Obstetrics and Gynecology, University of Michigan and University of Michigan Medical Center, 1500 East Medical Center Drive, WHL4602, Ann Arbor, Michigan 48109*

Janice A. Lyons, M.D. *Department of Radiation Oncology, Cleveland Clinic Foundation, 9500 Euclid Avenue, Cleveland, Ohio 44195*

Roger M. Macklis, M.D. *Professor and Chairman, Department of Radiation Oncology, Cleveland Clinic Foundation, 9500 Euclid Avenue, Cleveland, Ohio 44195*

F.J. Montz, M.D., K.M. *Director, Department of Gynecologic Oncology, Johns Hopkins Hospital, Baltimore, Maryland; Professor, Department of Gynecology and Obstetrics, Johns Hopkins University School of Medicine, 600 North Wolfe Street, Houck 248, Baltimore, Maryland 21287*

Seamus O'Reilly, M.D., Ph.D., M.R.C.P.I. *Consultant Medical Oncologist, Waterford Regional Hospital, Waterford, Ireland; Assistant Professor, Department of Oncology, Johns Hopkins University School of Medicine, 600 North Wolfe Street, Baltimore, Maryland 21287*

Brad Pohlman, M.D. *Director of Lymphoma Program, Department of Hematology and Medical Oncology, Taussig Cancer Center, Cleveland Clinic Foundation, 9500 Euclid Avenue, Cleveland, Ohio 44195*

Thomas C. Randall, M.D. *Clinical Fellow, Department of Obstetrics and Gynecology, Hospital of the University of Pennsylvania, 3100 Spruce Street, 1000 Courtyard, Philadelphia, Pennsylvania 19104*

Cornelia Liu Trimble, M.D. *Director of Colposcopy Clinics, Department of Gynecology and Obstetrics, Johns Hopkins Hospital, Baltimore, Maryland; Assistant Professor, Departments of Gynecology, Obstetrics, and Oncology, Johns Hopkins University School of Medicine, 600 North Wolfe Street, Harvey 319, Baltimore, Maryland 21287*

Edward L. Trimble, M.D., M.P.H. *Head of Surgery Section, Cancer Therapy Evaluation Program, National Cancer Institute, Bethesda, Maryland 20892; Associate Professor, Departments of Gynecology, Obstetrics, and Oncology, Johns Hopkins University School of Medicine, 600 North Wolfe Street, Houck 248, Baltimore, Maryland 21287*

Howard A. Zacur, M.D., Ph.D. *Director, Department of Gynecology and Obstetrics, Johns Hopkins Hospital and Johns Hopkins University School of Medicine, 600 North Wolfe Street, Houke 247, Baltimore, Maryland 21287*

Preface

When a woman is first diagnosed with cancer, she and her physicians often concentrate on treatment of the cancer. As discussions about therapeutic options unfold, however, women and their physicians must address how cancer treatment will affect ongoing health issues.

The main focus of this book is on the management of gynecologic and obstetric issues in cancer patients and cancer survivors. We devote chapters to various reproductive issues, such as sexuality, contraception, abnormal menstrual bleeding, assisted reproductive techniques, pregnancy, and menopause, as they affect the woman with cancer. In addition, we have included chapters addressing the obstetric and gynecologic issues associated with *specific* cancers.

Effective cancer care requires a multidisciplinary approach. We are grateful to our coauthors, who represent the disciplines of psychology, gynecologic oncology, medical oncology/hematology, internal medicine, radiation oncology, maternal-fetal medicine, and reproductive endocrinology, for their thoughtful contributions. We hope that this book will be useful to all those who care for women with cancer.

CANCER OBSTETRICS *AND* GYNECOLOGY

1

Ovulation, Menstruation, and Contraception in the Cancer Patient

Linda R. Duska, *Cornelia Liu Trimble, and *†Edward L. Trimble

*Department of Gynecologic Oncology, Massachusetts General Hospital, Gillette Center for Women's Cancer, Boston, Massachusetts 02114; *Departments of Gynecology, Obstetrics, and Oncology, Johns Hopkins University School of Medicine, Baltimore, Maryland 21287; and †Division of Cancer Treatment and Diagnosis, National Cancer Institute, Bethesda, Maryland 20892*

Normal ovulation and the menstrual cycle involve a complex interaction of the hypothalamus, pituitary, and ovary. Premenopausal patients who have survived cancer and cancer therapy or are currently undergoing cancer therapy are likely to suffer from disturbances of ovulation and the menstrual cycle for a variety of reasons. Physiologic consequences may include amenorrhea, dysfunctional uterine bleeding, premature ovarian failure, and infertility, as well as the loss of estrogenic benefits to the skeletal and cardiovascular systems. Whether or not the changes will be permanent depends on many factors, including type of treatment, length of treatment, and patient age.

The success of modern cancer therapy is perhaps best demonstrated by the number of people today who call themselves cancer survivors. One result of this success, however, is the number of women who are left with damage to their reproductive systems. The purpose of this chapter is to review normal ovulation and menstruation, disruption of both of these by cancer and cancer therapy, and contraception options for cancer patients.

First, it is appropriate to address some definitions of terms that will be used throughout this discussion. *Menopause* is defined as the permanent cessation of menstruation resulting from the loss of ovarian follicular activity. *Premature menopause,* also called premature ovarian failure, is defined as the cessation of menses before age 40 years. *Ovarian ablation* is defined as medically induced cessation of ovarian function. Ovarian ablation may be induced permanently through radiation, oophorectomy, or chemotherapy, or temporarily through luteinizing hormone–releasing hormone (LH-RH) agonists. *Amenorrhea* is defined as the absence or cessation of menstrual flow. Primary amenorrhea occurs in women who have never menstruated, and will not be discussed here. Secondary amenorrhea is defined as at least 3 months of amenorrhea in a woman who previously had menses. Finally, *dysfunctional uterine bleeding* is uterine bleeding that is abnormal for the patient.

NORMAL PHYSIOLOGY/EMBRYOLOGY OF THE OVARY

Development of the ovary begins in fetal life. Approximately 3 weeks following conception, the primordial germ cells arise from the yolk sac and migrate to the developing gonads. Beginning at gestational age 11 to 12 weeks, the fetal germ cells enter the first meiotic division and arrest in prophase, becoming oogonia.

By gestational age 16 to 20 weeks, the fetus will have 6 to 7 million oogonia, the most that it will have in its lifetime. The first meiosis will not be completed until adult life, when the primary oocyte completes the first meiotic division to become the secondary oocyte.

In fetal life, a continuous cycle of follicular formation, ripening, and atresia occurs, although full follicular maturity and ovulation are not achieved. Estrogen production does not begin until late in fetal life. As a result of fetal oocyte depletion, the neonate is born with only 1 to 2 million germ cells. Unlike spermatogenesis, which continues throughout a male's lifetime, no new germ cells will form in females after birth.

The two gonadotropins produced by the pituitary are follicle-stimulating hormone (FSH) and luteinizing hormone (LH). Release of these hormones is controlled by the ovary via a complicated feedback system, as well as by the hypothalamus via release of gonadotropin-releasing hormone (Gn-RH). During childhood, gonadotropin levels in the pituitary are low, and the hypothalamus is suppressed. The process of follicular atresia in the ovary, however, continues throughout childhood. By the onset of puberty, about 300,000 germ cells remain. From puberty until menopause, follicular growth occurs as a continuous process in a cyclic fashion. By menopause, only a few hundred germ cells remain. In the last 10 years to menopause, there is an acceleration of follicular loss.

MENSTRUAL CYCLE

Pulsatile secretion of Gn-RH by the hypothalamus results in the release of FSH and LH by the pituitary. The normal menstrual cycle is divided into three phases: the follicular phase, ovulation, and the luteal phase.

In the *follicular phase* of the cycle, multiple follicles are recruited through the action of FSH release from the pituitary. The granulosa cells surrounding the oocytes produce estrogen during this portion of the cycle. Together, estrogen and FSH increase the number of FSH receptors on the follicle. While many follicles are recruited for each cycle, in the majority of cycles only one follicle will reach complete maturity and progress to ovulation. High estrogen levels produced by the granulosa cells stimulate a hypothalamic Gn-RH pulse, which in turn results in a surge of LH from the pituitary. Concomitantly, the estrogen levels produced by the dominant follicle suppress FSH secretion. The length of the follicular phase may vary, accounting for the variability in the length of normal menstrual cycles.

Once *ovulation* occurs, the cycle enters the *luteal phase* dominated by the hormone progesterone, produced by the corpus luteum. The postovulatory phase is normally 11 to 14 days in length and is less varied than the follicular phase. If pregnancy does not occur, then the corpus luteum will undergo atresia and stop producing progesterone. Progesterone and estrogen withdrawal results in menstrual flow, and the cycle begins anew.

The regulation of the menstrual cycle depends on the regularity of ovulation. During the follicular phase, the endometrium becomes lush and thick under the influence of estrogen. During the luteal phase, the endometrium is stabilized and decidualized via the action of progesterone. Any disruption in the ovulatory cycle therefore will result in dysfunctional uterine bleeding. Anovulation can result in several bleeding patterns. Estrogen production unaccompanied by progesterone stabilization will result in an unstable endometrium subject to irregular sloughing. High levels of estrogen will result in a thick and unstable endometrium and therefore periodic, very heavy bleeding. Low levels of estrogen, on the other hand, will result in an atrophic but still unstable endometrium and light, irregular spotting. Withdrawal of progesterone support will also result in menstrual bleeding.

Finally, normal menstrual patterns depend on normal platelet and coagulation factors. If these functions are affected by drugs or systemic illness, abnormal bleeding may ensue.

The evaluation of women with amenorrhea or oligomenorrhea is made difficult by the inaccessibility of the ovary and the germ cells. In men, the testis is relatively accessible for biopsy. In contrast, the ovary is not as easily accessible for biopsy, and oocytes cannot be easily retrieved. Therefore, ovarian function must be inferred by analyzing menstrual history and measuring serum hormone and gonadotropin levels. Recording of a menstrual history alone is a crude measure of ovarian function, and amenorrhea is not synonymous with infertility. Moreover, the presence of menstrual cycles does not always imply fertility.

Menstrual disorders and infertility following both chemotherapy and radiation are believed to be the result of primary ovarian failure leading to a hypergonadotropic hypogonadism, similar to the menopause. Because there is no longer production of estrogen by the ovary, and therefore no negative feedback on the pituitary, the pituitary begins to produce large amounts of FSH and LH. Thus, in patients with primary ovarian failure, as in normal menopause, serum levels of estradiol are low and serum levels of FSH and LH are elevated.

An excellent illustration of the risk of premature menopause associated with cancer therapy is provided by Byrne et al. (1) They evaluated the risks of early menopause in 1067 women in whom cancer was diagnosed before age 20 years, who were at least 5-year survivors, and who were still menstruating at age 21. Self-reported menopause status was compared to 1599 controls. Women diagnosed with cancer before age 12 did not appear to be at increased risk for premature menopause. Women diagnosed with cancer between ages 13 and 19 years faced a relative risk of premature menopause of 2.32%, compared to controls. The relative risk of early menopause associated with radiotherapy alone was 3.7% and with alkylating agents alone 9.17%.

SINGLE-AGENT CHEMOTHERAPY

Chemotherapeutic agents have been used in the treatment of rheumatologic diseases since the 1950s (2). In particular, cyclophosphamide, an alkylating agent, is used not only for malignant conditions but also for several benign conditions, including nephrotic syndrome, chronic glomerulonephritis, rheumatoid arthritis, and systemic lupus erythematosus. Unfortunately, however, when given to ovulating women in a continuous manner for longer than 6 months, cyclophosphamide appears to be the most damaging of the commonly used chemotherapeutic agents (3). Alkylating agents cause cellular damage independent of cell cycle; they can thus affect the resting oocyte. In the 1970s, concerns began to be raised about the effects of cyclophosphamide on fertility and the menstrual cycle. In 1971, Miller et al. (4) reported on a child treated with cyclophosphamide for benign disease. At autopsy, the child was noted to have ovaries that totally lacked ova and follicles and consisted only of stromal cells. This histologic finding suggested that cyclophosphamide action on the ovary resulted in complete destruction of ova and primary follicles. This initial report was followed by a letter to the editors of *Lancet* in 1972 reporting that 18 (53%) of 34 women treated with cyclophosphamide for benign disease had amenorrhea as a result (5). Amenorrhea occurred on average 7 months after starting treatment, and only one patient had a return of menses following cessation of treatment. In addition, patients complained of menopausal symptoms that required estrogen. One year later, another series, involving 22 women receiving cyclophosphamide for glomerulonephritis or rheumatoid arthritis, was reported (6). The 22 women ranged in age from 20 to 43 years, and all had normal regular menses prior to treatment. Amenorrhea related to therapy developed in 17 (77%) of these 22 women. Fourteen (82%) of the 17 women had hormonal and gonadotropin patterns consistent with primary ovarian failure. In this study, there was no relationship between patient age and duration of therapy before development of amenorrhea. Notably, however, three women became pregnant during therapy, which emphasizes the importance of contraception during and following chemotherapy. Six patients with amenorrhea underwent ovarian biopsies. Ova were seen in only two of the six biopsies; the ova appeared abnormal, with no evidence of follicular development.

Prolonged daily oral administration of cyclophosphamide in one Japanese study of patients with breast cancer resulted in amenorrhea in 17 (94%) of 18 premenopausal patients (7). In contrast to the study just described (6), in this study the onset of amenorrhea was related to patient age, with older patients being more sensitive to cyclophosphamide. Patients who experienced permanent amenorrhea had received 4 g or more of cyclophosphamide. Urinary estrogens and progesterone, as well as serum LH and FSH, were measured. After the onset of amenorrhea, levels of estrogen and progesterone were noted to be suppressed, while FSH and LH levels were markedly elevated, again consistent with primary ovarian failure. Three patients underwent oophorectomy following cyclophosphamide therapy. Histologic evaluation of their ovaries revealed no ovarian follicles, again supporting the diagnosis of primary ovarian failure. In fact, the total absence of follicles in the ovaries examined histologically supported the diagnosis of a permanent, rather than temporary, ovarian failure. Cyclophosphamide treatment therefore resulted in chemical ovarian ablation. Permanent amenorrhea developed in all 13 patients older than 40 years.

Finally, cyclophosphamide treatment has been shown to be ablative to the ovary in a rat model (2). In a study by Montz et al. (3), rats were treated with varying doses of intraperitoneal cyclophosphamide. Histologic evaluation of the ovaries following treatment revealed that 80% or more of follicles were destroyed at cyclophosphamide doses of 8 and 12 mg/kg. Lower doses resulted in less follicular damage.

In summary, use of the single alkylating agent cyclophosphamide results in primary ovarian failure in 54% to 94% of patients treated, secondary to permanent destruction of oocytes. The effect of cyclophosphamide on the ovary depends on the total dose of drug used and the age of the patient being treated. Cyclophosphamide and other alkylating agents in combination regimens are thought to be responsible for ovarian ablation in many patients. Prior to the introduction of paclitaxel (Taxol) in the primary treatment of ovarian cancer, the combination of cyclophosphamide and cisplatin (Platinol) was the first-line treatment for ovarian cancer. Cyclophosphamide is also used in chemotherapy regimens for Hodgkin's disease and breast cancer. Other alkylating agents have been implicated in primary ovarian failure, including chlorambucil (Leukeran), busulfan (Myleran), mechlorethamine hydrochloride (Mustargen, nitrogen mustard), vinblastine sulfate (Velban), and mitomycin (Mutamycin).

Single-agent chemotherapy with etoposide (VePesid) has also been implicated in ovarian failure. Etoposide, a semisynthetic derivative of podophyllotoxin, interferes at the G_2 portion of the cell cycle. At a low level, it prevents cells from entering prophase; at higher levels, it can cause lysis of cells entering mitosis. Single-agent etoposide has successfully been used to treat young patients with gestational trophoblastic disease (GTD). In 1985, Choo et al. (8) reported on 22 patients with residual GTD treated with single-agent etoposide. Following an average dose of 5 g, temporary ovarian failure developed in five young patients, and two older patients experienced permanent ovarian failure as measured by serum gonadotropins. Matsui et al. (9). studied 47 patients with low-risk GTD treated with single-agent etoposide. Pituitary and ovarian function were assessed by measuring serum LH, FSH, estradiol, and progesterone levels, as well as by evaluating LH and FSH responses to LH-RH administration. Patients were divided into groups according to age. Women older than 40 years were noted to have significantly higher basal levels of LH and FSH following therapy. The interval between the cessation of chemotherapy and the return of ovulation increased with advanced patient age. Although ovulation returned in all 31 patients younger than age 40, only four of nine patients older than 40 resumed ovulation. The amount of etoposide administered did not appear to affect the return of ovulation.

COMBINATION CHEMOTHERAPY: HODGKIN'S DISEASE

In the United States, it has been estimated that in 1998 there will be 27,700 cases of Hodgkin's disease among women, with 12,600 deaths (10). Hodgkin's disease is a disease of young people. Treatment produces long-term remissions in more than 70% of patients. However, successful eradication of malignancy results in amenorrhea and infertility in more than 50% of premenopausal patients. One of the first reports of amenorrhea following treatment for Hodgkin's disease came from Yale–New Haven Hospital in 1971 (11). Ten female patients, ages 22 to 44 years, were treated for Hodgkin's disease with a variety of chemotherapeutic agents, including intravenous nitrogen mustard and chlorambucil. All patients had normal menstrual cycles prior to beginning treatment. No patient had prior pelvic or paraaortic radiation. All patients reported menstrual irregularities beginning 1 to 2 months following initiation of chemotherapy. Notably, once again, one patient who was treated with vinblastine alone became pregnant during chemotherapy—again emphasizing the need for contraceptive use in this population of patients. In eight patients, serum FSH and LH were measured, and in six of these patients the values were in the postmenopausal range. In two patients who had histologic evaluation of their ovaries, markedly atrophic ovaries were noted with an absence of follicular development.

Chapman et al. (12) reported 41 women with advanced Hodgkin's disease who underwent combination chemotherapy. All but one patient were treated with mechlorethamine, vinblastine, procarbazine hydrochloride (Matulane), and prednisolone (MVPP). The age range of patients was 20 to 51 years. Serum hormone levels were measured, and five patients underwent ovarian biopsy. On the basis of menstrual and fertility history, all the women had normal function prior to receiving chemotherapy. However, following therapy only 7 (17%) of 41 appeared to have unaffected gonadal function. In 20 (49%) of 41 women, LH and FSH levels were elevated, with estradiol levels in the postmenopausal range, consistent with primary ovarian failure. All 20 of these women were amenorrheic, and 17 reported postmenopausal symptoms, including hot flashes and vaginal dryness. The remaining 14 women reported oligomenorrhea. Notably, in this study, ovarian function observed over time became progressively impaired. The authors concluded that the majority of patients would eventually have complete ovarian failure by their early 30s.

A similar study from the National Cancer Institute was reported in 1981 (13). Twenty-four female patients with normal menstrual histories prior to treatment were selected for study. All patients were treated with methotrexate, vincristine sulfate (Oncovin), procarbazine, and prednisone (MOPP) chemotherapy and achieved complete remission. The median age at the time of evaluation was 30 years (range, 18 to 46 years). Patients were assessed via menstrual history, and serum FSH and LH levels were obtained. In this study, 48% were noted to menstruate regularly at a median of 9 years following chemotherapy. The remainder were amenorrheic. This group of patients was older than the menstruating patients, and the difference in age was statistically significant. In addition, the time from diagnosis to the occurrence of amenorrhea was significantly shorter for patients older than 25 years. Moreover, in seven patients, the onset of amenorrhea was gradual, occurring over 3 to 9 years. In fact, two of these patients were able to conceive prior to becoming amenorrheic. Total chemotherapy dose did not appear to be associated with amenorrhea. This study was unusual in the long-term follow-up of patients reported. Eighty percent of patients younger than 25 years had preserved ovarian function even 5 to 10 years following treatment. However, chemotherapeutic ovarian ablation seemed to be permanent. Women age 39 years or older became amenorrheic within 1 year of completing chemotherapy. Most of these women reported a gradual, rather than acute, change in their menstrual cycles.

A larger study of 103 women with Hodgkin's disease, most of whom received combination chemotherapy and irradiation, was reported in 1981 (14). The study was conducted via a mailed questionnaire, with questions related to menstrual history and pregnancy outcomes since chemotherapy. Patients were not examined, nor were serum gonadotropins measured. Thirty-two patients reported amenorrhea. A multivariate analysis was undertaken to determine factors predicting regular menses; the variables included interval after completion of treatment, stage of disease, number of cycles of chemotherapy, and dose of pelvic radiation Only age was found to be a significant predictor. The increased probability of regular menses was more striking in women younger than 30. Twenty of 26 women who attempted pregnancy were successful. Patients in this study became pregnant despite temporary amenorrhea and premature menopausal symptoms. However, no woman with permanent amenorrhea or menopausal symptoms became pregnant. Finally, women who received both pelvic irradiation and combination chemotherapy had a marked reduction in reproductive potential.

Seventy-four women treated with MOPP chemotherapy were reported by Andrieu and Ochoa-Molina (15). Again, the patients were evaluated via a mailed questionnaire. Sixty-eight patients were considered evaluable. Median age was 27 years. Follow-up ranged from 3 to 7.5 years. Sixteen women became amenorrheic, and two others reported oligomenorrhea (total, 26%). Again, the proportion of oligomenorrheic to amenorrheic women was significantly different, depending on patient age at the time of therapy. Fewer than 5% of patients younger than 30 were oligomenorrheic or amenorrheic, compared with 61.6% of women older than 30. Once again, the amount of chemotherapy given (three versus six cycles) was not found to be a significant predictor of ovarian failure.

In summary, then, primary ovarian failure occurred in at least 50% of women treated with MOPP. Ovarian failure following chemotherapy has consistently been shown to be related to patient age, with younger women more likely to maintain normal ovarian function. However, it is notable that premature menopause will eventually develop in many of these younger women if followed sufficiently long after chemotherapy. Therapy with doxorubicin hydrochloride (Adriamycin), bleomycin sulfate (Blenoxane), vinblastine, and dacarbazine (DTIC-Dome) (ABVD) was noted in one study to be less toxic to the gonads and thus should be considered as an alternative therapy for young women who wish to maintain their fertility (16)

COMBINATION CHEMOTHERAPY: BREAST CANCER

Breast cancer is the most common malignancy among American women. In the United States in 1998, it was predicted that there will be 178,000 new cases of breast cancer, with 43,500 deaths anticipated (10). Seven percent of breast cancers occur by age 40 years, and nearly 25% of women diagnosed with breast cancer are premenopausal (17). Ovarian ablation has frequently been noted in women who receive adjuvant combination chemotherapy.

In 1978, Samaan et al. (18) reported that amenorrhea developed in 39 (71%) of 55 premenopausal women with breast cancer treated with cyclophosphamide, doxorubicin (Adriamycin), and 5-fluorouracil (CAF) and BCG immunotherapy. The mean age of the 39 women in whom amenorrhea developed was 44.9 years, compared to a mean age of 33.5 years among the 17 patients in whom amenorrhea did not develop. Eleven of the 38 women in whom amenorrhea developed agreed to further endocrinologic testing. All had elevated levels of LH and FSH at baseline and after LR-RH stimulation, consistent with ovarian ablation. Rose and Davis (19) in 1980 reported permanent amenorrhea with elevated levels of LH and FSH in 13 of 15 patients treated with cyclophosphamide, methotrexate, and 5-fluorouracil (CMF), 8 of 10 patients treated with CMF and prednisone, and all 13 patients treated with CMF, prednisone, and tamoxifen. They noted an inverse relationship between patient age and the length of therapy required to produce amenorrhea.

Dnistrian et al. (20) reported a similar study of the effect of CMF adjuvant chemotherapy in 14 premenopausal women with breast cancer. Ten additional premenopausal patients with recurrent breast cancer who underwent bilateral salpingo-oophorectomy served as surgically castrated controls, while 10 premenopausal women without cancer served as normal controls. Baseline and monthly serum hormone and gonadotropin levels were obtained. Chemotherapy resulted in primary ovarian failure as documented by hormonal analysis in 80% of patients. Twelve of 14 premenopausal patients became amenorrheic sometime during therapy and remained amenorrheic during the study follow-up period. There was an inverse relationship between age and duration of treatment required to induce ovarian suppression. Amenorrhea occurred within 2 to 4 months in patients age 40 or older. Younger women required larger cumulative doses of drug to induce ovarian dysfunction. Two patients younger than 30 years showed no evidence of ovarian suppression after 24 cycles of CMF therapy.

Bonadonna and Valagussa (21) subsequently reported the incidence of amenorrhea following CMF among 549 menstruating women. Among women younger than 40 years, 31% developed permanent amenorrhea and 23% reversible amenorrhea. Among women older than 30, 92% developed permanent amenorrhea and 4% reversible amenorrhea. Among younger women, patient age at treatment was the most important factor in determining both amenorrhea incidence and reversibility. Ravdin et al. (22) measured ovarian function in 49 premenopausal breast cancer patients following chemotherapy and tamoxifen. Of these, seven were still menstruating, all of whom had normal estradiol levels. Interestingly, though, 9 of 14 patients with irregular menses and 2 of 23 patients who were amenorrheic also had evidence of ovarian function as measured by serum estradiol levels. These investigators measured serial blood samples weekly over a 10-week period and thus may have had more opportunity to document ovarian activity than researchers who sampled less often. This finding supports the concept that menstrual history is only a crude measure of ovarian function. Again, age was an important aspect of postchemotherapy endocrine status, with 11 (85%) of 13 patients younger than 40 years showing evidence of ovarian function but only 8 (22%) of 36 patients older than 40 showing evidence of ovarian function. Moreover, preservation of ovarian function was dose-dependent. More than one-half (56%) of patients treated with fewer than six cycles of therapy maintained ovarian activity, while only 23% of patients treated with more than six cycles of therapy continued to have ovarian function.

Hortobagyi et al. (23) reported on the toxicity of doxorubicin-based adjuvant chemotherapy in 796 women with operable breast cancer treated between 1974 and 1982 at the University of Texas M.D. Anderson Cancer Center. The regimens used included CAF for 2 years, CMF for 2 years, and CAF with vincristine and prednisone for 6 to 12 months. Around 80% of premenopausal patients became amenorrheic during chemotherapy. The incidence of amenorrhea was age-dependent. Of those women younger than 30 years, none had a change in menses. Amenorrhea during chemotherapy developed in one-third of those 30 to 39 years of age, 96% of those 40 to 49 years, and 100% of those older than 50. After completing chemotherapy, one-half of those younger than 40 resumed menstruation, while few over this age resumed menses.

Ovarian ablation has been used for the treatment of breast cancer for more than 100 years (24). Among premenopausal women with metastatic breast cancer, the response rate to ovarian ablation is about 33%. Ovarian ablation appears to be more effective in women older than 35 years and in those with estrogen receptor–positive tumors. In 1992, the Early Breast Cancer Trialists' Collaborative Group published a meta-analysis that included 1746 women younger than 50 years enrolled in various trials that evaluated ovarian ablation (25). At 15 years of follow-up, women who had undergone ovarian ablation experienced a 10.2% improvement in recurrence-free survival and a 10.6% improvement in overall survival, both of which were statistically significant. Survival benefits were seen in both node-negative and node-positive women. Adjuvant chemotherapy attenuated the effect of ovarian ablation, presumably because the chemotherapy rendered some women menopausal. Nonetheless, chemotherapy plus ovarian ablation decreased the annual rate of recurrence and death by 20%, compared to chemotherapy alone. Further study, however, is needed to define the role of ovarian ablation in conjunction with chemotherapy and hormonal therapy.

HORMONAL THERAPY: BREAST CANCER

Tamoxifen citrate (Nolvadex), a synthetic antiestrogen, has been shown to reduce the risk for recurrent and new breast cancers when used in the adjuvant setting after primary therapy (surgery with or without radiotherapy with or without chemotherapy) for breast cancer. More recently, it has been shown to decrease the incidence of primary breast cancer and carcinoma *in situ* among women at high risk for breast cancer (26). Tamoxifen, however, has been used to stimulate ovulation in therapy for infertility (27). It appears therefore to have a weak estrogenic effect on the ovary.

Sherman et al. (28) evaluated LH, FSH, estradiol, and progesterone levels in five healthy women who agreed to take tamoxifen, 20 mg per day for two to three menstrual cycles. All women continued to menstruate. Neither the mean cycle length nor the duration of the follicular or luteal phases was changed significantly by the tamoxifen. Mean estradiol and progesterone levels, however, were significantly elevated over normal values. Ravdin et al. (22) performed a similar study in premenopausal patients on adjuvant tamoxifen therapy following chemotherapy. Seven women who were having regular menses were identified in a cohort of 49 total women. These seven women, the remaining 42 women who were not regularly menstruating, and 12 healthy premenopausal controls had blood samples drawn for estradiol-17β and progesterone levels. Evidence of ovarian function was documented by normal estradiol-17β levels in all seven menstruating patients. Women taking tamoxifen who had ovarian function following chemotherapy were noted to have supraphysiologic serum levels of estradiol-17β. In fact, 12 of 21 patients who reported any recent menstrual activity while taking tamoxifen were noted to have supraphysiologic estradiol-17β levels. Jordan et al. (29) evaluated levels of LH, FSH, estradiol, estrone, progesterone, prolactin, and sex hormone–binding globulin (SHBG) in eight women with premenopausal stages I or II breast cancer. All eight were initially treated with mastectomy, followed by adjuvant tamoxifen without chemotherapy. All women continued to ovulate. They noted normal LH, FSH, and SHBG; elevated levels of estradiol, estrone, and progesterone; and decreased levels of prolactin.

Tamoxifen will therefore not affect ovulation in most premenopausal women. Women taking tamoxifen should use effective contraception.

MALIGNANT GERM CELL TUMORS OF THE OVARY

Malignant germ cell tumors of the ovary account for less than 5% of ovarian tumors and principally occur in young women and girls. Often, a secondary treatment objective is the preservation of fertility. Pektasides et al. (30) assessed gonadal function in 17 women with germ cell tumors treated with cisplatin, vincristine, methotrexate, bleomycin, actinomycin D (dactinomycin), cyclophosphamide, and etoposide. Although all patients had amenorrhea during chemotherapy, 16 of 17 had recovered menstrual function, with a median time of recovery of 4.5 months. Two women, however, were placed on oral contraceptives for irregular periods. Five women conceived after chemotherapy, with three full-term deliveries of healthy infants, two spontaneous abortions, one elective termination, and one continuing pregnancy. Gershenson (31) identified 40 patients with malignant germ cell tumors treated with surgery and combination chemotherapy with retention of the uterus and the normal contralateral ovary. Menstrual status was evaluated via a mailed questionnaire. The average age of patients at original diagnosis was 15 years, and various chemotherapeutic regimens were utilized, including vincristine, dactinomycin (Cosmegen), and cyclophosphamide (VAC); vincristine, bleomycin, and cisplatin (VBP); and bleomycin, etoposide, and cisplatin (BEP). All patients received combination chemotherapy. Ten patients were premenarchal at the time of diagnosis. Three of these patients experienced menarche during chemotherapy. Of the 33 patients who had menarche before or during chemotherapy, six (18%) had amenorrhea for the majority of the duration of chemotherapy. One patient became pregnant several months after beginning chemotherapy. After finishing chemotherapy, 27 patients (68%) maintained regular menses. Only two patients experienced amenorrhea: one for 6 months and the other for 9 months. Both had resumed regular menses at the time of the questionnaire. Only three patients had serious or persistent menstrual dysfunction. However, one of these three achieved a spontaneous pregnancy, indicating some level of ovarian function. Overall, patients in whom menstrual dysfunction developed after chemotherapy were older at diagnosis. However, the group of patients who had menstrual dysfunction did not differ from the group who continued normal menses with respect to cumulative alkylating agent doses, number of chemotherapy cycles, or duration of chemotherapy. Finally, nine patients conceived without difficulty following chemotherapy on one or more occasions. Four patients reported chronic infertility; however, only one of these four sought medical attention or seriously attempted pregnancy for more than one year. Only one patient had a long-term infertility problem. Eleven patients delivered 22 healthy infants, 21 of whom were born at term. Similar findings were reported by Wu et al. (32), who reported on 26 patients with germ cell tumors treated with conservative surgery followed by combination chemotherapy. The three patients in whom amenorrhea developed during chemotherapy all recovered to normal menstrual cycles after completion of therapy. One patient who received 11 courses of VAC remained amenorrheic. Of the 10 patients who desired pregnancy, seven achieved it and six achieved normal full-term deliveries.

HIGH-DOSE CHEMOTHERAPY WITH BONE MARROW TRANSPLANTATION

High-dose chemotherapy with bone marrow transplantation (BMT) is used primarily as a treatment for leukemia and lymphoma, although more recently it has been used for the treatment of solid tumors. High-dose chemotherapy often includes an alkylating agent. In patients with hematologic malignancies, total body irradiation (TBI) also may be administered. Gonadal damage from the high-dose regimens depends on the agents used, concomitant radiation therapy, the underlying disease, prior chemotherapy, and patient age (33).

Sarafoglou et al. (34) reported on 16 prepubertal girls who underwent BMT for acute leukemia. Cytoreduction before BMT included TBI in all patients. Of the 16 girls, nine (56%) had spontaneous pubertal development and regular menses. Six of these nine had elevated gonadotropins and three had normal levels of gonadotropins following treatment. While two of the six with elevated levels were noted to return to normal levels over 4 to 7 years, three others maintained elevated levels of gonadotropins despite regular menses. The remaining seven patients required estrogen replacement therapy because of delayed or arrested pubertal development. One patient developed regular menses after

5.5 years of estrogen replacement therapy. The girls with ovarian failure were older at the time of treatment than those with spontaneous puberty. There was no correlation between exposure to alkylating agents and loss of menstrual function. Keilholz et al. (35) reported on endocrine function and bone metabolism in 10 women following autologous BMT with high-dose chemotherapy. The mean age of the women was 37 years. Nine of 10 women reported secondary amenorrhea following BMT and received cyclic hormone replacement therapy for at least 2 years. One 25-year-old woman with Hodgkin's disease gave birth to two healthy children following autologous bone marrow stem cell transplant (ABSCT). She had secondary amenorrhea after transplantation, but spontaneous menstruation occurred 18 months following ABSCT. Thibaud et al. (36) reported on 31 girls following BMT. Again, chemotherapy was used both with and without TBI. Ovarian function was assessed by spontaneous breast development, onset of menses, and measurements of serum estradiol and gonadotropin. After a follow-up period of an average of 6 years, six patients had normal ovarian function. Two patients had oligomenorrhea with elevated gonadotropin, and 23 patients had no spontaneous estrogen activity. Sanders (37) recently reported on ovarian function in 65 women who underwent high-dose chemotherapy, which included cyclophosphamide, 200 mg/m^2, and BMT for aplastic anemia. All women younger than 26 years at time of chemotherapy recovered ovarian function, while 7 (39%) of the 18 women aged 26 to 38 years did not recover ovarian function.

In summary, premenopausal women receiving single or multiagent chemotherapy are at risk for short-term amenorrhea, as well as ovarian ablation. The risk of ovarian ablation appears to increase with advancing age, when ovarian reserve decreases. In addition, the risk of ovarian ablation increases with the dose of alkylating agents, notably cyclophosphamide. Even young women who resume menstruation after chemotherapy are at risk for early menopause. Women treated with chemotherapy in childhood and adolescence should be counseled that they may face an early menopause and should plan childbearing accordingly.

EFFECT OF RADIATION THERAPY ON OVARIAN FUNCTION AND MENSTRUATION

Radiation therapy is used in conjunction with chemotherapy in a number of clinical situations, including Hodgkin's disease and childhood leukemia and lymphomas. Ovarian damage is mediated by the total doses of radiation, as well as patient age at the time of exposure. The amount of radiation necessary to induce menopause in women older than 40 years is 600 rad (6 Gy), while women younger than 30 can tolerate 2000 to 3000 rad (20 to 30 Gy) in fractions without permanent sterility. Women who undergo abdominal and/or pelvic irradiation during childhood and adolescence, however, are at increased risk for premature menopause. Byrne et al. (1) reported that the relative risk of premature menopause associated with any radiotherapy treatment alone was 3.66%. If women had been treated with radiation below the diaphragm, as well as with alkylating agents, then the relative risk of premature menopause was 27.9%. These women reached menopause at a median age of 32 years. Women treated with subdiaphragmatic irradiation with or without chemotherapy in childhood or adolescence should be counseled that they may face an early menopause and should plan childbearing accordingly.

Studies with light and electron microscopes have shown that germ cells rapidly became pyknotic following irradiation (38). Initially, there is condensation of the chromosomes and damage to the nuclear envelope. Then, organelles become affected. Damaged oocytes can undergo either repair or atresia. The susceptibility of an oocyte to radiation depends on its developmental stage at the time of exposure. In the prenatal period, sensitivity is high. After birth, oocytes enter a resting phase of arrested development. In most species studied, the small primordial oocytes are more radiosensitive than developing oocytes (32). Unfortunately, the easiest model to study is the mouse model, and the mouse oocytes appear to be much more radiosensitive than human oocytes. In fact, it may be unreasonable to extrapolate from the mouse model to the human. Of necessity, most studies in humans evaluate menstrual history rather than ovarian histology.

PRESERVATION OF OVARIAN FUNCTION DURING RADIATION AND CHEMOTHERAPY

Patients treated with radiotherapy for advanced cervical and vaginal malignancies should be counseled that they will likely lose reproductive potential. Loss of reproductive potential in women treated for pelvic malignancies will be secondary to loss of ovulation, damage to the endometrium and myometrium, and cervical and vaginal stenosis.

Oophoropexy can be used to protect the ovaries from pelvic radiation. This technique involves surgically suspending the ovaries outside the anticipated radiation field. Oophoropexy can be performed via laparoscopy as well as laparotomy. The technique is useful in women who require pelvic irradiation for Hodgkin's disease, as well as for pelvic malignancies. Patients with Hodgkin's disease treated only with supradiaphragmatic radiation, however, have also been shown to have slightly decreased fertility rates, indicating some scatter effect to the ovaries.

Because chemotherapy, especially with alkylating agents, is known to cause premature ovarian failure, several authors have tried to identify ways to protect the ovaries from the cytotoxic effects of chemotherapeutic regimens. Many chemotherapeutic agents are more active against dividing cells. It has been hypothesized that nondividing oocytes might be protected from cytotoxicity. Chapman and Sutcliffe (39) considered the use of oral contraceptive pills in women undergoing chemotherapy for Hodgkin's disease. Six young women with untreated Hodgkin's disease were assessed prior to treatment via menstrual history, serum gonadotropin levels, and ovarian biopsy. Pretherapy gonadotropin levels and menstrual history were normal in five of the six women. The women ranged in age from 19 to 31 years. They were then all treated with six cycles of MVPP. At the beginning of chemotherapy, they were placed on combination oral contraceptives. Six to 12 weeks following the last cycle of chemotherapy, the menstrual cycles of all the women were reevaluated, and three women underwent repeat ovarian biopsy. Follow-up was repeated at intervals of 4 to 12 months. Posttherapy, five women reported normal menses. The three posttherapy ovarian biopsies were consistent in number of follicles to pretreatment biopsies, as well as to ovarian biopsies obtained from normal women not undergoing chemotherapy. The same authors had previously reported on women with Hodgkin's disease undergoing chemotherapy without oral contraceptives. Ovarian biopsies in these patients revealed a reduced number of follicles. From the results of these two small series, the authors thus concluded that oral contraceptives could protect the ovaries from follicular damage, and therefore from eventual ovarian failure. While the results of these studies are intriguing, one cannot conclude, without a large, randomized, controlled trial, that oral contraceptives confer protection to the ovary from chemotherapy.

Ataya et al. (40) used an animal model to test the effect of LH-RH agonists on the ovary following cyclophosphamide chemotherapy. Because LH-RH agonists are known to suppress gonadotropin receptors in the ovary, the authors' hypothesis was that the subsequent suppression of follicular development during cytotoxic chemotherapy would protect the dormant ovarian follicle from destruction. Multiple groups of rats were treated with varying doses of cyclophosphamide alone and cyclophosphamide plus LH-RH agonist. Cyclophosphamide treatment alone was noted to decrease the total number of follicles when compared with controls. The effect was noted mainly in medium to large follicles. When an

LH-RH agonist was administered with cyclophosphamide, it appeared to prevent the cyclophosphamide-induced reduction in total number of follicles. The decrease in follicular damage, however, was not statistically significant. When follicular size was considered, the number of large follicles was significantly lower in the cyclophosphamide and LH-RH groups than in the cyclophosphamide-alone group, while the number of small follicles was significantly higher. This finding is logical because the large follicles are the ones that are undergoing active development and the small follicles are thought to essentially be quiescent. Notably, accelerated atresia of follicles was noted in both groups.

Montz et al. (3) performed a similar study evaluating rats treated with cyclophosphamide and leuprolide acetate, a Gn-RH agonist. Animals were treated with cyclophosphamide alone and cyclophosphamide with either leuprolide or subcutaneous progesterone. Subsequently, fertility was measured by assessing mating and numbers of pups in the resulting litters. Cyclophosphamide-treated animals were noted to have decreased fertility rates following treatment. Once again, histologic evaluation of the ovaries demonstrated that higher doses of cyclophosphamide destroyed 80% or more of follicles. Lower doses of cyclophosphamide caused intermittent amounts of destruction. Progesterone was noted to protect the gonad from the negative effects of cyclophosphamide, maintaining fertility and fecundity not significantly different from those of control animals. Leuprolide, given once a day, however, failed to demonstrate any protective effect. However, the same dose of leuprolide given split on a 12-hour basis was able to protect fertility as by fecundity compared to controls. The authors concluded that progesterone was the most effective method in the rat model of protecting ovarian function as measured by fertility and fecundity. They suggested that a similar effect in women could be achieved via the use of medium-dosage oral contraceptives. They recommended that for suppression of the ovary prior to beginning chemotherapy, oral contraceptives should be started as soon as the decision to treat is made. Hormonal contraception should be continued uninterrupted until chemotherapy is completed.

Most recently, Blumenfeld et al. (41) reported on their experience with Gn-RH agonists in parallel with chemotherapy in women being treated for lymphoma. Eighteen women with lymphoma were studied. All women had regular cycles and normal pretreatment serum gonadotropins. A monthly injection of a 3.75-mg depot Gn-RH agonist was given in the early follicular phase of the menstrual cycle, starting 7 to 10 days prior to chemotherapy, and was continued until the conclusion of chemotherapy. Only 16 patients completed the treatment protocol. Thirteen of these were treated with MOPP and the remaining three with CHOP. A control group of 14 patients was used who received chemotherapy only without the Gn-RH agonist. Pretreatment hormone and gonadotropin levels were measured, and monthly levels were measured until spontaneous menses resumed. Hormonal and gonadotropin levels measured during chemotherapy with the Gn-RH agonist were consistent with ovarian suppression. Of the 16 women studied, 15 (94%) resumed spontaneous ovulation and menses within 3 to 8 months of completing therapy with the Gn-RH agonist. The oldest patient in the study group was age 40, and she experienced primary ovarian failure 4 months after treatment. In contrast, 7 (39%) of the 18 women in the control group resumed cyclic ovarian activity. The other 11 experienced premature ovarian failure. Notably, however, only 4 of the 16 patients in the study group received cyclophosphamide, while 10 of 18 in the control group received cyclophosphamide. However, of the four patients in the study group treated with cyclophosphamide, all resumed normal ovarian function, while only 4 of the 10 in the control group treated with cyclophosphamide resumed normal ovarian function. Finally, two patients (one in the study group and one in the control group) who underwent BMT and high-dose chemotherapy both became menopausal, consistent with the reports outlined above.

While the results of these studies of ovarian protection are promising, it must be remembered that the numbers are small and results in the animal model are not completely confirmatory. However, if oral contraceptives are not contraindicated, their use can be justified for reasons other than ovarian protection. Many reports in the literature have noted the occurrence of pregnancy during chemotherapy. Woman must face an agonizing choice when conception occurs while cytotoxic chemotherapy is being given: whether to continue with the pregnancy or undergo elective abortion. At the very least, the concurrent use of hormonal contraception would avoid this difficult situation. Moreover, Gn-RH agonists result in ovarian shutdown, or a temporary chemical menopause, and thus induce all the symptoms of an abrupt menopause, including hot flashes, impaired sleep, vaginal dryness, bone loss, and changes in lipid profiles. In the absence of firm data supporting a protective effect of Gn-RH agonists on ovarian function, hormonal contraception would appear to be a more acceptable method of preventing ovulation.

Ovarian function is essential for more than just fertility. The ovary is the primary source for estrogen, which has a major impact on skeletal and cardiovascular well-being. Moreover, loss of estrogen may cause disturbing symptoms in women, including but not limited to hot flashes, emotional swings, depression, vaginal dryness, dyspareunia, and decreased libido. It is vital that oncologists recognize the consequences of decreased or absent ovarian function.

DYSFUNCTIONAL UTERINE BLEEDING

The normal menstrual cycle depends on cyclic changes in estrogen and progesterone levels, as well as the integrity of the coagulation system, adequate platelets, and vasoconstriction of the spiral arterioles. Abnormalities in any of these components may cause abnormal uterine bleeding. Clinicians caring for women with cancer should understand the various etiologies of abnormal uterine bleeding, some of which may be associated with cancer therapy.

Normal menstrual bleeding occurs between menarche and menopause. The mean interval is every 28 days (range, 21 to 35 days). The mean duration of menstrual bleeding is 4 days (range, 1 to 8 days), with mean blood loss of 35 mL. When ascertaining a woman's history, a clinician should determine her normal menstrual pattern. Disruptions in an individual's normal menstrual pattern, even if within the overall range of normal for all women, should be considered abnormal. Patterns of abnormal bleeding include intermenstrual bleeding and postcoital bleeding, as well as cyclic bleeding that is heavier, lighter, or longer than normal. Up to 10% of women with regular menstrual cycles may experience idiopathic abnormal uterine bleeding. Empiric treatment includes nonsteroidal anti-inflammatory drugs (NSAIDs), oral contraceptive, and topical progesterone released from an intrauterine device (IUD).

The possibility of a congenital coagulation disorder would be considered in a young woman who presents with abnormal vaginal bleeding in the perimenarchal period. Up to 20% of adolescent girls requiring hospitalization for abnormal uterine bleeding are found to have coagulation disorders (42). Evaluation of a possible coagulation disorder includes personal and family history, physical examination, and a complete blood cell count, quantitative platelet count, template bleeding time, prothrombin time, partial thromboplastin time, and solubility of the fibrin clot in urea.

A variety of drugs, including phenothiazines, penicillins, and aminoglycosides, can affect coagulation factors. Many commonly used drugs, including penicillins, furosemide (Lasix), aspirin, ranitidine hydrochloride (Zantac), and acetaminophen, have been reported to cause thrombocytopenia, as have both cisplatin and cyclosporine (Sandimmune). Aspirin, the NSAIDs, and β-lactam antibiotics can alter platelet function. Disorders associated with thrombocytopenia include asplastic anemia and replacement of normal marrow by cancer. In addition, patients with cancer, sepsis, and systemic autoimmune disorders can undergo increased platelet destruction. Hypothyroidism can also cause menometrorrhagia. Recent and current medication history and concurrent medical conditions should be considered in evaluating a cancer patient with abnormal uterine bleeding.

In ovulating women, early miscarriage, threatened abortion, incomplete or missed abortion, and ectopic pregnancy may cause abnormal uterine bleeding. Evaluation of a premenopausal woman with abnormal vaginal bleeding should include a history, physical examination, and urinary pregnancy test. If the pregnancy test is positive, then a quantitative serum human chorionic gonadotropin (hCG) should be obtained. Serial hCG levels will help distinguish among an early miscarriage, an incomplete or missed abortion, an ectopic pregnancy, or an intrauterine pregnancy. Transvaginal ultrasound should be able to identify a gestational sac when the serum hCG level has risen above 1500 mIU/mL. The patient with an incomplete or missed abortion with heavy vaginal bleeding may require a dilation and curettage (D&C). An asymptomatic woman with an unruptured ectopic pregnancy less than 3.5 cm in diameter and a serum hCG less than 6000 mIU/mL may be treated with methotrexate, 50 mg/m^2 given intramuscularly, then followed with serial hCG levels. Symptomatic women with ectopic pregnancy should undergo emergent salpingectomy or salpingostomy.

Uterine leiomyomas are found in 40% of women older than 35 years. These benign tumors each arise from a single muscle cell. In many cases, estrogen stimulation causes growth of the tumors. Transvaginal ultrasound may help distinguish myomas from other causes of uterine or ovarian enlargement. In some cases, leiomyomas that impinge on the endometrial cavity appear to cause excessive and prolonged uterine bleeding. Symptomatic women may be treated with myomectomy or hysterectomy. In some women, leiomyomas shrink after menopause with the fall of estrogen levels. Conservative management without surgery may be appropriate therefore in certain perimenopausal women.

Another cause of abnormal uterine bleeding is infection of the endometrium. This may be acute, which is generally seen postpartum, or chronic. The diagnosis is generally made on the basis of the physical examination, when the uterus may be found to be boggy and tender, and by endometrial biopsy. Infectious endometritis is generally bacterial in origin. Appropriate antibiotic therapy generally corrects abnormal uterine bleeding.

Uterine polyps are generally asymptomatic. They can, however, cause menometrorrhagia. Polyps arise from focal hyperplasia of the basalis layer and are most commonly found in women aged 40 to 50 years. Tamoxifen use has been associated with an increased risk of endometrial polyps, particularly among postmenopausal women. They are best diagnosed with sonohysterography or hysteroscopy. The treatment of symptomatic uterine polyps is D&C under hysteroscopic guidance.

Neoplastic causes of abnormal vaginal bleeding include cervical carcinoma, endometrial hyperplasia, endometrial carcinoma, and uterine sarcomas. Gynecologic examination, together with routine Papanicolaou (Pap) smear screening, should be able to identify an etiology for bleeding from the ectocervix. Colposcopy with biopsies and endocervical curettage should be considered for women with a Pap smear demonstrating suspected intraepithelial lesions, including high-grade squamous intraepithelial lesion or atypical glandular cells. Endocervical curettage, endometrial biopsy, and transvaginal ultrasound should be considered in a woman with abnormal uterine bleeding of unknown etiology. Hysteroscopy and D&C may also be necessary to establish the etiology of abnormal bleeding in certain patients.

Endometrial hyperplasia is caused by an excess of estrogenic stimulation without progestational counterbalance. Risk factors for endometrial hyperplasia include obesity, nulliparity, diabetes mellitus, and use of exogenous estrogens, including tamoxifen. The pathologist who diagnoses endometrial hyperplasia should also comment on the presence or absence of cellular atypia. Endometrial hyperplasia without atypia has a very low risk (1%) of becoming carcinoma. Women with atypical endometrial hyperplasia, however, have a risk for endometrial carcinoma as high as 29%. Endometrial hyperplasia without atypia can be effectively treated with progestins, whether administered orally (megestrol acetate [Megace], 40 mg twice daily, or medroxyprogesterone acetate, 10 mg daily), via intramuscular injection (medroxyprogesterone acetate [Depo-Provera], 150 mg every 3 months), or via a progesterone-releasing IUD (Progestasert). The same hormonal therapy can also be used to treat atypical endometrial hyperplasia, although the success of such an intervention may only be as high as 50%. If atypical endometrial hyperplasia persists despite 3 to 12 months of progestin therapy, then hysterectomy should be considered. Women in whom endometrial hyperplasia has been reversed with progestins or who remain at risk for recurrent hyperplasia due to unopposed estrogen should be considered for intermittent progestin therapy. The risk for the development of endometrioid endometrial carcinoma among women taking tamoxifen appears to be 1 per 1000 women per year (43). This risk appears to be increased among women with a history of estrogenic stimulation before commencing tamoxifen.

Leiomyosarcoma, carcinosarcoma, and adenocarcinoma of the uterus should be treated in most cases with primary hysterectomy. Decisions as to adjuvant radiotherapy or chemotherapy are best made after hysterectomy and surgical staging. Well differentiated endometrioid endometrial adenocarcinoma has been treated successfully with the same progestin regimens used for endometrial hyperplasia. The success rates for such hormonal therapy are about 50%, in the same range as those for atypical endometrial hyperplasia. Hormonal therapy of endometrial cancer may take from 6 to 12 months for neoplastic changes to resolve.

In all women, however, including those undergoing cancer therapy, the most common causes of abnormal uterine bleeding are hormonal. A women who undergoes withdrawal of either estrogen or progesterone will develop uterine bleeding. Estrogen withdrawal may occur with spontaneous natural menopause, ovarian ablation from chemotherapy or radiation therapy, or stopping exogenous estrogen, including tamoxifen. Progesterone withdrawal bleeding may occur in women who have experienced a miscarriage, elective abortion, treatment of an ectopic pregnancy, delivery, or stopping exogenous progesterone.

Prolonged exposure to progesterone can result in minimal endometrial thickness. This can occur in women with prolonged oral contraceptive use or with the use of depot progesterones, such as Depo-Provera and levonorgestrel implants (Norplant System). This thinned endometrium, which lacks estrogenic support, is fragile and can bleed easily. In addition, if the myometrial arteries become exposed, heavy uterine bleeding can develop. Treatment should include estrogen replacement either with high-dose-estrogen oral contraceptives, such as norgestrel and ethinyl estradiol (Ovral), or intravenous estrogen. If a high-dose oral contraceptive is used, it should be given every 8 to 12 hours for 24 to 48 hours and then tapered over the course of several days. Patients will also require a prophylactic antiemetic. Intravenous estrogen is given at a dose of 25 μg every 4 hours for three doses. Once the bleeding has subsided, consideration should be given to intermittent supplemental estrogen.

As discussed above, anovulation and amenorrhea often develop in women undergoing treatment with chemotherapy or abdominopelvic radiotherapy, which may lead to the growth of a thickened endometrial lining. As these women are not exposed to cyclic progestins, they often may have irregular vaginal spotting or bleeding. In addition, without the stabilizing influence of progesterone, the endometrium does not shear off in orderly fashion. Necrosis and hemorrhage may occur randomly in the endometrium. If the basal endometrium is exposed, then the myometrial arteries may cause heavy bleeding.

Preliminary evaluation should include history, physical examination, and a complete blood cell count, as well as a urine pregnancy test and evaluation of coagulation if indicated. If the pregnancy test is negative, the hematocrit is in the normal range, and the patient does not have profuse bleeding, then the clinician may wish to consider oral contraceptives to restore menstrual regularity. Rhythmic cycling of estrogen and progesterone will help establish a normal menstrual pattern. If oral contraceptives are contraindicated, then a short course of an oral progestin, such as medroxyprogesterone acetate, 10 mg a day for 10 days every month for 3 months, may help stabilize a friable endometrium. Another possibility is a progestin-releasing IUD.

Should the patient experience heavy vaginal bleeding with a symptomatic drop in hematocrit, then consideration should be given to a short course of a high-dose-estrogen oral contraceptive. A typical regimen would be Ovral four times a day (every 6 hours) for 4 days, then one pill three times a day (every 8 hours) for 3 days, then one pill twice a day (every 12 hours) for 2 days, then one pill daily. This high dose of estrogen and progesterone may cause nausea and vomiting, so patients should be pretreated with an antiemetic. Another possibility would be intravenous conjugated estrogens (Premarin), 25 μg every 4 hours for three doses, followed by daily Ovral.

In general, the treatment of dysfunctional uterine bleeding is empiric, based on the clinical history. If there is inadequate response to the treatment approaches outlined above, then workup should include further evaluation of coagulation and platelet function, a transvaginal ultrasound to rule out structural abnormalities in the uterus, and possibly an endometrial biopsy. Patients with thrombocytopenia may need platelet transfusions to stop or slow endometrial bleeding. Control of abnormal bleeding is almost always possible via hormonal methods. D&C may be performed as a last resort, if the patient is considered stable for the operating room. Often, this procedure will require a platelet transfusion to establish a platelet count of at least 50,000/mm^3, as manipulation of the cervix and myometrium with penetrating instruments will be required.

CONTRACEPTION DURING AND AFTER CANCER THERAPY

The need for effective contraception during and after cancer treatment cannot be overemphasized. As noted above, normal menstrual cycles do not imply normal fertility; the inverse of this statement is also true. Women in whom irregular menses or even amenorrhea develop during or after therapy are still capable of spontaneous ovulation and conception. Multiple reports in the literature attest to this potential.

The most reliable form of birth control for any population of women is injectable progestins. These rely on progestins to suppress LH secretion. Depo-Provera, 150 mg injected intramuscularly, will effectively block ovulation for 4 months. The first-year failure rate for Depo-Provera is 0.4% (44). Norplant System consists of six silicon rubber capsules sealed with dimethylsiloxane. The capsules, which slowly release levonorgestrel, are placed under local anesthesia in the subcutaneous tissue of the upper arm just above the antecubital fossa. Norplant will effectively block ovulation for 5 years. The first year failure rate for Norplant is 0.09% (44). The most common side effects of both technologies are breakthrough bleeding, breast tenderness, weight gain, and depression. As neither technology relies on estrogen, they are not associated with an increased risk of thromboembolism. Therefore, they can be used in women with congenital heart disease, sickle cell anemia, or a prior history of thromboembolism, or in women older than 30 years who smoke cigarettes or have other risk factors. In general, these progestin-containing injectable contraceptives have not been prescribed for women with a history of breast cancer. In theory, an injectable contraceptive might be an option for a woman with an estrogen and progesterone receptor–negative breast cancer.

Sterilization is currently the most popular form of contraception in the United States. Tubal ligation can be performed as an outpatient procedure under general or local anesthesia. Vasectomy can be performed as an outpatient procedure under local anesthesia. Men and women should be informed that success rates for reversal of sterilization are less than 50%. The 1-year failure rate for tubal ligation is 0.4% and for vasectomy 0.15% (44).

Another contraceptive option for cancer patients is an IUD, which functions by making the endometrium less receptive to ovum implantation. The presence of a foreign body in the endometrial cavity, attached to a string that passes through the cervical canal, does increase the risk of endomyometritis in women with multiple sexual partners. An IUD therefore should only be prescribed for women in a mutually monogamous relationship. IUDs currently available in the United States include the copper TCU 380A (ParaGard) and the Progestasert. The ParaGard, consisting of 310 mg of copper wire wound about a T-shaped polyethylene body, is thought to work by setting up a mild inflammatory reaction in the endometrium. In addition, copper ions change the composition of cervical mucus. The ParaGard has been approved for use up to 10 years. The first-year failure rate for the ParaGard is 0.8% (44). The Progestasert contains 38 mg of progesterone, which it releases at a rate of 65 μg per 24 hours within the endometrial cavity. In clinical studies, no systemic absorption of the progestin has been reported. The first-year failure rate for the Progestasert is 2% (44).

Oral contraceptives, although less effective than injectable contraception, IUDs, or sterilization, are generally acceptable to most women. Oral contraceptives combine progestins, which suppress LH secretion, and estrogens, which suppress FSH secretion. The estrogen also stabilizes the endometrium, preventing breakthrough bleeding and potentiating the action of progestins. In addition, progestins make the endometrial lining unreceptive to ovum implantation and the cervical mucus hostile to sperm penetration. Absolute contraindications to the use of oral contraceptives are thromboembolic disease, markedly impaired liver function, congenital hyperlipidemia, and cigarette smoking (more than 15 cigarettes per day) over age 35 years. Due to the presence of both estrogenic and progestin components in oral contraceptives, they are generally not prescribed for women with a history of breast cancer. Relative contraindications to the use of oral contraceptives are migraine headaches, hypertension, sickle cell disease, diabetes mellitus, and gallbladder disease. In general, oral contraceptives with the lowest possible estrogen dose should be prescribed. These include the multiphasic preparations, as well as the menophasic preparations with an estrogen dose of 20 to 35 μg. As discussed above, however, short-term administration of high-dose-estrogen pills (Ovral) may be appropriate for women undergoing high-dose chemotherapy who are at risk for thrombocytopenia. The failure rate per year for oral contraceptives with usual use is 2.4% (44). In addition, a short course of high-dose-estrogen (50 μg of ethinyl estradiol) pills is also effective at blocking implantation ("the morning-after pill") (45). With this regimen, two pills are taken within 72 hours of unprotected intercourse, followed by another two pills 12 hours later. This regimen may be useful for the woman who reports recent unprotected intercourse and does not desire pregnancy. The failure rate for this regimen appears to be about 3%.

Barrier methods include condoms, diaphragm, and spermicides (foam, cream, jelly, and vaginal suppository). As none of these affects a woman's hormonal milieu, they may be appropriate for women with hormonally sensitive cancers such as breast cancer. Because the failure rates per year of normal use are relatively high (male condoms alone, 12%; diaphragm with spermicidal cream or jelly, 18%; spermicides, 21%), these barrier methods are best used in combination (44). Condoms and diaphragms will also decrease the transmission of infectious agents such as

Chlamydia, Neisseria gonorrhoeae, human immunodeficiency virus, and hepatitis B virus. Barrier methods will not block transmission of human papillomavirus.

SUMMARY

Damewood et al. (46) reported on a case of successful induction of ovulation and pregnancy following lateral oophoropexy for Hodgkin's disease. The patient was a 31-year-old who was diagnosed at age 23 with Hodgkin's disease. At the time of her diagnosis, she was experiencing regular menses. She was treated with radiation therapy following a wide lateral displacement of the ovaries at the time of staging laparotomy. Following her treatment, the patient was noted to have elevated levels of gonadotropins despite regular menses. Induction of ovulation was achieved with human menopausal gonadotropins. Conception occurred after the second cycle, and an uneventful pregnancy and delivery ensued. This case illustrates several points:

- Regular menses does not imply normal ovulation and fertility.
- Even after oophoropexy (or any other measure utilized to preserve ovarian function during cancer therapy), there can be unexpected ovarian damage resulting in loss of fertility.
- Despite previous cancer therapy, be it radiation or chemotherapy, a genotypically and phenotypically normal infant can be expected.
- Even in the face of ovarian compromise, there is hope for women previously treated for cancer to successfully achieve pregnancy via assisted reproductive technologies (ARTs). Further advances in ARTs, including use of donor eggs, the possibility of freezing embryos, and eventual oocyte pretreatment, will offer more options to young women anticipating impending cancer chemotherapy.

Cancer therapy in young people, while becoming more successful, causes disruption of normal ovarian function, often leading to amenorrhea or irregular, dysfunctional uterine bleeding. Premenopausal women undergoing cancer treatment should use effective contraception. Finally, as both malignancy and treatment of malignancy can compromise immune and hematologic functions, clinicians must be hypervigilant to structural and infectious causes of dysfunctional uterine bleeding.

REFERENCES

1. Byrne J, Fears TR, Gail MR, et al. Early menopause in long-term survivors of cancer during adolescence. *Am J Obstet Gynecol* 1992;166:788–793.
2. Gradishar WJ, Schilsky RL. Ovarian function following radiation and chemotherapy for cancer. *Semin Oncol* 1989;16:425–436.
3. Montz FJ, Wolff AJ, Gambone JC. Gonadal protection and fecundity rates in cyclophosphamide-treated rats. *Cancer Res* 1991;51:2124–2126.
4. Miller JJ, Williams GF, Leissring JC. Multiple late complications of therapy with cyclophosphamide, including ovarian destruction. *Am J Med* 1971;50:530–535.
5. Uldall PR, Kerr DN, Tacchi D. Sterility and cyclophosphamide [Letter]. *Lancet* 1972;1:693–694.
6. Warne GL, Fairley KF, Hobbs JB, Martin FI. Cyclophosphamide-induced ovarian failure. *N Engl J Med* 1973;289:1159–1162.
7. Koyama H, Wada T, Nishizawa Y, Iwanaga T, Aoki Y. Cyclophosphamide-induced ovarian failure and its therapeutic significance in patients with breast cancer. *Cancer* 1977;39:1403–1409.
8. Choo YC, Chan SY, Wong LC, Ma HK. Ovarian dysfunction in patients with gestational trophoblastic neoplasia treated with short intensive courses of etoposide (VP-16-213). *Cancer* 1985;55:2348–2352.
9. Matsui H, Seki K, Sekiya S, Takamizawa H. Reproductive status in GTD treated with etoposide. *J Reprod Med* 1997;42:104–110.
10. Landis SH, Murray TM, Bolden S, Wingo PA. Cancer statistics, 1998. *CA Cancer J Clin* 1998;48:6–29.
11. Sobrinho LG, Levine RA, DeConti RC. Amenorrhea in patients with Hodgkin's disease treated with antineoplastic agents. *Am J Obstet Gynecol* 1971;109:135–139.
12. Chapman RM, Sutcliffe SB, Malpas JS. Cytotoxic-induced ovarian failure in women with Hodgkin's disease. I. Hormone function. *JAMA* 1979;242:1877–1881.
13. Schilsky RL, Sherins RJ. Hubbard SM, Wesley MN, Young RC, De Vita VT. Long-term follow-up of ovarian function in women treated with MOPP chemotherapy for Hodgkin's disease. *Am J Med* 1981;71:552–556.
14. Horning SJ, Hoppe RT, Kaplan HS, Rosenberg SA. Female reproductive potential after treatment for Hodgkin's disease. *N Engl J Med* 1981;304:1377–1382.
15. Andrieu JM, Ochoa-Molina ME. Menstrual cycle, pregnancies and offspring before and after MOPP therapy for Hodgkin disease. *Cancer* 1983;52:435–438.
16. Viviani S, Santoro A, Ragni G, Bonfante V, Bestetti O, Bonadonna G. Gonadal toxicity after combination

chemotherapy for Hodgkin's disease: comparative results of MOPP vs. ABVD. *Eur J Cancer Clin Oncol* 1985;21:601–605.
17. Bines J, Oleske DM, Cobleigh MA. Ovarian function in premenopausal women treated with adjuvant chemotherapy for breast cancer. *J Clin Oncol* 1996;14: 1718–1729.
18. Samaan NA, DeAsis DN Jr, Buzdar AU, Blumenschein GR. Pituitary-ovarian function in breast cancer patients on adjuvant chemoimmunotherapy. *Cancer* 1978;41: 2084–2087.
19. Rose DP, Davis TE. Effects of adjuvant chemohormonal therapy on the ovarian and adrenal function of breast cancer patients. *Cancer Res* 1980;40:4043–4047.
20. Dnistrian AM, Schwartz MK, Fracchia AA, Kaufman RJ, Hakes TB, Currie VE. Endocrine consequences of CMF adjuvant therapy in premenopausal and postmenopausal breast cancer patients. *Cancer* 1983;51: 803–807.
21. Bonadonna G, Valagussa P. Adjuvant systemic therapy for resectable breast cancer. *J Clin Oncol* 1985;3: 259–275.
22. Ravdin PM, Fritz NF, Tormey DC, Jordan VC. Endocrine status of premenopausal node-positive breast cancer patients following adjuvant chemotherapy and long-term tamoxifen. *Cancer Res* 1988;48:1026–1029.
23. Hortobagyi GN, Buzdar AU, Marcus CE, Smith TL. Immediate and long-term toxicity of adjuvant chemotherapy regimens containing doxorubicin in trials at J.D. Anderson Hospital and Tumor Institute. *NCI Monogr* 1986;1:105–109.
24. Davidson NE. Ovarian ablation as treatment for young women with breast cancer. *J Natl Cancer Inst Monogr* 1994;16:95–100.
25. Early Breast Cancer Trialists' Collaborative Group. Systemic treatment of early breast cancer by hormonal, cytotoxic, or immune therapy. *Lancet* 1992;229:1–15, 71–85.
26. Fisher B, Costantino JP, Wickerham DL, et al. Tamoxifen for prevention of breast cancer: report of the National Surgical Adjuvant Breast and Bowel Project P-1 study. *J Natl Cancer Inst* 1998;90:1371–1388.
27. Gerhard I, Runnebaum B. Comparison between tamoxifen and clomiphene therapy in women with anovulation. *Arch Gynecol* 1979;227:279–288.
28. Sherman BM, Chapler FK, Crickard K, Wycoff D. Endocrine consequences of continuous antiestrogen therapy with tamoxifen in premenopausal women. *J Clin Invest* 1979;64:398–404.
29. Jordan VC, Fritz NF, Langan-Fahey S, Thompson M, Tormey DC. Alteration of endocrine parameters in premenopausal women with breast cancer during long-term adjuvant therapy with tamoxifen as the single agent. *J Natl Cancer Inst* 1991;83:1488–1491.
30. Pektasides D, Rustin GJ, Newlands ES, Begent RH, Bagshawe KD. Fertility after chemotherapy for ovarian germ cell tumors. *Br J Obstet Gynaecol* 1987;94:477–479.
31. Gershenson DM. Menstrual and reproductive function after treatment with combination chemotherapy for malignant ovarian germ cell tumors. *J Clin Oncol* 1988;6: 270–275.
32. Wu PC, Huang RL, Lang JH, Huang HF, Lian LJ, Tang MY. Treatment of malignant ovarian germ cell tumors with preservation of fertility: a report of 28 cases. *Gynecol Oncol* 1991;40:2–6.
33. Chatterjee R, Goldone AH. Gonadal damage and effects on fertility in adult patients with haematological malignancy undergoing stem cell transplantation. *Bone Marrow Transplant* 1996:17:5–11.
34. Sarafoglou K, Boulad F, Gillio A, Sklar C. Gonadal function after bone marrow transplantation for acute leukemia during childhood. *J Pediatr* 1997;130: 210–216. [See comments *J Pediatr* 1997;130:175–175; 1997;131:651–652.]
35. Keilholz U, Max R, Scheibenbogen C, Wuster C, Korbling M, Haas R. Endocrine function and bone metabolism 5 years after autologous bone marrow/blood-derived progenitor cell transplantation. *Cancer* 1997;79; 1617–1622.
36. Thibaud E, Rodriguez-Macias K, Trivin C, Esperou H, Michon J, Brauner R. Ovarian function after bone marrow transplantation during childhood. *Bone Marrow Trans* 1988;21:287–290.
37. Sanders JE. Growth and development after bone marrow transplantation. In: Forman SJ, Blume KG, Thomas ED, eds. *Bone marrow transplantation.* Oxford: Blackwell Science, 1994:527–551.
38. Baker TG. Radiosensitivity of mammalian oocytes with particular reference to the human female. *Am J Obstet Gynecol* 1971;110:746–761.
39. Chapman RM, Sutcliffe SB. Protection of ovarian function by oral contraceptives in women receiving chemotherapy for Hodgkin's disease. *Blood* 1981;58:849–851.
40. Ataya KM, McKanna JA, Weintraub AM, Clark MR, LeMaire WJ. A luteinizing hormone-releasing hormone agonist for the prevention of chemotherapy-induced ovarian follicular loss in rats. *Cancer Res* 1985;45: 3651–3656.
41. Blumenfeld Z, Avivi I, Linn S, Epelbaum R, Ben-Shahar M, Haim N. Prevention of irreversible chemotherapy-induced ovarian damage in young women with lymphoma by a gonadotrophin-releasing hormone agonist in parallel to chemotherapy. *Hum Reprod* 1996;11:1620–1626.
42. Claessens EA, Colwell CA. Acute adolescent menorrhagia. *Am J Obstet Gynecol* 1981;139:277–281.
43. Fisher B, Costantino JP, Redmond CK, Fisher ER, Wickerham DL, Cronin WM. Endometrial cancer in tamoxifen-treated breast cancer patients: findings from the National Surgical Adjuvant Breast Project (NSABP) B 14. *J Natl Cancer Inst* 1994;86:527–537.
44. Hatcher RA, et al. *Contraceptive technology,* 16th rev ed. New York: Irvington Publishers, 1994.
45. Glasier A, Baird D. The effects of self-administering emergency contraception. *N Engl J Med* 1998;339:1–4.
46. Damewood MD, Hesla HS, Lowen M. Schultz MJ. Induction of ovulation and pregnancy following lateral oophoropexy for Hodgkin's disease. *Int J Gynaecol Obstet* 1990;33:369–371.

2

Sexuality for the Woman with Cancer

Barbara L. Andersen

Departments of Psychology and Obstetrics and Gynecology, Ohio State University, Columbus, Ohio 43210-1222

Cancer patients often experience sexual difficulties following treatment. In fact, it is the area most likely to undergo disruption, more so than other major areas of life such as interpersonal relations and employment (1). Review of disease-site data suggests that disease and treatment factors may in large measure account for much of the sexual dysfunction that occurs. Women treated for gynecologic cancer are particularly vulnerable to sexual dysfunction (2). Across sites, estimates range from 30% (e.g., women treated with surgery only, such as radical hysterectomy) to 70% to 90% (e.g., women with vulvar cancer treated with modified radical vulvectomy). Although sexual function has been studied more closely in women with breast and gynecologic cancers, women with other malignancies, such as lung cancer, colon cancer, and leukemia, are also at risk for sexual dysfunction.

Cancer treatments can affect a woman's sexuality in several ways. For example, gynecologic changes (e.g., vaginal discharge) have been associated with long-term adjuvant tamoxifen therapy for breast cancer (3), and so-called female androgen deficiency syndrome has been seen in association with cytotoxic agents and/or bilateral salpingo-oophorectomy (4). Additionally, controlled longitudinal studies of breast cancer patients (5,6) and gynecologic cancer patients (7) have indicated that if sexual problems develop, they do so as soon as intercourse resumes, and, if untreated, they are unlikely to resolve. Thus, a significant number of female cancer survivors will experience sexual problems of either an acute or chronic nature, often as a direct result of the disease and/or its treatment.

This chapter reviews the central findings regarding sexuality in women with cancer. Three sections are included. First, available data on sexual morbidity for women and their partners are reviewed. Predicting which women are at risk for sexual dysfunction is the focus of the second section. In particular, a model for identifying which women will be at risk for mild, moderate, or severe sexual difficulty is described, together with discussion of the individual difference variable—sexual self schema—that can predict sexual outcomes. The third and final section presents a conceptual model for understanding the processes of sexual problem development and discusses various options currently available for the treatment of sexual dysfunctions in cancer patients.

COMMON FEMALE MALIGNANCIES AND ASSOCIATED SEXUAL MORBIDITY

Breast

Breast cancer accounts for 32% of all cancers in women, and no other cancer site among women or men approaches this percentage. In the last 40 years, there have been dramatic changes in the recommended therapies for breast cancer. In this regard, the type of treatment and the extent of reconstructive surgery are the two most influential variables in determining sexual outcome for those treated for local or regional breast disease. More recent clinical trials have compared modified radical mastectomy with lumpectomy and radiotherapy. Studies generally find no psychologic benefit *per se* yet do find more positive sexual outcomes for women receiving lumpectomy (8–10). For example, lumpectomy patients report less alteration in body image and greater comfort with nudity and discussion of sexuality with one's partner, with few changes in intercourse frequency and a lower incidence of sexual dysfunction.

Women who receive systemic adjuvant chemo- or hormonal therapy may confront a variety of other sexual difficulties from regimens that adversely affect their interest in and ability to engage in sexual activity. For instance, chemotherapy can lead to estrogen deficiency, in which vaginal mucosa can thin and dry and in some cases the vagina may shrink or close completely (11); it can also lead to female androgen deficiency syndrome (decreases in testosterone related to orgastic responsivity), resulting in loss of sexual desire and diminished sexual pleasure (4,11).

Cervix, Endometrium, and Ovary

Sexual outcomes for patients with cervical, endometrial, or ovarian malignancies are combined, as the treatment modalities (and therefore the sexual outcomes) have similarities. Treatment strategies typically consist of radical surgery (e.g., radical hysterectomy, total abdominal hysterectomy), pelvic irradiation with or without vaginal irradiation, or a combination of these. Ovarian patients of course are vigorously treated with chemotherapy. For those with recurrent disease or extensive cervical disease at diagnosis, the scenario is much more difficult and may include radical pelvic surgery such as pelvic exenteration. This is an accepted strategy for cure despite the occurrence of considerable behavioral, psychologic, and sexual morbidity.

Sexual Disruption before Diagnosis

Clinical studies have noted that postcoital bleeding or pelvic pain, for example, may alert a woman to the need for medical care. For instance, Andersen et al. (12) found that prior to the onset of cancer signs and symptoms, gynecologic cancer patients reported similar patterns of sexual activity and responsiveness as healthy women, but with the appearance of disease signs and symptoms (e.g., fatigue, postcoital bleeding, vaginal discharge, pain), they experienced significant sexual difficulties. In fact, women have reported that they have initiated changes in intercourse frequency because of bleeding (or fear of it), pain, and anxiety (13). Thus, it appears that women who experience a substantial change in sexual functioning tend to negatively interpret this disruption and seek medical attention.

Surgery or Radiation with or without Chemotherapy

The three primary treatments for localized or regional pelvic disease have potentially different effects on sexuality. With radical hysterectomy and related surgeries, controlled prospective longitudinal data confirm that even simple hysterectomy for benign disease produces significant sexual disruption (7,14). Thus, vaginal shortening with radical hysterectomy, in which approximately one-third of the upper vagina is removed, can contribute to subjective feelings that the vagina is too short for intercourse. Nerve and vascular disruption to the pelvis, as may occur with lymphadenectomy, may also result in loss of sensitivity and orgasmic disruption. Premature menopause with the direct effects of atrophic vaginitis from estrogen deprivation can also result in sexual difficulties (e.g., vaginal narrowing or closing). For women also receiving chemotherapy, there are the general toxicities (e.g., nausea/vomiting, bladder/kidney toxicity, and bone marrow suppression), but some agents may also induce menopause or at least suppress ovulation during the therapy period.

Radiation therapy destroys ovarian functioning and thus induces menopausal symptomatology for premenopausal women, leading to vaginal atrophy and stenosis for all women. These outcomes are most severe for women treated with vaginal irradiation (intracavitary radium or cesium implants; see Andersen et al. [15] for a discussion of the psychologic aspects of this difficult treatment) used alone or in combination with external-beam irradiation (16). Estrogen therapy following treatment can control symptoms such as hot flushes and aid in the healing of the vaginal epithelium (17); vaginal dilators can reduce or eliminate fibrosis (18). However, due to the magnitude of the vaginal changes, dyspareunia may still occur.

In general, the rates of sexual behavioral disruption and dysfunction are comparable between surgery and radiation treatments (see Andersen et al. [19] for a review). Following cancer treatment, women have reported awareness of fewer signs of sexual excitement and lower arousability for sexual activities with their partner (7), especially women who have received radiation (20). The most likely reason for the arousal deficits is the simultaneous occurrence of significant disruptors (e.g., dyspareunia due in part to radiation effects and/or induced menopause). Data consistent with these results have been reported by others (14,18,20). Additionally, Krumm and Laberti (18) noted that poor compliance with treatment may lead to sexual avoidance and ultimately to sexual difficulties (e.g., older women who do not feel comfortable using vaginal dilators). As it has been estimated that radiation-induced tissue changes continue for 36 months following the completion of therapy, the need to adhere to treatment recommendations is critical.

Combined Therapies

Patients treated with combination therapy (surgery and radiation) may receive a lower total dose of radiation than those treated with radiotherapy only. In addition, depending on the surgical procedure, the apex of the vagina, which is exposed to the largest dose of radiation when intracavitary treatment is included, is removed during surgery. Thus, the remaining portion of the vagina is less affected, and perhaps less vulnerable to problems of dyspareunia. These patients would be expected to be at lower risk for sexual morbidity because of the combination therapy.

Radical Surgery (Pelvic Exenteration)

This surgery has been used for extensive but resectable disease at diagnosis and for centrally recurrent disease in some women. It is a disfiguring and life-altering surgery. Clinical reports, not surprisingly, have noted the cessation of sexual activity for many women: from 15% in Corney et al. (21) to 80% to 90% in Andersen and Hacker (22). For the majority of women and couples, the prospect of ending their sexual life (as most couples cease all sexual activity when intercourse becomes impossible) is distressing and may be a source of continuing marital discord.

Vaginal reconstruction (e.g., with a loop of bowel or portions of inner thigh or rectus muscle) is a possibility for some and enables them to maintain sexual activity that includes intercourse. However, many sexual difficulties often remain, including problems with the physical characteristics of the new vagina (e.g., the cavity is too large, too narrow), arousal and/or orgasm, or dyspareunia and/or bleeding with intercourse. The presence of ostomies for urine and/or stool may also adversely affect body image. Regardless of whether or not women with pelvic exenteration undergo vaginal reconstruction, these women face the greatest disruption to their sexual body and functioning of any women with cancer.

Vulva

Vulvar cancer is rare and occurs most commonly among older women, with a median age of 65 years for white women and 55 years for black women. Treatment has previously included modified radical vulvectomy, which removes labial tissue and often the clitoris and typically includes groin surgery to assess nodal disease, with radiation therapy playing a more limited role. Treatments such as these produce extreme genital disfigurement, and so there has been more interest among physicians to individualize treatment and potentially reduce the extent of surgery without compromising survival (23).

Even though the population of women diagnosed with vulvar cancer is older than the average patient with pelvic disease, there are no data to suggest that they will be less distressed by changes to their sexuality. Not surprisingly, the reports of women who are treated with radical vulvectomy versus wide local excision are dramatically different, with the former patients becoming nonorgasmic and the latter maintaining orgasm and other sexual responses (24). Andersen et al. (59) also provided data on the sexual outcomes for women treated with wide local excision and related treatments for *in situ* disease. Overall, it appears that patients with *in situ* disease as a group are more likely to be sexually inactive at follow-up, whether or not they have available sexual partners, than age-matched healthy counterparts. However, the outcomes for women with *in situ* disease contrast markedly with those for women with invasive disease, many of whom are treated with modified radical vulvectomy with or without groin dissection. The general trend is consistent: At least 30% to 50% of patients become sexually inactive, and of the women remaining active, 60% to 70% have multiple sexual dysfunctions. For the women who become sexually inactive, many factors may be contributory, including negative feelings (by the women or their partners) about the physical changes to the body or severe dyspareunia related to a narrowed introitus. However, despite poorer sexual responsiveness (25), the majority of women would have preferred to remain sexually active rather than have all intimacy end (22).

PREDICTING RISK FOR SEXUAL MORBIDITY

Sufficient psychosocial research has been conducted in the last two decades to make it possible to predict which women will be at risk for psychologic or behavioral morbidity. For example, Schag et al. (26) noted the importance of identifying characteristics of women at risk for psychosocial distress. In a test of predictors for women with breast cancer, women who were at moderate to high risk for problem development at diagnosis had concerns such as continuing psychologic distress, difficult communication with marital partners, negative body image, and disrupted sexuality at the 12-month follow-up.

This section provides a model and identifies variables, both medical and psychologic, that predict sexual difficulties following cancer treatment. The majority of the variables identified are ones known at the times of diagnosis and early recovery.

Medical Contributors

The preceding section makes clear the significant role that medical factors such as disease extent and magnitude of treatment appear to play in determining sexual outcomes for women with breast or gynecologic cancers. A model of disease and treatment pathways has been formulated that can yield differential levels of risk for sexual morbidity (27) (Fig. 1). Variables are introduced according to a disease time line—from cancer appearance to the immediate posttreatment recovery period—as disease-relevant events provide a meaningful framework to understand psychologic adjustment to cancer (28).

With reference to this model, disruptive signs and symptoms may occur at the onset of cancer (see Fig. 1). When the disease is detected and produces sexual disruption, this is the first point of psychologic/behavioral morbidity. It is clear that such early disruption occurs for women eventually diagnosed with gynecologic cancer (12). With the appearance of indications of disease (e.g., fatigue, postcoital

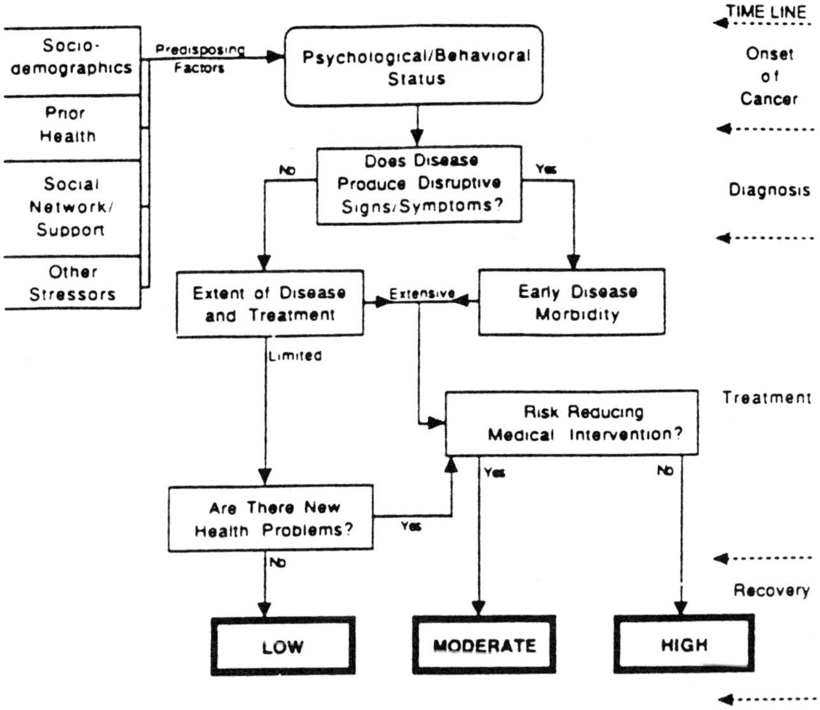

FIG. 1. Sociodemographic, psychologic, behavioral, and disease and treatment elements leading to low, moderate, and high levels of psychologic and behavioral morbidity risk. (From ref. 27. Copyright ©1993, American Cancer Society. Reprinted by permission of Wiley-Liss, Inc., a subsidiary of John Wiley & Sons, Inc.)

bleeding, vaginal discharge, pain), women report a dramatic change in sexual functioning that can include loss of desire, lowered excitement, and dyspareunia. A four- to fivefold increase in the frequency of sexual dysfunctions may be found from pre- to postappearance of cancer signs and symptoms. This early change is included because of its role in increasing women's emotional distress and alerting them to the potential for subsequent life changes.

The model indicates that disease extent and treatment are major determinants of risk. As indicated, the disease and treatment statuses are summarized into routes of "limited" versus "extensive"; these alternatives should have supporting medical endpoint data, as well as stage and magnitude-of-treatment information. The limited/extensive distinction is based in part on the classification of disease stage—localized versus regional or metastatic—and its direct relationship to survival for most disease sites; for example, for breast cancer, 5-year relative survival rates are 97%, 76%, and 21%, for localized, regional, and distant disease, respectively (29). The model goes one step further and suggests that the extent of disease be considered in the context of the magnitude of treatment received. For example, women with localized or regional vulvar cancer often receive the same disfiguring surgical treatment—radical vulvectomy—and might only differ in the provision of radiotherapy for the groin nodes in the case of regional disease. Thus, even though the women differ in disease extent, they both receive the same (or closely related) radical surgical therapy. Across cancer sites, there is support for the correlation between the magnitude of disease/treatment and psychologic/behavioral endpoints. For example, Cella et al. (30) examined emotional distress in patients with lung cancer and found that a composite score for the extent of disease and physical impairment from treatment best predicted the magnitude of mood disturbance.

For women whose therapy cannot be modified, the model next considers the availability of risk-reducing medical interventions. For those with extensive disease/treatment, the availability of such interventions might reduce the level of risk from high to moderate. Examples of rehabilitative medical efforts include vaginal reconstruction for pelvic exenteration patients, labia preservation for vulvar cancer patients, or breast reconstruction for women treated with a modified radical mastectomy. For women who have had such interventions, psychologic/behavioral and sexual outcomes are significantly better, although the interventions are not panaceas (22,31) (see Berek and Andersen [32] for a review).

For those with limited disease/treatment, the availability of medical interventions could reduce their risk from low to approximately that of healthy individuals undergoing related experiences (e.g., the base rate). For example, some women experiencing a surgical menopause following treatment for localized cervical cancer can be treated with hormone replacement therapy, just as healthy women who experience a natural menopause with its attendant difficulties are treated (33).

The final contributor to risk is new health problems (e.g., hormonal changes and/or continuing stressors from the disease/treatment). Consideration of hormonal changes includes two issues: induced menopause and infertility. As just mentioned, many women undergo premature menopause because of their treatment. Menopausal changes produce significant sexual effects (see Walling et al. [17] for a review). In addition, ovary removal/sterilization ends child bearing—a potential stressor for young women with cancer.

Continuing stressors can be heterogeneous. Examples include chronic fatigue or nausea/vomiting from toxic and/or lengthy chemotherapy regimens (34) or late morbidities from treatments (e.g., a bowel fistula following pelvic irradiation). Should such problems arise, the model considers the availability of effective treatments. As can be seen, multiple pathways can lead to high or moderate morbidity risk, but only those individuals who have limited disease/treatment and no new or continuing problems are hypothesized to have the lowest risk.

Sexual Schema and Other Psychologic Contributors

Whereas medical factors contribute to morbidity, psychologic/behavioral variables may be the most important. The model in Fig. 1 begins with baseline psychologic/behavioral factors: age, sexual status (active/inactive), and prior frequency of important sexual activities (e.g., intercourse). These factors have emerged as important predictors of sexual activity in the earliest research on sexuality (35), as well as in contemporary variants (36–38). These variables are important predictors in studies of healthy individuals, but their predictive utility is also found in studies of individuals with chronic conditions and illnesses (39,40). Thus, we note these variables in preface to the discussion below.

In an effort to identify a psychologically relevant variable, Cyranowski and I (41) have proposed a woman's view of herself as a sexual person—her sexual self-concept or sexual self schema—as a predictor of sexual morbidity. A sexual self schema is a cognitive view about sexual aspects of oneself; it is derived from past experience and manifest in current experience, and guides the processing of domain-relevant social information (41). With this conceptual formulation, extensive psychometric work was done to operationalize the construct and develop a measure of sexual self schema. Using the trait-adjective methodology, the brief, 36-item Sexual Self Schema Scale assesses a cognitive self-view of sexuality. It includes two positive aspects—an inclination to experience romantic/passionate emotions and a behavioral openness to sexual experiences and/or relationships—and a negative aspect—embarrassment and/or conservatism—that appears to be a deterrent to sexual expression. The construct is related to intrapersonal and interpersonal aspects of sexuality. It is distinguishable from related constructs, such as self-esteem, and is unhampered by emotional negativity or social desirability biases. Finally, the measure reliably demonstrates these properties, consistent with a stable, individual difference metric.

Prior studies have demonstrated that the sexual self schema predicts sexual behavior, attitudes, and responsiveness in healthy women, and is an important individual-difference measure of female sexuality (41). In addition, its predictive power has been tested in the context of risk for sexual morbidity following gynecologic cancer. Consistent with the definition of the construct, my colleagues and I have found that women with a more negative sexual self-concept in contrast to women with a more positive sexual self-concept are at greatest risk for sexual difficulty following gynecologic cancer treatment (42). Moreover, the effect of a sexual self schema was important after other factors in the model (i.e., age, menopausal status, extent of treatment/disease) were controlled for. Thus, women with negative views of themselves as sexual persons have more sexual difficulties, as they generally report that they are less romantic/passionate in their emotions, less open to sexual experiences, and more likely to have difficulties becoming sexually aroused.

DEVELOPMENT OF SEXUAL DYSFUNCTION FOLLOWING TREATMENT

This section provides a process model of sexual-activity and sexual-response-cycle problem development among women with cancer (43,44). It details the differences between "dysfunctional" and "nondysfunctional" response patterns. The dysfunctional pattern, based on empiric findings (7), is characterized by low arousal, behavioral inhibition, and negativity—a constellation of responses relevant to sexual self schema.

The model begins with an explicit initiation of sexual activity, as couples attempt to return to their prior routines for sex. Longitudinal data indicate that from the beginning couples make few changes to accommodate to the fact that the woman has had cancer (7). The only accommodation usually made is "waiting"—and usually not long enough—to resume intercourse. The model includes the interactions of behavioral, cognitive, affective, and physiologic processes.

Regarding sexual behavior—the frequency and context for sexual activity—we have found that the frequency of intercourse declines significantly during the early posttreatment recovery period and remains at a lowered level during the first year of recovery. This general effect of reduction in intercourse frequency has been replicated across gynecologic and breast cancer patients, although the reductions are more extreme (intercourse occurring rarely or never) for women receiving the most radical genital surgeries (22,31). Global behavioral disruption usually does not occur; that is, when couples engage in intercourse, albeit less often, they continue the same pattern of sexual behaviors that had occurred prior to the cancer diagnosis. This suggests that no prompting of the sexual behavior repertoire is needed, but it also shows that couples do not spontaneously vary their sexual behavior. Indeed, couples continue to engage, perhaps unadvisedly, in the same range and type of sexual activities, even when the result is significant sexual disruption or even intercourse pain for the woman.

Regarding sexual desire, many data suggest that up to 50% of women will be diagnosed with a sexual desire disorder during the early posttreatment period (2). One-half of these cases will resolve during the first posttreatment year; however, there will be a comparable number of new, late cases by 1 year posttreatment. The higher rate of desire problems early in the posttreatment year may be due in part to the emotional crisis surrounding the cancer diagnosis and treatment. This suggests that interventions to reduce affective distress would be important and that lowered distress might enhance sexual desire.

Of all the phases of the sexual response cycle, sexual excitement, including cognitive, affective, behavioral, and physiologic responses, undergoes the greatest disruption with cancer treatment. This disruption takes the form of women's viewing themselves as dysfunctional, reporting lowered arousability and reduced awareness of physiologic signs of arousal (e.g., body/pelvic warmth, lubrication). The lowered arousability is specific to foreplay and intercourse (7), suggesting that women's ability to focus on erotic cues is significantly impaired. Some women, particularly those treated for pelvic tumors (e.g., cervix, ovary, colon) may also have dyspareunia, the most significant and distracting sensation to sexual arousal. In addition, women also report negative cognitions about their body, with a narrowing of negative thoughts and evaluations for the body part that has undergone change (e.g., breast, pelvis, genitals) (45).

In view of these difficulties, it is not surprising that orgasm can be impaired. For example, there is a fourfold increase (7% to 25%) in the frequency of orgasmic dysfunction from pre- to posttreatment (7) among women treated for gynecologic cancer. Orgasmic difficulty for women produces moderate distress and provides a salient indicator to them that their sexual responses are significantly impaired. For some, the high levels of dyspareunia during intercourse is a probable contributor to orgasmic dysfunction.

Finally, the resolution phase is also disrupted for many women. There may be residual pain following intercourse. In addition, women have a general feeling that their sexual life is significantly worse. Again, data indicate that this evaluation worsens with the magnitude of disease/treatment: For women with cervical, endometrial, ovarian, or breast cancer, these evaluations are "below average" (7), for women with vulvar disease "inadequate" (31), and for women treated with pelvic exenteration "poor" (22).

Data suggest that the problems described above are most severe in the earliest posttreatment months, beginning as soon as intercourse is resumed. Further, the development of sexual problems for the male partner (e.g., delayed ejaculation in particular) may be a sequela to the woman's problems. For couples who abandon sexual activity, longitudinal data indicate that the typical scenario is that a couple will resume intercourse in the early months, experience significant sexual problems, and then not make future attempts. Thus, for both the woman and her partner, the sexual interaction is initially problematic, and the situation can become more difficult and may worsen with the lack of knowledge or failed efforts to change. Thus, we hypothesize that the response to subsequent sexual opportunities after these initial, difficult times may be avoidance. The avoidance mechanism then results in further reduction in the frequency of sexual activity, resulting in a negative-feedback loop.

INTERVENTIONS FOR SEXUAL MORBIDITY

Psychologic interventions can reduce distress, hasten resumption of routine activities, and improve social outcomes for groups at high risk for psychologic or behavioral morbidity, such as those with disseminated or recurrent disease, as well as those at low or moderate risk (see Andersen [46] for a review). When controlled studies have been reviewed, effective therapy components have included the following:

- An emotionally supportive context to address fears and anxieties about the disease (47–49)
- Information about the disease and treatment (48–51)
- Behavioral coping strategies (e.g., role-playing difficult discussions with family or the medical staff) (50,52)
- Cognitive coping strategies (47,52–54)
- Relaxation training to lower "arousal" and/or enhance sense of control (50,53)

Clinical services for sexuality might best be offered within a broad-based stress-and-coping framework (46). Such interventions might be designed, for example, to reduce stress, enhance coping and effective problem solving, provide information regarding the effects of disease and treatment, enhance social adjustment, and address gynecologic-specific sexual concerns—sexual self-concept, sexual behavior, and sexual functioning. Selection of specific therapeutic techniques and content for sexual interventions can be guided by the literature in psychosocial intervention research with cancer patients (55) (see Andersen [46] for a review), behavioral sex therapy techniques, clinical experience in the treatment of women during health crises or for sexual dysfunction, and of course empiric literature. For the sexuality portions, one can rely on many of the same sexual therapy principles and techniques that have documented effectiveness with healthy individuals (56,57), as many of the sexual problems described above are common (e.g., anticipatory concerns about resuming sexual activity following abstinence, arousal deficits, orgasmic dysfunction). However, other problems are unique (e.g., dyspareunia due to radiation-induced vaginal atrophy or stenosis), more severe (e.g., orgasmic dysfunction due to nerve and/or vascular disruption/removal rather than a skills deficit), or more distressing or difficult to overcome (e.g., permanent body disfigurement). Thus, development of some new techniques may be necessary, although the basic principles of social learning interventions (e.g., graduated assignments, development of a nondemanding performance environment) will be important. Finally, an often preferred strategy for conducting a sexual intervention involves partners who are available and interested in participating; however, it is clear that significant gains can be achieved by treating the individual, whether a woman has cancer or is healthy (58).

There are six components to interventions that can be helpful.

1. Information on coping with cancer and the potential impact on one's body can include didactic information on the specific disease, treatment modality, and changes anticipated or received for body parts and functions. Therapy sessions can include dialogue regarding the woman's feelings about the didactic information, problem solving for immediate concerns (e.g., recuperation from surgery, coping with menopausal symptoms, fear of recurrence), and role-playing of communication skills for facilitating problem solving and soliciting the support or assistance of others.

2. It is useful to consider the context for physical and sexual (body) changes and attempt to enhance sexual self-esteem. Didactic components can review the bodily changes brought by treatment, with emphasis on female sexual anatomy and physiology (coverage of the sexual response cycle and expected changes), sexual activity as a natural function, identifying and relabeling pain/discomfort or other difficult-to-control symptoms that may occur following treatment, and learning about one's body through touch. Homework components are often necessary and will need to be individualized depending on the disease site and treatment. Regardless of the site, however, assignments often include self-exploration of the body in bath or shower with or without including the breasts/genitals, a clinical look at the genitals/breasts, and Kegel (vaginal) exercises, for example.

3. Broadening the contexts for sexual activity and facilitating and enhancing sexual communication are important. Didactic/therapy sessions can include consideration of optimal timing for sexual activity given current health status, broadening the behavioral repertoire (e.g., sexual activities in lieu of intercourse, alternative intercourse positions), sexual desire as an "appetite," and strategies to facilitate desire (e.g., fantasy, erotic materials). Role-playing of negotiation with one's partner for changes in sexual routines and sharing information about anticipated changes (e.g., diminished lubrication, intercourse pain, difficulty with orgasm) are useful for women. Homework sessions might include body explorations with erotic focus, making choices about the contexts and types

of sexual activities, and information sharing with one's partner.

4. Efforts must be taken to manage dyspareunia (or other symptom/sign distractors during sexuality). Didactic information can include discussion of the causes (specific and general) of the sexually disruptive symptoms and signs with regard to the woman's disease/treatment. For vaginal pain, a multimodal strategy is often useful, combining behavioral strategies (e.g., use of vaginal dilators to gauge pain and decide about advisability of intercourse), the use of aids such as artificial lubricants, and relaxation procedures. For women with severe vaginal atrophy/stenosis, a regimen of dilator usage may be necessary. Homework sessions can include the use of dilators and the above treatments/aids with the continuation of vaginal Kegel exercises. In all cases, however, it is important to assess the advisability of sexual activity in the context of pain, vaginal or otherwise.

5. Discovering a partner's sexuality concerns and communicating one's own sexual concerns and needs are important. Didactic sessions can include discussion of male anatomy/physiology and anticipated partner reactions to the woman's illness, body changes, and sexual changes. Therapy may also include discussion of the woman's concerns about the partner's reaction to disease, illness, and changes in health and sexuality, and role-playing a discussion with the partner on topics of concern to the woman can be very comforting. For women without partners, one can discuss strategies for sharing information about one's cancer and treatments to a prospective partner, if the woman wishes. Homework, if appropriate, could be specific discussions with the partner.

6. Specific efforts to enhance arousal and orgasm may be needed. Strategies to facilitate orgasm, if disrupted by treatment, can be suggested, such as including additional manual stimulation. Therapeutic efforts need to encourage a woman's experimentation with alternative sexual activities, as well as engaging in activities to maintain interpersonal intimacy.

SUMMARY

For approximately one-half of women who receive a diagnosis of cancer, cancer is a survivable disease. Available data suggest cautious optimism that psychologic and sexual outcomes can be improved through general psychologic interventions, but it is likely that even greater gains could be achieved if sexuality-specific interventions were a central part of a therapeutic effort. As illustrated in Fig. 1, a strategy is offered for considering the medical factors that may contribute to risk for sexual morbidity. Moreover, a foundation of clinical research in cancer and basic research in sexuality have led to the discovery of an important individual-difference variable—a sexual self schema—that can be used to predict which women will be at risk for significant sexual morbidity. Consideration of both factors would be an important step forward in intervention research. Longitudinal data have highlighted the early trajectory of sexual problem development. A clinical model for the design of interventions for sexual rehabilitation is provided, and it suggests specific intervention strategies that can be of assistance for female cancer survivors.

REFERENCES

1. Welch-McCaffrey D, Hoffman B, Leigh SA, Loescher LJ, Meyskens FL. Surviving adult cancers. Part 2: psychosocial implications. *Ann Intern Med* 1989;111: 517–524.
2. Andersen BL, van der Does J. Sexual morbidity following gynecologic cancer: an international problem. *Int J Gynecol Cancer* 1994;4:225–240.
3. Wolf DM, Jordan VC. Gynecologic complications associated with long-term adjuvant tamoxifen therapy for breast cancer. *Gynecol Oncol* 1992;45:118–128.
4. Kaplan HS, Owett T. The female androgen deficiency syndrome. *J Sex Marital Ther* 1993;19:3–24.
5. Maguire GP, Lee EG, Bevington DJ, Kuchemann CS, Crabtree RJ, Cornell CE. Psychiatric problems in the first year after mastectomy. *BMJ* 1978;1:963–965.
6. Morris T, Greer HS, White P. Psychological and social adjustment to mastectomy: a two-year follow-up study. *Cancer* 1977;40:2381–2387.
7. Andersen BL, Anderson B, deProsse C. Controlled prospective longitudinal study of women with cancer: I. Sexual functioning outcomes. *J Consult Clin Psychol* 1989;57:683–691.
8. Margolis G, Goodman RL, Rubin A. Psychological effects of breast-conserving cancer treatment and mastectomy. *Psychosomatics* 1990;31:33–39.

9. Holmberg L, Omne-Ponten M, Burns T, Adami HO, Bergstrom R. Psychosocial adjustment after mastectomy and breast-conserving treatment. *Cancer* 1989;64:969–974.
10. Schover LR. Sexuality and body image in younger women with cancer. *J Natl Cancer Inst Monogr* 1994;6:177–182.
11. Kaplan HS. A neglect issue: the sexual side effects of current treatments for breast cancer. *J Sex Marital Ther* 1992;18:1–19.
12. Andersen BL, Lachenbruch PA, Anderson B, deProsse C. Sexual dysfunction and signs of gynecologic cancer. *Cancer* 1986;57:1880–1886.
13. Harris R, Good RS, Pollack L. Sexual behavior of gynecologic cancer patients. *Arch Sex Behav* 1982;11:503–510.
14. Weijmar Schultz WCM, van de Wiel HBM, Bouma J. Psychosexual functioning after treatment for cancer of the cervix: a comparative and longitudinal study. *Int J Gynecol Cancer* 1991;1:37–46.
15. Andersen BL, Karlsson JA, Anderson B, Tewfik HH. Anxiety and cancer treatment: response to stressful radiotherapy. *Health Psychol* 1984;3:535–551.
16. Karlsson JA, Andersen BL. Radiation therapy and psychological distress: outcomes and recommendations for enhancing adjustment. *J Psychosom Obstet Gynaecol* 1986;5:283–294.
17. Walling MK, Andersen BL, Johnson SR. Hormonal replacement therapy for postmenopausal women: sexual outcomes and related gynecologic effects. *Arch Sex Behav* 1990;119:119–137.
18. Krumm S, Lamberti J. Changes in sexual behavior following radiation therapy for cervical cancer. *J Psychosom Obstet Gynaecol* 1993;14:51–63.
19. Andersen BL, van der Does J, Anderson B. Sexual outcomes following gynecologic cancer. In: Coppelson M, Morrow P, Tattersall M, eds. *Gynecologic oncology*, 2nd ed. Edinburgh: Churchill Livingstone, 1992:1481–1497.
20. Cull A, Cowie VJ, Farquharson DIM, Livingstone JRB, Smart GE, Elton RA. Early-stage cervical cancer: psychosocial and sexual outcomes of treatment. *Br J Cancer* 1993;68:1216–1220.
21. Corney RH, Crowther ME, Everett H, Howells A, Shepherd JH. Psychosexual dysfunction in women with gynaecological cancer following radical pelvic surgery. *Br J Obstet Gynaecol* 1993;100:73–78.
22. Andersen BL, Hacker NF. Psychosexual adjustment following pelvic exenteration. *Obstet Gynecol* 1983;61:331–338.
23. Hacker NF. Treatment of cancer of the vulva. *Cancer* 1992;71:863–869.
24. DiSaia PJ, Creasman WT, Rich WM. An alternate approach to early cancer of the vulva. *Am J Obstet Gynecol* 1979;33:825–832.
25. Weijmar Schultz WCM, van de Wiel HBM, Bouma J, Janssens J, Littlewood J. Psychosexual functioning after treatment for cancer of the vulva: a longitudinal study. *Cancer* 1990;66:402–407.
26. Schag CAC, Ganz PA, Polinsky ML, Fred C, Hirji K, Petersen L. Characteristics of women at risk for psychosocial distress in the year after breast cancer. *J Clin Oncol* 1993;11:783–793.
27. Andersen BL. Predicting sexual and psychological morbidity and improving quality of life for women with gynecologic cancer. *Cancer* 1993;71:1678–1690.
28. Andersen BL. *Health Psychology's* contribution to addressing the cancer problem: update on accomplishments. *Health Psychol* 1989;8:683–703.
29. *Cancer facts and figures—1998.* New York: American Cancer Society, 1998.
30. Cella DF, Orofiamma B, Holland JC, et al. The relationship of psychological distress, extent of disease, and performance status in patients with lung cancer. *Cancer* 1987;60:1661–1667.
31. Andersen BL, Hacker NF. Psychosexual adjustment after vulvar surgery. *Obstet Gynecol* 1983;62:457–462.
32. Berek J, Andersen BL. Sexual rehabilitation: surgical and psychological approaches. In: Hoskins WJ, Perez CA, Young RC, eds. *Gynecologic oncology:* principles and practice, 2nd ed. Philadelphia: Lippincott–Raven Publishers, 1997:551–568.
33. Matthews KA, Wing RR, Kuller LH, et al. Influences of natural menopause on psychological characteristics and symptoms of middle-aged healthy women. *J Consult Clin Psychol* 1990;58:345–351.
34. Meyerowitz BE, Watkins IK, Sparks FC. Psychosocial implications of adjuvant chemotherapy: a two-year follow-up. *Cancer* 1983;52:1541–1545.
35. Kinsey AC, Pomeroy WB, Martin CE, Gebhard PH. *Sexual behavior in the human female.* Philadelphia: WB Saunders, 1953.
36. Newcomb ME. Notches on the bedpost: generational effects of sexual experience. *Psychology* 1986;23:37–46.
37. Wyatt GE, Peters SD, Guthrie D. Kinsey revisited, part I: comparisons of the sexual socialization and sexual behavior of white women over 33 years. *Arch Sex Behav* 1988;17:201–239.
38. Wyatt GE, Peters SD, Guthrie D. Kinsey revisited, part II: comparisons of the sexual socialization and sexual behavior of black women over 33 years. *Arch Sex Behav* 1988;17:289–331.
39. Curry SL, Levine SB, Jones PK, Kurit DM. Medical and psychosocial predictors of sexual outcome among women with systemic lupus erythematosus. *Arthritis Care Res* 1993;6:23–30.
40. Keil JE, Sutherland SE, Knapp RG, Waid LR, Gazes PC. Self-reported sexual functioning in elderly blacks and whites: the Charleston Heart Study experience. *J Aging Health* 1992;4:112–125.
41. Andersen BL, Cyranowski JC. Women's sexual self schema. *J Personal Soc Psychol* 1994;67:1079–1100.
42. Andersen BL, Woods XA, Copeland LJ. Sexual self-schema and sexual morbidity among gynecologic cancer survivors. *J Consult Clin Psychol* 1997;65(2):221–229.
43. Andersen BL, Elliott ML. Sexuality for women with cancer: assessment, theory, and treatment. *Sex Disabil* 1993;11:7–37.
44. Andersen BL, Golden-Kreutz D. Sexual self-concept for the women with cancer: implications for women and partners. In: Baider L, Cooper CL, De-Nour AK, eds. *Cancer and the family.* New York: John Wiley and Sons, 1996:337–366.
45. Andersen BL, LeGrand J. Body image for women: conceptualization, assessment, and a test of its importance to sexual dysfunction and medical illness. *J Sex Res* 1991;28:457–477.
46. Andersen BL. Psychological interventions for cancer

patients to enhance the quality of life. *J Consult Clin Psychol* 1992;60:552–568.
47. Cain EN, Kohorn EI, Quinlan DM, Latimer K, Schwartz PE. Psychosocial benefits of a cancer support group. *Cancer* 1986;57:183–189.
48. Capone MA, Good RS, Westie KS, Jacobson AF. Psychosocial rehabilitation of gynecologic oncology patients. *Arch Phys Med Rehabil* 1980;61:128–132.
49. Maguire P, Brooke M, Tait A, Thomas C, Sellwood R. The effect of counselling on physical disability and social recovery after mastectomy. *Clin Oncol* 1983;9: 319–324.
50. Fawzy FI, Cousins N, Fawzy N, Kemeny ME, Elashoff R, Morton D. A structured psychiatric intervention for cancer patients: I. Changes over time in methods of coping and affective disturbance. *Arch Gen Psychiatry* 1990;47:720–725.
51. Jacobs C, Ross RD, Walker IM, Stockdale FE. Behavior of cancer patients: a randomized study of the effects of education and peer support groups. *Am J Clin Oncol* 1983;6:347 353.
52. Houts PS, Whitney CW, Mortel R, Bartholomew MJ. Former cancer patients as counselors of newly diagnosed cancer patients. *J Natl Cancer Inst* 1986;76: 793–796.
53. Davis H. Effects of biofeedback and cognitive therapy on stress in patients with breast cancer. *Psychol Rep* 1986;59:967–974.
54. Telch CF, Telch MJ. Group coping skills instruction and supportive group therapy for cancer patients: a comparison of strategies. *J Consult Clin Psychol* 1986;54: 802–808.
55. Schover LR. *Sexuality and fertility after cancer.* New York: John Wiley and Sons, 1997.
56. Masters WH, Johnson VE. *Human sexual inadequacy.* Boston: Little, Brown and Company, 1970.
57. Rosen RC, Beck JG. *Patterns of sexual arousal.* New York: Guilford, 1988.
58. Andersen BL. A comparison of systematic desensitization and directed masturbation in the treatment of primary orgasmic dysfunction in females. *J Consult Clin Psychol* 1981;49:568–570.
59. Andersen BL, Turnquist D, LaPolla J, Turner D. Sexual functioning after treatment of *in-situ* vulvar cancer: Preliminary report. *Obstetrics and Gynecology* 1988; 71:15–19.

3

Hormone Therapy, Menopause, and Malignancy

Howard A. Zacur

Department of Gynecology and Obstetrics, Johns Hopkins Hospital and Johns Hopkins University School of Medicine, Baltimore, Maryland 21287

Management of menopause in a patient diagnosed with cancer requires an understanding of the physiology of menopause, as well as the known etiology of the malignancy. This information may then be shared with the patient, allowing her and her physician to formulate the best plan of future management.

MENOPAUSE AND HORMONE REPLACEMENT: BENEFITS AND RISKS

Menopause is clinically defined as the absence of menses for 1 year in women of appropriate age. In general, the average age of menopause is 50 years, although menopause may occur as early as age 43 or as late as age 57. Loss of oocytes within the ovaries causes menopause. Oocytes within the ovaries are fixed in number at birth. Oocytes with their surrounding granulosa cells are located in structures named follicles and form the follicular apparatus. The follicular apparatus is responsible for the secretion of estradiol-17β prior to ovulation. After ovulation, the follicular apparatus becomes the corpus luteum, which secretes estradiol-17β and progesterone. Estradiol and progesterone are responsible for causing menstruation by their actions on the endometrium. Absence of oocytes results in low levels of estradiol and progesterone and absence of menses.

Menopause is a biologic condition resulting in part from an increase in age. Aging is a risk factor for heart disease and cancer, which are the leading causes of death in the United States. On average, this means that each year more than 400,000 women will die from heart disease, while 250,000 will die from cancer (1). The population of the United States is aging, and it is estimated that by 2000 one-third of all women in the United States will be menopausal (2). One method of medical treatment of menopause is to administer estrogen or estrogen and progesterone. This has been called estrogen replacement therapy (ERT) when only estrogen is given and hormone replacement therapy (HRT) when both estrogen and progesterone are given.

After reviewing the data from many studies of menopause and hormone replacement, Bush et al. (3) reported in the 1980s that menopausal women receiving ERT experienced a 50% reduction in risk of being diagnosed with heart disease and dying from heart disease. Other investigators soon confirmed these findings. No study to date has failed to corroborate the beneficial effects of ERT on prevention of heart disease. Reports describing risk of heart disease and death from heart disease appear to be consistent with sex differences. Men have higher rates of heart disease and death from heart disease at all ages prior to the average age of menopause in women. Following menopause, the rates of heart disease and death from heart disease in women increase and become similar to those found in men.

In the initial studies of hormone replacement, women were given unopposed estrogen therapy. While a reduction in risk of heart disease was seen in these women, an increase in the risk of endometrial cancer was also observed (4,5). This risk was diminished when progestogen therapy was given with estrogen (6), which led to the recommendation that menopausal women with a uterus receiving hormone replacement be given progestogens with estrogens.

Initially, it was believed that ERT prevented heart disease by causing an increase in high-density lipoprotein coupled with a decrease in low-density lipoprotein (LDL). Subsequent research revealed that estrogen may affect coronary artery blood flow directly at the level of the vessel and prevent abnormal vasospasm (7). Because results from previous epidemiologic studies showed a reduction in risk of heart disease in menopausal women who took unopposed conjugated equine estrogens, concern was raised as to whether progestogens given with estrogen as part of a replacement regimen would be antagonistic to estrogen's actions. Recent studies in humans and subhuman primates show that progestogens (steroids that act like progesterone) given with estrogens worsen the lipid profile and increase the likelihood of abnormal coronary artery vasospasm. These adverse effects are not seen when progesterone (a progestin) alone is used (8,9). Unfortunately, mortality rates from long-term estrogen and progestogen-progestin therapy are not yet available to compare with mortality rates obtained after long-term use of estrogen replacement only.

In addition to its ability to protect against heart disease, ERT has also been shown to protect against bone loss and prevent osteoporosis. Bone loss occurs in both men and women after 30 years of age but is accelerated at the time of menopause in women. The rate of bone loss may be reduced in women with the administration of exogenous estrogens. Osteoporosis is not a leading cause of death, but it is believed to be responsible for more than 1.3 million fractures occurring annually in people age 45 years and older (10). Consequences of vertebral and hip fractures include preventing otherwise productive individuals from working while also increasing their utilization of nursing home care (11).

With aging comes an increase in the risk of being diagnosed with Alzheimer's disease, a neurodegenerative process affecting the brain and resulting in a progressive loss of mental function. It is a leading cause of loss of independence and institutionalization. The incidence of Alzheimer's disease is higher in women than in men, even when adjusted for age (12). Preliminary data appear to indicate that HRT reduces the risk of Alzheimer's disease by 30% to 40% (12,13). The mechanism by which estrogen is protective remains unknown, but reports have demonstrated the ability of estrogen to stimulate neurotrophic factors, as well as axonal regeneration and synaptogenesis (15,16). Positive effects on cerebral blood flow have also been reported following exogenous estrogen treatment (17).

The third leading cause of cancer death in women is colon cancer. The incidence of this disease begins to rise at age 40 and peaks between 60 and 75 years. Colon cancer is more common in women than men. Preliminary data appear to indicate a 30% to 40% reduction in risk of colon cancer in women using hormone replacement (18,19). The mechanism by which estrogen accomplishes this remains unknown, but alteration in bile salts has been suggested as one possibility. Unfortunately, the reduction in risk is lessened after cessation of hormone use.

The most common cancer diagnosed in women and the second leading annual cause of cancer death in women is breast cancer. It is estimated that breast cancer will develop in 180,000 women in the United States in 1998 and 44,000 will die from it (21). A relationship between menopausal estrogen use and risk for breast cancer has been reported by some authorities but not by others.

The leading cause of cancer death in women is lung cancer. At present, information is not available on any relationship between lung cancer, menopause, and HRT. Almost all believe that there is no relationship between ovarian cancer and estrogen use. The purpose of this chapter is to focus on the relationships between hormone use and cancer in menopausal women.

CAUSE OF CANCER

To better interpret the results of studies investigating the relationship between hormone replacement and malignancy in menopausal women, it is important to briefly review what is currently known about how cancer develops. After many years of intensive research, a general outline of how a malignancy arises has taken shape. An excellent review of this process, presented by Weinberg (22), is briefly summarized below.

Cellular function governed by a cell's genome is quite complex and has evolved to allow orderly cellular growth and differentiation. Many factors controlling cellular division exist for the purpose of either stimulating or inhibiting. Cell division is best described in terms of the cell cycle composed of four stages: G_1, S, G_2, and M. In the G_1 (gap 1) phase, the cell synthesizes proteins in preparation for its upcoming division. At a certain point in the G_1 phase, the cell passes a point of no return and it is committed to division. This is called the cell's *restriction point.* Once this is passed, the cell enters its S (synthesis) phase, during which duplication of its deoxyribonucleic acid (DNA) occurs. After this phase is completed, the cell enters the G_2 (gap 2) phase, during which proteins are synthesized in preparation for its mitosis (M) phase. After mitosis, two daughter cells are formed that now may enter the G_1 phase or may undergo cell rest, in which the cell remains at what is called its G_0 stage.

Integral to the process of successful cellular division is the synthesis of key proteins. Of particular importance are the cyclins—D, E, B, and A—and the cyclin-dependent kinases (CDK). During G_1 when sufficient levels of cyclins D and E are present, CDK activity increases, resulting in phosphorylation of the retinoblastoma protein that allows transcription factors bound to this protein to become activated. These factors in turn lead to additional gene activation and subsequent synthesis of additional proteins that ultimately leads to DNA synthesis and cell division.

Mechanisms within the cell regulate the cell cycle. Inhibiting proteins known as p27 or p15, whose production is affected by growth factors, may block the CDK activity. Production of proteins known as p53 or p21 may result in inhibition of CDK activity or stimulation of cell death (apoptosis). Well known growth-factor-protein genes include *erb B* and *erb B2*, which code for the receptors for epidermal growth factor and growth factor, respectively. *Myc* genes, that is, C-*myc*, N-*myc*, and L-*myc*, code for transcription factors that activate growth-promoting genes, while the *ras* genes, that is, Ki-*ras* and N-*ras*, are involved in stimulatory cell signaling. The gene *Bc*1-2 codes for a protein that blocks cell suicide. Many steps must be taken before a cell begins to divide. Mutations in the genes responsible for controlling cellular division have been identified in malignancies. These mutations may either be inherited or acquired during life. When genetics plays a major role in the development of certain malignancies such as colon or brain cancer, the most differentiated and least aggressive forms of these cancers contain only a few gene mutations, whereas the undifferentiated and most aggressive malignancies possess these same mutations and many others as well. As a consequence of this observation, the clonal selection theory of malignancy has been proposed. In this model, when a gene mutation occurs within a cell capable of dividing, its daughter cells will be similarly affected (23). When these daughter cells are exposed to additional insults, other gene mutations may occur; and when these cells divide, all their daughter cells will consist of all of these mutations and so forth. Eventually, cellular control mechanisms are circumvented, and unregulated cell growth occurs. For example, in breast cancer cells, excessive production of cyclins D and E has been reported. In many human tumors, absence or nonfunction of the p53 protein has been observed. Loss or mutation of an allele or alleles responsible for specifying the synthesis of a tumor-suppressor protein may initiate the process. If the gene mutation involves the cellular processes involved in adhesion, invasive metastatic cells may be created.

Estrogen is well known as a mitogen (a hormone that stimulates cell division). This action may result from the ability of estrogen to stimulate transcription of the protein cyclin D responsible for stimulating cellular division (24). No scientific report exists proving that estrogen is mutagenic or carcinogenic. Progesterone will stimulate differentiation of cells, for example, the decidualization of an endometrial stromal cell. Progesterone is not mutagenic. Agents believed to act as carcinogens by causing mutations of genes include tobacco smoke and chemicals such as polychlorinated biphenyls and benzene. Mechanisms by which these agents actually cause mutagenesis remain to be determined.

MANAGEMENT OF MENOPAUSAL WOMEN DIAGNOSED WITH CANCER

It is important for menopausal patients diagnosed with cancer to be informed about the known benefits and risks of and alternatives to HRT. Until quite recently, healthy menopausal patients were treated with estrogen solely for quality-of-life reasons. These included suppression of hot flushes, amelioration of vaginal dryness, and improvement in skin tone and appearance. For many healthy menopausal women, these aforementioned changes are not of sufficient benefit to cause them to request ERT. In fact, many women have believed, as many still do, that menopause is a natural physiologic event that should not be reversed or treated by hormones.

Since it is now known that the risk of heart disease may be reduced along with the risk of osteoporosis, health benefits may be afforded those willing to take HRT. But does taking HRT cause any medical problems? Increased risks for breast cancer and thrombosis from HRT are of concern to menopausal women. These risks are of even greater concern to menopausal women who have already been diagnosed with cancer or another medical problem. But when one is discussing the management of menopause with a patient who has already been diagnosed with cancer, or with a patient who is concerned that hormone replacement could cause cancer, the discussion should place emphasis on the treatment of a whole or complete individual and not a specific organ. That is to say the fear of acquiring cancer within a particular organ should be assessed in context with the knowledge that HRT could prolong life even while causing cancer.

Alternatives to HRT do exist for menopausal patients. These include specific drugs to treat bone loss or hot flushes. Exercise, weight loss, and medications to lower cholesterol and blood pressure may all be used to reduce the risk and/or recurrence of heart disease and stroke. Menopausal women concerned about risks of HRT should be counseled as to alternatives to it.

Bone Loss

Bone accretion is governed by bone-forming osteoblasts, while osteoclasts are responsible for bone resorption. Before age 30 years, bone formation exceeds bone resorption in men and women. After age 30, a gradual loss in bone thickness occurs. Once a critical threshold of bone density is reached, the likelihood of fracture increases significantly. A fracture threshold may never be reached in individuals who have very dense bones at age 30, but may be rapidly reached in individuals whose bones are quite thin when active bone loss begins. African-American women in general have denser bones than white women. Lindsay (25) provides an excellent review of bone formation and loss.

Bone density may be estimated by one of several techniques, but the current gold standard is dual-energy x-ray absorptiometry.

With this method, x-rays with two different photon energies are used to penetrate the body, allowing the density of bone to be differentiated from the density of adjacent soft tissue (26). Densities of trabecular bone (vertebrae) and cortical bone (head and neck of femur) are calculated and compared to the respective bone densities found in a young reference population of women 20 to 35 years of age who presumably have maximal bone density.

If a patient's bone density measurement is more than 1 standard deviation less than that of the reference population (T score), osteopenia is present, as defined by a working group of the World Health Organization (27). If the T score is 2.5 standard deviations below peak bone mass, osteoporosis is said to exist.

If a menopausal patient's baseline bone density is equivalent to that of a younger woman, her chances of experiencing a bone fracture are reduced. HRT would be less likely to be recommended to this patient for the purpose of reducing bone loss and fracture risk. Serial bone density measurements at 1- to 2-year intervals could be ordered, and consideration of HRT entertained if bone density markedly declined. Current recommendations to preserve bone mass that do not involve hormone replacement include daily ingestion of adequate amounts of calcium and vitamin D. Daily intakes of 1000 to 1500 mg of calcium (28) and 800 IU of vitamin D are suggested. Calcium citrate maleate has better bioavailability than calcium carbonate and has been recommended by Dawson-Hughes (29). Weightbearing exercise should also be encouraged, but exercise alone will not improve bone mass in women with low bone density.

Bisphosphonate compounds such as alendronate sodium (Fosamax), taken orally in daily doses of 10 mg after awakening and before eating or drinking, has been found to prevent bone loss and increase bone mass in women with osteoporosis (30). Bisphosphonates inhibit osteoclastic activity. A major side effect of bisphosphonate use is gastrointestinal irritability, which prevents many women from taking this medication. There are no data yet on adverse consequences after long-term use of bisphosphonates.

Changes in personal life habits may also affect bone loss. Women who smoke cigarettes have lower bone densities than nonsmokers. Smoking accelerates the metabolic clearance of endogenous estrogens and may inhibit gastrointestinal absorption of calcium. All men and women who smoke cigarettes should be encouraged to stop. Alcohol intake impairs absorption of vitamin D. Nutrient absorption may also be inhibited by excessive alcohol intake that has caused liver damage and/or gastrointestinal irritation. Individuals who drink excessive amounts of alcohol should be encouraged to stop.

Hot Flushes/Flashes

Hot flushes or flashes are manifestations of withdrawal of estrogen from the central nervous system (CNS). Typically, a hot flush is described as a sensation of warmth beginning in the area of the face and spreading down toward the neck and chest, followed by erythema and perspiration in those areas.

Events that trigger the onset of hot flushes remain undetermined. A hot flush begins because the body's core temperature has been reset to a lower value (31). Heat loss occurs as the body attempts to achieve a lower core temperature through vasodilation of blood vessels beneath the skin. As heat escapes, a hot flush is experienced. When the brain's temperature regulator resets the core body temperature to its normal value, heat loss stops and a chill may occur. When a hot flush occurs at night, the woman is often awakened and has difficulty in going back to sleep. Sleep deprivation over time may be responsible for some changes in mood or behavior observed or complained of during the perimenopause or early menopausal years. Hot flushes are experienced by almost all women during the first year of menopause and are most intense for those who have experienced surgical menopause. After the first year of menopause, 20% of women will continue having hot flushes indefinitely. Cessation of hot flushes will almost certainly occur following administration of the appropriate estrogen dose. Failure to prevent a hot flush after appropriate estrogen administration usually implies that the hot flush is due to a cause other than estrogen deficiency. For women with cancer who have been advised not to take hormonal therapy or who are afraid to take hormonal therapy, alternatives to estrogen treatment of hot flushes are limited (Table 1).

Behavioral therapy, that is, deliberate deep breathing, has been reported to reduce the frequency of hot flushes by 40% (32). Women who exercise regularly have reported having fewer hot flushes than women who do not exercise (33). Anecdotally, some women have reported that the use of various herbs or acupuncture is of benefit in treating hot flushes, but definitive scientific studies proving this are lacking. In a recent double-blind, randomized, placebo-controlled study, dong quai failed to produce biologic estrogen-like responses and did not relieve menopausal symptoms (34). Patients must be urged to use caution when considering herbal therapies to treat hot flushes; possibly severe risks may exist from this therapy. A recent report evaluated the hormonal potential of the herbal preparation known as PC-SPES (35). This had been used by men with prostate cancer. PC-SPES consists of chrysanthemum, isatis, licorice, *Ganoderma lucidum, Panax,* pseudoginseng, *Rabdosia rubescens,* saw palmetto, and scutellaria. From *in vitro* studies, PC-SPES was found to have potent estrogenic activity and, when taken by men, caused breast tenderness, loss of libido, and venous thrombosis (35). Other herbal preparations have been found to cause liver damage and to act as anticoagulants when taken by men or women.

TABLE 1. *Alternatives to estrogen for treatment of hot flushes*

Behavioral therapy (deep breathing)
Exercise
Clonidine HCl (Catapres) 0.2–0.4 mg/d
Lofexidine
Veraliperide, 100 mg/d
Phenobarbital/ergotamine tartrate/belladonna (Bellergal-S)
Ethamsylate
Soy, 60 g/d
Danazol (Danocrine), 100 mg/d
Medroxyprogesterone acetate, 20 mg/d

Alpha-adrenergic agonists have been recommended as treatment for hot flushes. Clonidine hydrochloride (Catapres), given in doses up to 0.4 mg per day, has been reported to significantly reduce the frequency of hot flushes (46% decline). Use of a 0.2-mg dose reduced the frequency of hot flushes to a value almost as low as that seen with a 0.4-mg dose. Dry mouth, insomnia, syncopal episodes, severe headaches, nausea, and dizziness have been reported as significant side effects (36). Lofexidine, another adrenergic agonist, has also been used to reduce hot flushes, but side effects have been reported as well (37).

An antidopaminergic drug, veraliperide, 100 mg per day given orally, has been used by women to significantly reduce the frequency of hot flushes. Side effects have included prolactin elevation and mastodynia (38). An open 6-month comparison between veraliperide and transdermal estrogen showed that estrogen treatment was significantly superior to veraliperide with regard to quality of life (39).

A medication consisting of ergotamine tartrate, belladonna alkaloids, and phenobarbital (Bellergal-S) has also been used to reduce the frequency of hot flushes. This is the United States Food and Drug Administration (FDA)–approved indication for this drug. Side effects include paresthesias, palpitations, and dry mouth. Use of phenobarbital may be habit forming as well (40).

Another nonhormonal agent is ethamsylate (41–43). Use of dietary supplements has also been recommended to control hot flushes. In a recent report, it was shown that daily ingestion of 60 g of soy protein reduced the frequency of hot flushes by 45%. However, women ingesting 60 g of casein daily (placebo) had a 30% reduction of hot flushes. Over 10% of the subjects in each group of this study (70 in each group) dropped out because of gastrointestinal symptoms (44). Use of either soy or wheat flour has also been reported to reduce hot-flush frequency by 40% and 25%, respectively, after 12 weeks (45). Certain dietary supplements contain phytoestrogens. Common phytoestrogens include the isoflavones genistein and daidzein found in soy beans, the lignins enterolactone and enterodiol (formed in the colon as metabolites of matairesinol and secoisolariciresinol), and the coumestans, which are flavonoid molecules (e.g., coumestrol) found in legumes (46).

Hormones other than estrogens or phytoestrogens have been used to treat hot flushes. Androgens and progestogens have been utilized for this purpose. Danazol (Danocrine), a 17α-ethinyl derivative of testosterone has been shown to be effective in low doses (100 mg/day) (47). Testosterone given alone has not proven effective for this purpose (48). Medroxyprogesterone acetate, given orally in a dose of 20 mg daily or intramuscularly as monthly injection of up to 150 mg, has been shown to markedly reduce the frequency of hot flushes (49,98).

For women with a past history of ovarian or endometrial malignancy, androgen or progestogen therapy to treat hot flushes would not appear to be controversial in view of the fact that high-dose progestin therapy is used to treat endometrial cancers. Patients should be informed that data do not exist on the actual risk of malignancy recurrence when these hormones are taken. Use of androgens and estrogens to suppress hot flushes in women previously treated for breast cancer is problematic, given the knowledge that duct and alveolar growth within the breast may respond to progestogens and the effect of androgens on breast cancer has not been well studied.

CARDIOVASCULAR DISEASE

Reductions in risk of heart disease and in death from heart disease are two reasons frequently given for advocating ERT or HRT for menopausal women. Detrimental effects from HRT include the risk of causing a malignancy, recurrence of a malignancy, or a life-threatening side effect (e.g., venous thromboembolism).

Reduction in heart disease risk without HRT may be accomplished by many methods (Table 2). Dietary habits need to be altered to reduce caloric intake to levels necessary to maintain ideal body weight. Decreased fat with increased fiber intake should be emphasized. Smoking and excessive alcohol intake should be curtailed and exercise encouraged. A more precise estimate of how these changes in lifestyle may affect survival in menopausal women will hopefully be determined when results from the National Institutes of Health–funded Women's Health Initiative are published.

For individuals unable or unwilling to change their diet or adopt changes in their lifestyle, further reduction in cardiovascular disease risk may be obtained through appropriate drug therapy. While it is known that ERT is associated with an improvement in the lipid profile, this favorable change is not as great as that resulting from use of cholesterol-lowering drugs i.e. "statin" therapy (50). Identification of individuals with carbohydrate intolerance and institution of therapy designed to improve or replace endogenous insulin activity are of obvious benefit. So too are the diagnosis and appropriate treatment of hypertension. If hypertensive menopausal patients cannot undertake a weight loss and exercise regime, antihypertension medication is well known to reduce cardiovascular risk.

Data collected from the Nurses' Health Study indicated that after adjustments for age and other risk factors, the overall relative risk of major coronary disease in women currently

TABLE 2. *Reduction in heart disease risk without hormone therapy*

Dietary change
Cessation of smoking
Curtailment of excessive alcohol intake
Use cholesterol-lowering drugs
Prevention/treatment of hypertension
Treatment of diabetes
Intake of vitamin E

taking estrogen was 0.56. There was no evidence of an increased risk of stroke in this study (51).

It has been hypothesized that oxidized LDL plays an important role in causing atherosclerosis. It is believed that oxidized LDL is readily taken up by macrophages to create foam cells (52,53). Vitamin E is carried in LDL particles and prevents the oxidation of LDL (54). Results of the Nurses' Health Study showed that women taking vitamin E supplements at higher levels (average, 208 IU per day; range, 21.6 to 1000 IU/day) experienced an age- and smoking-adjusted relative risk of major coronary heart disease of 0.66. This value is not dissimilar to that found with use of estrogen alone (55). A lower risk for heart disease in vitamin-E users remained even after adjustment for coronary risk factors and use of other dietary antioxidants. It should be mentioned, however, that other prospective epidemiologic studies did not show a beneficial effect of vitamin E in all instances (14).

Results from the Heart and Estrogen/Progestin Replacement Study (HERS) indicate that the cardioprotective effects of estrogen may not be as great for women with known heart disease (56). In this study, women with documented heart disease were followed for 4 years, during which they were given either placebo or 0.625 mg of conjugated equine estrogens with 2.5 mg of medroxyprogesterone acetate (Prempro). This study was prospective, randomized, and double-blind. At its conclusion, no difference in the number of heart attacks or deaths was observed between study groups. A trend of reduced number of heart attacks was noted over time in the estrogen users, and a follow-up study of these women is currently in progress. Women who were already taking medications for treatment of heart disease, hypertension, and hypercholesterolemia were not excluded from this study. As a consequence, the cardioprotective effect of estrogen might have been masked, as its beneficial effects may not have been additive to those of the other medications that these women were taking.

Of some concern was the observation that during the first year of the study, women taking hormone replacement experienced more adverse cardiac events and venous thromboembolic events (56). The reason for this remains undetermined. A relationship between estrogen dosage and thromboembolic events has previously been noted from studies of women taking the combination oral contraceptive pill. An increase in idiopathic venous thromboembolism in hormone replacement users (approximately 1 extra case per 5000 users) has now been reported (57,58). Risk of venous thromboembolism appears to be restricted to current use and is not increased by past use of either oral contraceptives or hormone replacement (20).

BREAST CANCER AND HORMONE REPLACEMENT

There is no question that a relationship exists between estrogen and cancer of the breast. Breast cancer rarely occurs in men who have low levels of estradiol circulating in their blood stream. Exposure to higher levels of estrogen at puberty in women results in breast gland development and growth of breast tissue because the breast is a target tissue for estrogen. Existence of breast tissue is therefore correlated with an increased risk of breast cancer. Thus, it is not surprising to learn of associations between breast cancer risk and estrogen exposure.

However, a *causal* relationship between estrogen and breast cancer has never been demonstrated. Breast cancer is a disease associated with aging. Most breast cancers occur after menopause, when estrogen levels are lowest. During the years of peak estrogen levels (i.e., after menarche and before menopause), the risk of developing breast cancer is extremely low. Use of high-dose exogenous estrogen (i.e., contraceptive pills) by women who already have high endogenous estrogen levels between the ages of menarche and menopause is not associated with an increased risk of breast cancer (59). To implicate estrogen in causing breast cancer epidemiologically, it would be necessary to demonstrate from the medical literature a very strong association between hormone use and development of breast cancer, a dose–response effect, consistency between studies, and biologic plausibility. This has not yet been accomplished.

Breast cancer is the most common cause of cancer in women and is the second leading cause of cancer death in women. While the incidence of breast cancer appears to be increasing, fatalities from this disease have actually declined slightly since 1990 (60). At age 50 years, a woman's risk for breast cancer is 1 in 50 (2%). If a woman lives to be older than age 85, her risk for breast cancer is 1 in 8 (12.5%) (61). Women at greater risk for breast cancer are those who have the following factors (62):

- Family history of breast cancer
- Earlier age of menarche
- Older age at first childbirth
- Later age of menopause
- Nulliparity
- Previous radiation therapy
- Obesity
- Increased height
- Alcohol use

The magnitude of the increased risk from each of these predisposing factors is frequently expressed as a relative risk, and ranges from 1.1 to 1.5 for most factors but may be as high as 4 to 6 for other factors. A relative risk is the ratio between the rate of disease in a population exposed to a suspected cause of the disease and the rate of disease identified in a similar patient population not exposed to the disease. For example, this would be the rate of breast cancer in menopausal women taking hormone replacement versus the rate of breast cancer in menopausal women not taking hormone replacement. Calculation of the true relative risk must be obtained from prospective, controlled studies. Retrospective, case–control studies produce an odds ratio that is used to estimate the relative risk, but this is not the true relative risk. To be statistically significant, the confidence interval (CI) for the value of the relative risk must exceed 1. Relative risks are often announced to the public as increased risks of 10%, 20%, 30% or more, instead of the values 1.1, 1.2, and 1.3, respectively. This frequently causes confusion. Another way of describing increased risk is to use the relative risk in conjunction with the age-dependent rate of disease diagnosis. For example, after living to age 50, a woman's normal risk for breast cancer by that age is 1 in 50 (2%). If a particular factor increases a woman's risk for breast cancer by 40% to 50%, which is equivalent to a relative risk of 1.4 or 1.5, her risk for breast cancer would be 1.4 or 1.5 divided by 50, or a 2.8% or 3% risk, instead of 1.0 divided by 50 (2%). One predisposing factor that increases a woman's risk for breast cancer by 40% to 50% is alcohol use, that is, one or two drinks per day. This risk is as great as that ascribed to estrogen use. Obesity also produces a comparable increased risk. Despite the identification of risk factors for breast cancer, it should not be forgotten that women may develop breast cancer without having risk factors or they may never develop breast cancer while having many risk factors.

During the past 70 years, the rate of breast cancer has been steadily increasing in the United States, with the greatest increase being seen in older women. This should not seem surprising, since life expectancy has also increased during the past 70 years. Methods used to detect breast cancer have also changed during this time. Modern-day breast-imaging techniques such as mammography are capable of detecting malignancies not detectable by palpation. The effect of improved screening as an explanation for the overall increased incidence of breast cancer has been disputed, however.

To adequately discuss relationships between estrogen/progesterone hormone use and breast cancer, it is essential to discuss the anatomy of the breast, the response of the breast to hormonal stimulation, and the types of malignancies that may arise within the heart. Breast tissue is composed of ducts, glands, connective tissue, and fat (Fig. 1).

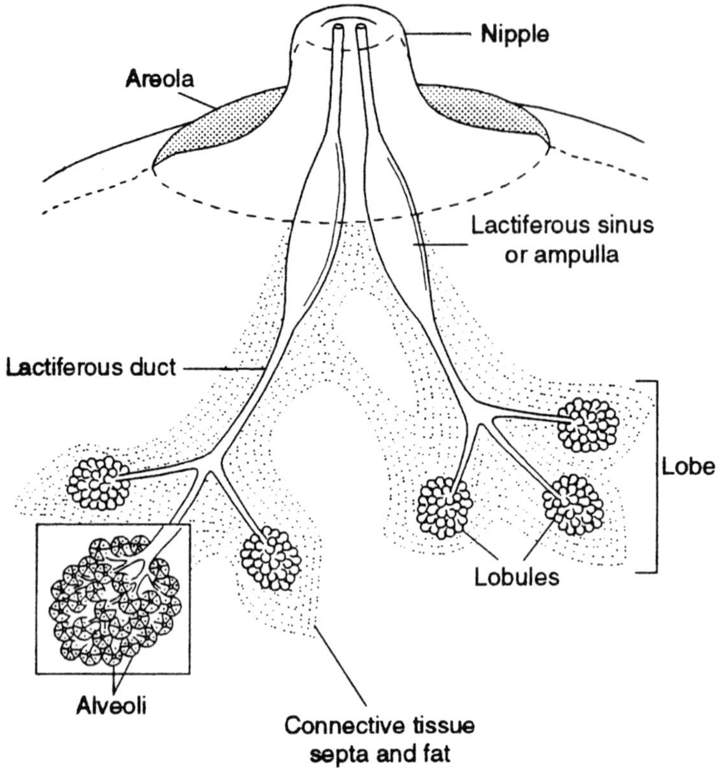

FIG. 1. Ducts, sinuses, lobes, lobules, and alveoli of the human breast depicted schematically. Each lactiferous sinus or ampulla drains one of 15–25 breast lobes. (From ref. 97, with permission.)

Each breast is divided into 10 to 15 lobes that are separated by connective tissue and fat. Each lobe is identified by a common duct that ultimately discharges its fluid from an opening located on the nipple. Small ductules or ductuli emanate from this common duct and are directed into the outer regions of the breast lobe, ending in small sacs or alveoli. Alveoli are lined by acinar cells that secrete proteins found in breast milk. The alveolar cells represent the glandular component of the breast. In response to estrogen secreted into the blood stream in increasing amounts at puberty, the duct system of the breast begins to arborize. In response to progesterone secreted into the blood stream after ovulation begins to occur, the glandular cells of the breast begin to enlarge and divide. As a consequence of exposure to estrogen and progesterone, the human breast enlarges and matures throughout puberty. Complete maturation of the breast is not thought to take place until pregnancy, when the breast is exposed to very high concentrations of both estrogen and progesterone, as well as to other steroids and proteins secreted from the placenta. After childbirth, the breast, having already been primed by high levels of estrogen and progesterone, is exposed to prolactin, insulin, and growth hormones. This causes breast-milk synthesis and secretion. Breast milk is composed of the proteins casein and α-lactalbumin, produced by the acinar cells of the breast. Electrolytes and fluid secreted into the duct lumen across acinar cells also contribute to the formation of breast milk. In the absence of pregnancy, small amounts of fluids, electrolytes, steroids, and proteins are continually secreted into the breast duct system and reabsorbed by acinar cells.

BREAST CARCINOMA

Breast cancers arise from neoplastic changes occurring in the ducts and alveolar units. The most common malignancies are ductal and lobular carcinomas, which may either be *in situ* or invasive.

Ductal carcinoma *in situ* (CIS) or intraductal breast cancer is characterized by malignant cells that do not invade adjacent stromal tissue. This type of breast cancer accounts for 20% to 30% of all newly diagnosed breast cancers (63) and is commonly diagnosed by mammography, as its presence is made known by microcalcifications. Microcalcifications result from necrosis of atypical ductal cells that have accumulated in ductal lumina. A fourfold increase in incidence of ductal CIS has been reported since 1980 (64). The probability that superficial ductal breast cancer will progress to invasive cancer remains unknown, with some authorities suggesting that this will never occur and others suggesting that there is a 30% chance of invasive disease arising within 6 to 10 years of the initial diagnosis of CIS (62,63). In a recent review of autopsy reports, the median prevalence of ductal CIS was 8.9% (range, 0 to 14.7%) (67). This prevalence rate was based on autopsy data of women not previously known to have breast cancer. It may therefore be argued that since mortality from breast cancer has not increased, there is less likelihood that ductal CIS of the breast will cause death (67).

Lobular CIS refers to disease found within breast lobules that rarely includes the ducts. This type of cancer rarely becomes invasive and is often multicentric. It is a histologic diagnosis because distinctive features of this malignancy are not found on mammography or by gross inspection. Its true prevalence is uncertain because it is only detected incidentally by breast biopsies performed for other reasons.

Invasive breast cancers are adenocarcinomas that are classified as ductal or lobular based on histologic appearance. Most of these tumors are found in distal ducts near the lobules. The most common invasive breast cancer is infiltrating ductal carcinoma, which accounts for 75% of malignancies. Infiltrating lobular breast cancer accounts for 5% to 10% of malignancies. Invasive breast cancers are most apt to metastasize to ipsilateral axillary nodes (68).

Estrogen Effect

Estrogen is a term used to describe a class of steroid hormones that act on specific target organs. The dictionary definition of an estrogen is a substance that will produce estrus. This is an effect seen in murine species. Commonly accepted actions of estrogen in humans include producing tissue effects within the breasts, uterus, and vagina. More recently, effects of estrogen on the brain, heart, bones, and colon of humans have also been identified. The most potent endogenous estrogen is estradiol-17β, produced principally by the follicular apparatus within the ovaries. The next most potent endogenous estrogen is estrone, formed within fat cells after the aromatization of the A ring of androstenedione. Least potent of the biologic estrogens is estriol, secreted from the fetal-placental unit during pregnancy. The definition for the potency of an estrogen may be debated. Traditionally, estrogenic potency was determined by the change in weight of uterine horns in immature rats exposed to varying doses of the estrogenic steroid of interest. This type of definition is species- and organ-specific and may be of limited usefulness when determination of the potency of an estrogen within another species or within another organ is attempted.

Initial efforts to identify how estrogen produces its biologic response in different tissues resulted in the identification of an estrogen receptor (ER). Later, it was found that the ER existed within the cell nucleus. Following the binding of one estrogen molecule to one receptor, pairs of receptors with their estrogen molecules join together and then attach to the genome at a specific site known as an estrogen-response element.

Following binding of ERs to the gene, a transcription complex forms, allowing ribonucleic acid (RNA) polymerase to transcribe the DNA into messenger RNA. At one time, it was believed that all actions of estrogens could be explained on the basis of this aforementioned ER-gene binding concept. Weaker estrogens were said to bind less tightly to the ER than more potent estrogens.

At present, the actions of estrogens appear to be far more complex then initially believed. A second ER, termed beta, has been identified (69). The first ER is known as alpha. The ability of estrogen to affect cell wall permeability of Ca^{2+} and K^{+} has been reported, as well as the ability of estrogen to stimulate adenylate cyclase activity using mechanisms independent of binding to either the nuclear alpha- or beta-ER. As a consequence of this new knowledge, care must be exercised in trying to interpret data from previous studies that attempted to show how estrogen might or might not affect a target organ because of its ability or lack of ability to bind to the alpha-ER.

The relationship between estrogen and breast cancer has been one of guilt by association. The majority of invasive breast cancers are ductal cancers. Growth of breast ducts is a biologic response of the mammary gland to estrogen exposure. If estrogen exposure does not occur, breast duct development will be limited. Therefore, it is not surprising that almost all breast cancers occur in women, since women possess more ductal breast tissue than men. A similar explanation may be used to explain the other well known associations between estrogen and breast cancer. Early menarche, late menopause, nulliparity, obesity, and alcohol use have all been associated with heightened estrogen production (62). With increased estrogen exposure, increased breast duct growth is expected. Therefore, an increase in the risk of breast cancer would also not seem surprising because of this biologic response. Estrogen is a mitogen. Numerous studies have not shown estrogen to be a carcinogen (70). That is to say, exposure of normal cells to estrogen does not result in malignant transformation of a normal cell, which is one response that might be seen after radiation exposure. Basic research studies have shown that estrogen may increase the amount of cyclins within cells. Cyclins are responsible for triggering cell division. This is again consistent with the mitogenic activity of estrogen and inconsistent with carcinogenic activity.

Administration of estrogen and progesterone to breast cancer cells in culture has yielded conflicting results. Increase in tumor cell growth and inhibition in cell growth have both been reported. Cellular growth is dependent on changes in the cell cycle that cause cells to go from resting or G_0 phase into the G_1 phase and beyond. Triggering factors for this process include growth factors or inhibitors, such as transforming growth factors α or β. These factors are frequently presented to tumor cells from adjacent cells, which are often not included in *in vitro* experiments. As a consequence, the usefulness of trying to interpret results from *in vitro* cultures of breast cancer cells may be quite limited.

Overview

Recently, a rereview of 51 previously published epidemiologic studies on breast cancer was published (72). The authors of this study were given the raw data from each of the 51 original studies reported in the literature. The authors then used these data to perform a reanalysis of all the combined data. Involved were 54,000 menopausal women, of whom 18,000 had breast cancer and 36,000 did not. The median age at diagnosis was 60 years. Even use of hormone replacement was associated with a relative risk of 1.1 for breast cancer, while hormone use for more than 15 years was associated with a relative risk of 1.6. If hormone was used 5 years or more in the past, there was no increased risk for breast cancer. This would imply a recency-of-use effect or that exposure to estrogen stimulates or promotes the growth of preexisting disease, rather than stimulating the formation of a new cancer. It would also appear to be an argument that one could use to refute the hypothesis that prolonged exposure to estrogen increases the risk of being diagnosed with breast cancer. Results from this study also reveal an effect of estrogen that is dependent on body mass index (BMI). For women with a high BMI, there was a decrease in breast cancer risk with estrogen use. For women with a low BMI, the relative risk following estrogen use was 1.7 (70%).

Biases favoring a higher rate of identifying breast cancer in ERT users include greater utilization of mammography services, higher socioeconomic status, and more frequent use of alcohol. Biases lowering the risk of breast cancer include increased physical activity and lower bone density. Controversy about the risk of breast cancer in hormone replacement users exists. This was recently made most evident by the publication of two epidemiologic studies with different conclusions. In 1995, Colditz et al. (73) published a report in which there was an increased relative risk of breast cancer of 1.46 in women using hormone replacement for more than 5 years. At the same time, another report indicated that there was no increased risk of breast cancer in women using estrogen alone or estrogen and progestin as replacement for longer than 5 years (74). As previously mentioned, biases that could have existed in these studies include enrolling women who were thinner, had fewer children, drank more alcohol, and had more mammograms.

One apparent paradox exists from all epidemiologic studies, except for the Nurses' Health Study. This paradox is that while an increase in the diagnosis of breast cancer is reported in hormone replacement users, there is either no change or a decrease in mortality from breast cancer when diagnosed in these same individuals. The better survival for women who have used estrogen and have been diagnosed with breast cancer could be the result of a different type of breast cancer, earlier detection, or decreased risk of death from other causes.

In summary, there is little risk of breast cancer following ERT for less than 5 years. Long-term use does appear to increase risk, but this risk disappears 5 years after cessation of hormone use.

HORMONE REPLACEMENT REGIMENS

Hormone replacement for menopausal cancer patients should be made available to well informed women who are unable to tolerate alternative regimens or who feel strongly that the benefits of hormone replacement outweigh the risks. The willingness of both a menopausal patient with cancer and her physician to proceed with hormone replacement will frequently depend on the type of malignancy diagnosed.

Data are lacking on the negative aspects of hormone replacement given to women diagnosed with nonreproductive tract malignancies, including lung, skin, or CNS malignancies. As previously mentioned, there may be a protective effect of estrogen therapy on reduction in the risk for colon cancer, but no data exist on whether ERT given to women already diagnosed with colon cancer will prevent recurrence or further spread the disease.

Absence of data on hormone replacement and development or worsening of malignancies other than those related to the reproductive tract necessitates that physicians and their patients recognize the limitations of current medical knowledge and the uncertain risk that HRT could pose.

For women previously diagnosed with endometrial cancer, data do exist to help in deciding whether or not to take systemic hormone replacement. Creasman et al. (75) demonstrated that for women previously treated for endometrial cancer, HRT utilizing 0.0625 mg of conjugated equine estrogens does not appear in short-term follow-up studies to shorten survival. In fact, women diagnosed with endometrial cancer in the 1970s while taking unopposed estrogen were actually shown to live longer than their peers who were not diagnosed with endometrial cancer and did not take HRT (76). This surprising statistic may well be due to the cardioprotective effect of estrogen that would remain despite the coexistence of a malignancy.

Most authorities believe that it is safer to use HRT in individuals previously diagnosed with limited and well differentiated disease, that is, stage I/II and grade 1 endometrial cancer (77). Use of progestogen therapy with estrogen in these women who do not possess a uterus has been suggested as well, but the need for this remains to be determined because of the possible adverse impact of progesterone on estrogen's cardioprotective effect.

Whether or not to give ERT to women previously diagnosed and treated for breast cancer is a topic of great current controversy (78,79). Only a few studies exist in the literature in which women previously treated for breast cancer have been given ERT. Results from these few studies are encouraging in that they do not report an increased risk of disease recurrence or shortened survival (80,81). One must be careful not to be overly enthusiastic about these results due to their small numbers and possible inclusion of bias. In one of these studies, a very large dose of progestogen (20 to 40 mg of medroxyprogesterone acetate) was given with 0.625 mg of conjugated equine estrogens (81). An increased risk of recurrence of breast cancer was not seen in the study, but the dose of progestogen used greatly exceeds that commonly prescribed in the United States.

HORMONE REPLACEMENT AND OVARIAN CANCER

Lifetime risk for the development of ovarian cancer in the United States is 1.4% (82). Ovarian cancer is also a disease associated with aging, with median ages at diagnosis of 54 years for early-stage disease and 62 years for advanced disease (83). Results from the few studies on estrogen use and risk for ovarian cancer have been controversial. Rodriguez et al. (84) surveyed women enrolled in the American Cancer Society's Cancer Prevention Study. They found that over-use of HRT was associated with a rate ratio for fatal ovarian cancer of 1.15 (95% CI: 0.94 to 1.42). A ratio of 1.71 (95% CI: 1.06 to 2.77) was reported with more than 11 years of use. Hempling et al. (85) in a case–control study with 491 women with ovarian cancer were unable to document a specific association between HRT and epithelial ovarian cancer. Using metaanalysis, Garg et al. (86) reported an odds ratio of 1.15 for the development of invasive epithelial ovarian cancer with over-use of HRT with a 95% CI of 1.05 to 1.27. Prolonged hormone use (more than 10 years) was associated with an ovarian cancer risk of 1.27 in this study with a 95% CI of 1.00 to 1.61.

Of interest is the fact that younger women using high-dose combined hormone therapy (combination birth-control pill) experience a 40% reduction in the risk for ovarian cancer (59). It is surmised that this may be due to suppression of ovulation, but a definite answer remains to be reported. High-dose ERT has even been given to 14 women with advanced ovarian cancer, with two patients having an improved response and one a worsening (87).

SELECTIVE ESTROGEN RECEPTOR MODULATORS

Recent studies have revealed that estrogen-like compounds are of benefit in increasing the survival of women treated for ER-positive breast cancer, with tamoxifen citrate (Nolvadex) being the best example (88). This steroid has both estrogen antagonist and agonist actions. When given to women with breast cancer for 5 years after initial diagnosis and treatment, tamoxifen has improved their survival and increased their bone density (89). Use of tamoxifen for longer than 5 years has not proven to be of additional benefit in increasing survival (88). The rationale given for the usefulness of tamoxifen is that this drug acts as an antiestrogen at the level of the breast. Yet this steroid exerts estrogen-like activity on the human endometrium. Since a comparison between tamoxifen and estrogen replacement in women previously treated for breast cancer has never been performed, it remains uncertain whether all of tamoxifen's beneficial actions can be attributed only to its antiestrogen actions.

Diethylstilbestrol (DES) is a very potent synthetic estrogen that has successfully been used for the treatment of advanced breast cancer when given either above or with chemotherapy (90,91). Clinical trials comparing tamoxifen with DES for the treatment of breast cancer have been conducted, and results have been comparable, although more side effects were experienced by women taking DES (92). This again could imply that the estrogenic activity of tamoxifen may be just as important as its antiestrogenic activity in the treatment of breast cancer.

Steroids that are related in structure to tamoxifen and have similar biologic activity have recently been introduced. Raloxifene (Evista), given as a 60-mg daily oral dose, is the most recent to be made available (93). This drug has antiestrogenic action at the breast, while also having estrogenic activity on the skeleton. It remains entirely speculative as to whether or not this medication may be used safely in women previously treated with breast cancer. Results from prospective, randomized clinical trials using raloxifene in this manner do not exist. A major side effect of raloxifene is hot flushes.

LOCAL ESTROGEN THERAPY

A major complaint of menopausal women is vaginal dryness. This condition may be treated using systemic estrogen therapy, but this may produce unwanted side effects. While this condition may be alleviated by use of vaginal lubricants, this is often not well accepted. An alternative is highly regulated local estrogen therapy provided by vaginal insertion of an estradiol-impregnated Silastic ring (94). Placed in the vagina for 90 days, this ring is designed to release very low concentrations of estradiol-17β to the vaginal mucosa. Minimal to no steroid is released into the systemic circulation (94). Use of estrogen-containing creams applied locally to the vaginal mucosa results in variable amounts being absorbed systemically (95). For a patient concerned about the risk of malignancy or recurrence of malignancy from systemic estrogen treatment, the estrogen-containing Silastic ring could be considered as a reasonably safe alternative therapy for treatment of vaginal dryness, as long as her oncologist is in agreement.

For other menopausal symptoms experienced by menopausal women with breast cancer, the alternatives to hormonal therapy previously discussed may be considered. If one is going to use standard hormone replacement, it should be mentioned that there are no data on the appropriateness of a particular type or dose of estrogen or progestogen to be given.

HORMONE REPLACEMENT THERAPY AND BREAST CANCER IN WOMEN WITH POSITIVE FAMILY HISTORY OF BREAST CANCER

Menopausal women who have a positive family history of breast cancer and are trying to make an informed decision about HRT/ERT use often wonder whether their risk of breast cancer will be further increased if they use hormone replacement. Few studies have been conducted to answer this question. When data have been published, some authors reported that use of conjugated estrogens for 5 years or more was associated with a 3.9-fold increased risk of breast cancer in women with a positive family history of breast cancer, compared to a risk of only 1.6 in women without a positive family history (96). Other studies have shown not only no increased risk but a reduced total mortality rate (71).

HORMONE REPLACEMENT REGIMENS

Estrogen Replacement

Orally administered conjugated equine estrogens are currently the most widely used estrogens for hormone replacement and are provided in the product known as Premarin. There is no generic substitute. Premarin contains a mixture of estrogens (Table 3). The predominant steroid is estrone sulfate. Premarin may be dispensed in strengths of 0.3, 0.625, 0.9, and 1.25 mg. The proportions of the estrogens in each strength are similar but not identical. Previous epidemiologic studies revealed that 0.625 mg or more of Premarin was required to protect against heart disease and bone loss.

TABLE 3. *Composition of conjugated estrogens in 1.25-mg and 0.625-mg formulations*

Estrogen conjugated to sodium sulfate (%)	Formulation 1.25 mg (%)	Formulation 0.625 mg (%)
Estradiol-17α (0.6)	4.1	1.2
Estradiol-17β (0.4)	0.58	0.67
A) Dihydroequilin-17α (1.1)	14.3	10.6
Dihydroequilenin-17α (<0.1)	1.8	1.5
B) Dihydroequilenin-17α (0.1)	1.2	0.8
Dihydroequilenin-17β (<0.1)	0.46	Not detected
Sodium/sulfate estrone (74)	49.3	81.5
A) Sodium/sulfate equilin (15.1)	26.1	3.7
Sodium/sulfate equilenin (7.9)	1.8	Not detected

From Johnson R, Masserano R, Haring R, Kho B, Schilling G. Quantitative GLC determination of conjugated estrogens in raw materials and finished dosage forms. *J Pharm Sci* 1975;64:1007–1011; with permission.

Many other types of estrogens may be prescribed orally for hormone replacement. Esterified estrogens consisting of sodium estrone sulfate (7.5% to 85%) or sodium equilin sulfate (6% to 15%) are marketed as Estratab and Menest, respectively, in 0.3-, 0.625-, 1.25-, and 2.5-mg tablets. Estropipate (formerly piperazine estrogen sulfate) is available as Ogen or Ortho-Est. Ethinyl estradiol, marketed as Estinyl in a 20-µg strength, may also be taken orally. This steroid is identical to that found in combination oral contraceptive pills. Estradiol-17β in a micronized formulation known as Estrace is available for oral use as 0.5-, 1-, and 2-mg tablets. The patented process of micronization refers to dispersion of crystalline steroids to tiny particles, improving absorption.

Orally administered estrogen results in a complex and variable pharmacokinetic pattern (97). This causes difficulty when one is trying to correlate plasma or serum steroid levels with a particular dosage strength.

Estrogens may be administered by routes other than the mouth. These include use of transdermal, intramuscular, or vaginal routes. An estradiol transdermal system, pioneered by the Ciba-Geigy Corporation (Summit, NJ), is available as Estraderm. An alcohol solvent within this patch facilitates the passage of estradiol-17β across the skin, but the patch must be replaced every 3 to 4 days due to evaporation. Incorporation of estradiol-17β into the adhesive of a patch, enabling replacement at weekly intervals, is marketed as Climara. An advantage of a transdermal patch is the delivery of a relatively constant amount of steroid into the general circulation over time. Measurement of the steroid level in the blood stream will correlate with the strength of patch used.

Estrogen replacement may also be provided vaginally by use of creams, tablets, or rings. Depending on dosage, vaginal estrogen administration can result in measurable plasma concentrations of hormone. Vaginal administration of the same estrogen dose given orally will result in plasma levels that are 25% to 70% of those found after the oral dose.

Progestin/Progestogen Replacement

Exposure of the human endometrium to unopposed estrogen results in endometrial hyperplasia. In the recently completed PEPI study, a 30% risk of endometrial hyperplasia was detected within 3 years of unopposed estrogen treatment (8).

Protection against endometrial hyperplasia, which is a precursor to atypical hyperplasia and malignancy, is offered by progestin/progestogen treatment. Progesterone may be provided orally in micronized form at 200 mg per day for 10 to 14 days during estrogen administration. Recently, the FDA approved Prometrium, a formulation containing micronized progesterone in 100-mg capsules. Alternatively, medroxyprogesterone acetate in 5- to 10-mg doses may be provided orally for 10 to 14 days or daily as a 2.5-mg oral dose. Due to the amount of progesterone required to be absorbed transdermally, a progesterone-containing patch is not currently available. However, a combined estrogen and progestogen patch using estradiol and norethindrone has been introduced as the Combi-patch.

SUMMARY

Life expectancy for women is increasing, and with aging there is an increase in the incidence of malignancy. Cardiovascular disease remains the major cause of mortality, accounting yearly for roughly twice as many deaths as those due to cancer. Use of exogenous hormones during the menopause has been advocated as one pharmacologic means of markedly reducing the risk of cardiovascular disease and death from cardiovascular disease. An increase in the risk of causing or promoting a malignancy, particularly breast cancer, from using HRT during the menopause has also been suggested. For menopausal women who fear being diagnosed with cancer or who already have been treated for cancer, the decision whether to use hormone therapy to reduce the risk of heart disease or treat menopausal symptoms creates a tremendous conflict. An informed decision about this matter may be made by a patient and her physician(s) only when all possess or are given complete and accurate information. It is hoped that this chapter has helped in this regard.

REFERENCES

1. National Center for Health Statistics. Annual summary of births, marriages, divorces, and deaths: United States, 1993. *Mon Vital Stat Rep* 1994;42(13).
2. Campbell PR. *Population projections for states, by age, race and sex: 1993 to 2020.* US Bureau of the Census, Current population reports, P25-1111. Washington, DC: US Government Printing Office, 1994.
3. Bush TL. Noncontraceptive estrogen use and risk of cardiovascular disease: an overview and critique of the literature. In: Korenman SG, ed. *The Menopause: biological and clinical consequences of ovarian failure: evolution and management.* Norwell, MA: Serono Symposia, 1990:211–224.
4. Smith DC, Prentice R, Thompson DJ, Herrmann WL. Association of exogenous estrogens and endometrial cancer. *N Engl J Med* 1975;293:1164–1167.
5. Ziel HK, Finkle WD. Increased risk of endometrial carcinoma among users of conjugated estrogens. *N Engl J Med* 1975;293:1167–1170.
6. Gambrell RD Jr. Sex steroids and cancer. *Obstet Gynecol Clin North Am* 1987;14:191–206.
7. Reis SE, Gloth S, Blumenthal RS, et al. Ethinyl estradiol acutely attenuates abnormal coronary vasomotor responses to acetylcholine in postmenopausal women. *Circulation* 1994;89:52–60.
8. Writing Group for the PEPI Trial. Effects of estrogen/progestin regimens on heart disease risk factors in postmenopausal women: the Postmenopausal Estrogen/Progestin Interventions (PEPI) trial. *JAMA* 1995;273:199–208.
9. Miyagawa K, Rosch J, Stanczyk F, Hermsmeyer K. Medroxyprogesterone interferes with ovarian steroid protection against coronary vasospasm. *Nature Med* 1997;3:324–327.
10. Office of Medical Applications, National Institutes of Health. Consensus conference: osteoporosis. *JAMA* 1984;252:799–802.
11. Melton LJ III, Riggs BL. Epidemiology of age-related fractures. In: Avioli LV, ed. *The osteoporotic syndrome.* New York: Grune & Stratton, 1983:45–72.
12. Birge SJ. Is there a role for estrogen replacement therapy in the prevention and treatment of dementia? *J Am Geriatr Soc* 1996;44:865–870.
13. Paganini-Hill A, Henderson VW. Estrogen replacement therapy and risk of Alzheimer disease. *Arch Intern Med* 1996;156:2213–2217.
14. Diaz N, Frei B, Vita JA, Keaney JF. Antioxidants and atherosclerotic heart disease. *N Engl J Med* 1997;337: 408–416.
15. Brinton RD. 17β-Estradiol induction of filopodial growth in cultured hippocampal neurons within minutes of exposure. *Mol Cell Neurosci* 1993;4:36–46.
16. Brinton RD, Tran J, Profitt P, Kahil M. 17β-Estradiol increases the growth and survival of cultured cortical neurons. *Neurochem Res* 1997;22:1339–1351.
17. Belfort MA, Saade GR, Anabes M, et al. Hormonal status affects the reactivity of the cerebral vasculature. *Am J Obstet Gyencol* 1995;172:1273–1278.
18. Calle EE, Miracle-McMahill HL, Thun MJ, Heath CW Jr. Estrogen replacement therapy and risk of fatal colon cancer in a prospective cohort of postmenopausal women. *J Natl Cancer Inst* 1995;87:517–523.
19. Grodstein F, Martinez E, Platz EA, et al. Postmenopausal hormone use and risk for colorectal cancer and adenoma. *Ann Intern Med* 1998;128:705–712.
20. Grodstein F, Stampfer MJ, Manson JE, et al. Postmenopausal estrogen and progestin use and the risk of cardiovascular disease. *N Engl J Med* 1996;335: 453–461.
21. Landis SH, Murray T, Bolden S, Wingo PA. Cancer statistics, 1998. *CA Cancer J Clin* 1998;48:6–27.
22. Weinberg RA. How cancer arises. *Sci Am* 1996; 275:62–70.
23. Nowell PC. The clonal evolution of tumor cell populations. *Science* 1976;194:23–28.
24. Baldin V, Lukas J, Marcole MJ, Pagano M, Draetta G. Cyclin D_1 is a nuclear protein required for cell cycle progression in G_1. *Genes Dev* 1993;7:812–821.
25. Lindsay R. Osteoporosis in the postmenopausal women in reproductive medicine and surgery. In: Wallach EE, Zacur HA, eds. *Reproductive medicine and surgery.* St Louis, MO: Mosby–Year Book, 1995:993–1018.
26. Blake GM, Fogelman I. Applications of bone densitometry for osteoporosis. *Endocrinol Metab Clin North Am* 1998;27:267–288.
27. Kanis JA, Melton LJ III, Christiansen C, Johnston CC, Khaltaev N. The diagnosis of osteoporosis. *J Bone Miner Res* 1994;9:1137–1141.
28. Heaney RP. Lifelong calcium intake and prevention of bone fragility in the aged. *Calcif Tissue Int* 1991; 49(suppl):S42–S45.

29. Dawson-Hughes B, Dallal GE, Krall EA, Sadowski L, Sahyoun N, Tannenbaum S. A controlled trial of the effect of calcium supplementation on bone density in post-menopausal women. *N Eng J Med* 1990;323: 878–883.
30. Liberman UA, Weiss SR, Broll J, et al. Effect of oral alendronate on bone mineral density and the incidence of fractures in postmenopausal osteoporosis. *N Engl Med* 1995;333:1437–1443.
31. Lomax P, Schonbaum E: Postmenopausal hot flushes and their management. *Pharmacol Ther* 1993;57:347–358.
32. Freeman RR, Woodward S: Behavioral treatment of menopausal hot flushes: Evaluation by ambulatory monitoring. *Am J Obstet Gynecol* 1992;167:436–439.
33. Hamar M, Berg G, Lingren R: Does physical exercise influence the frequency of postmenopausal hot flushes? *Acta Obstet Gynecol Scand* 1990;69(5):409–412.
34. Hirata JD, Swiersz L, Zell B, Small R, Ettinger B. Does dong quai have estrogenic effects in postmenopausal women. *Fertil Steril* 1997;68:981–986.
35. DiPaola RS, Zhang H, Lambert G, et al. Clinical and biologic activity of an estrogenic herbal combination (PC-SPES) in prostate cancer. *N Engl J Med* 1998;339: 785–791.
36. Laufer LR, Erlik Y, Medrum DR, Judd HL. Effect of clonidine on hot flushes in postmenopausal women. *Obstet Gynecol* 1982;60:583–586.
37. Jones KP, Ravnikar V, Schiff I. A preliminary evaluation of the effect of lofexidine on vasomotor flushes in post-menopausal women. *Maturitas* 1985;7:135–139.
38. Melis GB, Gambacciani M, Cagnacci A, Paoletti AM, Mais V, Floretti P. Effects of the dopamine antagonist veraliperide on hot flushes and luteinizing hormone secretion in postmenopausal women. *Obstet Gynecol* 1988;72:688–692.
39. Limouzin-Lamothe M, Mairon N, Joyce CRB, Le Gal M. Quality of life after the menopause: influence of hormonal replacement therapy. *Am J Obstet Gynecol* 1994;170:618–624.
40. Lebherz TB, French LT. Non-hormonal treatment of the menopausal syndrome: a double-blind evaluation of an autonomic system stabilizer. *Obstet Gynecol* 1969;33: 795–799.
41. Harrison RF. Ethamsylate in the treatment of climacteric flushing. *Maturitas* 1981;3:31–37.
42. Alcoff JM, Campbell D, Tribble D, Oldfield B, Cruess D. Double-blind, placebo-controlled, cross-over trial of propranolol as treatment for menopausal vasomotor symptoms. *Clin Ther* 1981;3:356–364.
43. Tulandi T, Kinch RA, Guyda H, Mazella L, Lal S. Effect of methyldopa on menopausal flushes, skin temperature, and luteinizing hormone secretion. *Am J Obstet Gynecol* 1984;150(6):709–712.
44. Albertazzi P, Pansini I, Bonaccorsi G, Zanotti L, Forini E, DeAloysio D. The effect of dietary soy supplementation on hot flushes. *Obstet Gynecol* 1998;91:6–11.
45. Murkies AL, Lombard C, Strauss BJG, Wilcox G, Burger HG, Morton MS. Dietary flour supplementation decreases post-menopausal hot flushes: effect of soy and wheat. *Maturitas* 1995;21:189–195.
46. Murkies AL, Wilcox G, Davis SR. Clinical Review 92: Phytoestrogens. *J Clin Endocrinol Metab* 1998;83: 297–303.
47. Foster GV, Zacur HA, Rock JA. Hot flushes in post-menopausal women ameliorated by danazol. *Fertil Steril* 1985;43:401–404.
48. Sherwin BB, Gelfand MM. Effects of parenteral administration of estrogen and androgen on plasma hormone levels and hot flushes in the surgical menopause. *Am J Obstet Gynecol* 1984;148:552–557.
49. Schiff I, Tulchinsky D, Cramer D, et al. Oral medroxyprogesterone acetate in the treatment of post-menopausal symptoms. *JAMA* 1980;244:1443–1445.
50. Darling GM, Johns JA, McCloud PI, Davis SR. Estrogen and progestin compared with simvastatin for hypercholesterolemia in postmenopausal women. *N Engl J Med* 1997;337:595–601.
51. Stampfer MJ, Colditz GA, Willet WC, et al. Postmenopausal estrogen therapy and cardiovascular disease: ten-year follow-up from the Nurses Health Study. *N Engl J Med* 1991;325:756–762.
52. Steinberg D. Antioxidants and atherosclerosis: a current assessment. *Circulation* 1991;84:1420–1425.
53. Kugiyama K, Kerns SA, Morrisett JD, Robert R, Henry PD. Impairment of endothelium-dependent arterial relaxation by lysolecithin in modified low-density lipoproteins. *Nature* 1990;344:160–162.
54. Esterbauer H, Dieber-Rotheneder M, Striegl G, Waeg G. Role of vitamin E in preventing the oxidation of low density lipoprotein. *Am J Clin Nutr* 1991;53(1 Suppl): 314S–321S.
55. Stampfer MJ, Hennekens CH, Manson J, Colditz GA, Rosner B, Willett WC. Vitamin E consumption and the risk of coronary disease in women. *N Engl J Med* 1993; 328:1444–1449.
56. Hulley S, Grady D, Bush T, et al. Randomized trial of estrogen plus progestin for secondary prevention of coronary heart disease in postmenopausal women. *JAMA* 1998;280:605–613.
57. Jick H, Derby LE, Myers MW, Vasilakis C, Newton KM. Risk of hospital admission for idiopathic venous thromboembolism among users of postmenopausal oestrogens. *Lancet* 1996;348(9033):981–983.
58. Daly E, Vessey MP, Hawkins MM, Carson JL, Gough P, Marsh S. Risk of venous thromboembolism in users of hormone replacement therapy. *Lancet* 1996;348(9033): 977–980.
59. Schlesselman JJ. Net effect oral contraceptive use has on the risk of cancer in women in the United States. *Obstet Gyencol* 1995;85(5 pt 1):793–801.
60. Chu KC, Tarone RE, Kessler LG, et al. Recent trends in U.S. breast cancer incidence, survival and mortality rates. *J Natl Cancer Inst* 1996;88:1571–1579.
61. Feuer EJ, Won LM, Boring CC, Flanders WD, Timmel MJ, Tong T. The lifetime risk of developing breast cancer. *J Natl Cancer Inst* 1993;85:892–897.
62. Harris JR, Lippman ME, Veronesi U, Willett W. Breast cancer (Part 1). *N Engl J Med* 1992;327:319–328.
63. Silverstein MJ, Cohlan BF, Gierson ED, et al. Duct carcinoma *in situ:* 227 cases without microinvasion. *Eur J Cancer* 1992;28:630–634.
64. Ernster VL, Barclay J, Kerlikowske K, Grady D, Henderson IC. Incidence of and treatment for ductal carcinoma *in situ* of the breast. *JAMA* 1996;275:913–918.
65. Rosen PP, Braun DW Jr, Kinne DE. The clinical significance of preinvasive breast carcinoma. *Cancer* 1980; 46(suppl):919–925.
66. Page DL, Dupont WD, Rogers LW, Landenberger M. In-

traductal carcinoma of the breast: follow-up after biopsy only. *Cancer* 1982;49:751–758.
67. Welch HG, Black WC. Using autopsy series to estimate the disease reservoir for ductal carcinoma of the breast: how much more breast cancer can we find? *Ann Intern Med* 1997;127:1023–1028.
68. Harris JR, Lippman ME, Veronesi U, Willett W. Breast cancer (2). *N Engl J Med* 1992;327:390–398.
69. Kuiper GCJM, Enmark G, Pelto-Huikko M, Nilsson S, Gustaffson J-A. Cloning of a novel estrogen receptor expressed in rat prostate and ovary. *Proc Natl Acad Sci U S A* 1996;93:5925–5930.
70. Theriault RL, Sellin RV. A clinical dilemma: estrogen replacement therapy in postmenopausal women with a background of primary breast cancer. *Ann Oncol* 1991;2:709–717.
71. Sellers TA, Mink PJ, Cerhan JR, et al. The role of hormone replacement therapy in the risk for breast cancer and total mortality in women with a family history of breast cancer. *Ann Intern Med* 1997;127:973–980.
72. Collaborative Group on Hormonal Factors in Breast Cancer. Breast cancer and hormone replacement therapy: collaborative reanalysis of data from 51 epidemiological studies of 52,705 women with breast cancer and 108,411 women without breast cancer. *Lancet* 1997; 350:1047–1059.
73. Colditz GA, Hankinson SE, Hunter DJ, et al. The use of estrogens and progestins and the risk of breast cancer in postmenopausal women. *N Engl J Med* 1995;332: 1589–1593.
74. Stanford JL, Weiss NS, Voigt LF, Daling JR, Habel LA, Rossing MA. Combined estrogen and progestin hormone replacement therapy in relation to risk of breast cancer in middle-aged women. *JAMA* 1995;274:137–179.
75. Creasman WT, Henderson D, Hinshaw W, Clarke-Pearson D. Estrogen replacement therapy in the patient treated for endometrial cancer. *Obstet Gynecol* 1986;67:326–330.
76. Collins J, Allen LH, Donner A. Oestrogen use and survival in endometrial cancer. *Lancet* 1980;2:961–963.
77. Chapman JA, DiSaia PJ, Osann K, Roth PD, Gillotte DL, Berman ML. Estrogen replacement in surgical stage I and II endometrial cancer survivors. *Am J Obstet Gynecol* 1996;175:1195–2000.
78. DiSaia PJ. Estrogen replacement therapy for the breast cancer survivor: a reappraisal. *J Surg Oncol* 1997;64: 175–180.
79. DiSaia PJ, Grosen EA, Odicino F. Replacement therapy in breast cancer survivors: a pilot study. *Cancer* 1995; 76:2075–2080.
80. Wile AG, Opfel RW, Murgileth DA. Hormone replacement therapy in previously treated breast cancer patients. *Am J Surg* 1993;165:371–375.
81. Eden JA, Bush T, Nand S, Wren BG. The Royal Hospital for Women Breast Cancer Study: a case-controlled study of combined continuous estrogen-progestogen replacement therapy amongst women with a personal history of breast cancer. *Menopause* 1995;2:67–72.
82. Trimble EL. The NIH Consensus Conference on Ovarian Cancer: screening, treatment and follow-up. *Gynecol Oncol* 1994;55(3 pt 2):S1–S3.
83. Yancik R, Ries LC, Yates JW. Ovarian cancer in the elderly: an analysis of surveillance, epidemiology and end results program data. *Am J Obstet Gynecol* 1986;154: 639–647.
84. Rodriquez C, Calle EE, Coates RJ. Miracle-McMahill HL, Thun MJ, Heath CW. Estrogen replacement therapy and fatal ovarian cancer. *Am J Epidemiol* 1995;141: 828–835.
85. Hempling RE, Wong C, Piver MS, Natarajan N, Mettlin CJ. Hormone replacement therapy as a risk factor for epithelial ovarian cancer: results of a case-control study. *Obstet Gynecol* 1997;89(6): 1012–1016.
86. Garg PP, Kerlikowske K, Subak L, Grady D. Hormone replacement therapy and the risk of epithelial ovarian carcinoma: a meta-analysis. *Obstet Gynecol* 1998;92: 472–479.
87. Long RTL, Evans AM. Diethylstilbestrol as a chemotherapeutic agent for ovarian carcinoma. *Mo Med* 1963;60:1125.
88. Osborne CK. Tamoxifen in the treatment of breast cancer. *N Engl J Med* 1998;339:1609–1618.
89. Love RR, Mazess RB, Barden HS, et al. Effects of tamoxifen on bone mineral density in postmenopausal women with breast cancer. *N Engl J Med* 1992;326: 852–856.
90. Boyer MJ, Tattersall MH. Diethylstilbestrol revisited in advanced breast cancer management. *Med Pediatr Oncol* 1990;18:317–320.
91. Kiang DT, Gay J, Goldman A, Kennedy BJ. A randomized trial of chemotherapy and hormonal therapy in advanced breast cancer. *N Engl J Med* 1985;313: 1241–1246.
92. Ingle JN, Ahmann DL, Green SJ, et al. Randomized clinical trial of diethylstilbestrol versus tamoxifen in postmenopausal women with advanced breast cancer. *N Engl J Med* 1981;304:16–21.
93. Delmas PD, Bjarnason NH, Mitlak BH, et al. Effects of raloxifene on bone mineral density, serum cholesterol concentrations and uterine endometrium in postmenopausal women. *N Engl J Med* 1997;337: 1641–1647.
94. Schmidt G, Andersson SB, Nordle O, Johansson CJ, Gunnarsson PO. Release of 17-beta estradiol from a vaginal ring in postmenopausal women—pharmacokinetic evaluation. *Gynecol Obstet Invest* 1994;38: 253–260.
95. Mandel F, Geola F, Meldrum DR, et al. Biological effects of various doses of vaginally administered conjugated equine estrogens in postmenopausal women. *J Clin Endocrinol Metab* 1983;57:133–139.
96. Hoover R, Glass A, Finkle WD, Azevedo D, Milne K. Conjugated estrogens and breast cancer risk in women. *J Natl Cancer Inst* 1981;67:815–820.
97. Zacur HA, Burkman RT, Kimball AW, Kiviterovich P, Bell WR. Existence of multiple peaks in plasma ethinyl estradiol and norethindrone after oral administration of a contraceptive pill. *J Clin Endocrinol Metab* 1992;75: 1268–1272.
98. Zacur HA, Chapanis NP, Lake CR, Ziegler M, Tyson JE. Galactorrhea-amenorrhea: psychological interaction with neuroendocrine function. *Am J Obstet Gynecol* 1976; 125:859–862.
99. Morris JC, Martin DC, Blair RA, et al: The use of medroxyprogesterone acetate for relief of climacteric symptoms. *Am J Obstet Gynecol* 1980;138:99–104.

4

Fertility After Cancer Treatment

Jairo E. Garcia

Department of Reproductive Endocrinology, Johns Hopkins Hospital and Johns Hopkins School of Medicine, Baltimore, Maryland 21287

Since the birth of the world's first *in vitro* fertilization (IVF) baby in 1978 (1), extraordinary advances in reproductive medicine have made biologic parenthood possible for many individuals suffering from infertility or desiring to avoid the risk of passing inherited illnesses or genetic disabilities. Such advances have also extended reproductive potential to men who have congenital or acquired azoospermia, as well as to women with a history of premature ovarian failure and physiologic menopause. The scope of assisted reproductive technologies (ARTs) has broadened to include patients who survive different types of cancer treatment.

REPRODUCTIVE PROCESS—OVERVIEW

Reproduction is a complex, highly ordered process, in which the male and female gametes unite to form a new individual. The fundamental principle of reproduction in humans and other mammals is based in the interaction of two mature cells: spermatozoon and oocyte. Human reproduction alone is an inefficient process that requires thousands of oocytes and millions of spermatozoa before the selected oocyte is fertilized by a spermatozoon. Furthermore, 60% of embryos never implant or are rejected during the first trimester of pregnancy. Chromosome abnormalities are the primary reason for miscarriages. Although most chromosome abnormalities occur *de novo,* they are the result of abnormal gametogenesis during the process of chromosomes' crossing over during meiosis (e.g., nondisjunction) (2). Other, equally important factors, such as immunologic problems, mechanical factors, infections, and toxic substances, among others, may also cause miscarriages. Irradiation and chemical substances may interfere with the normal development of an early pregnancy or account for congenital malformations.

To understand the effects of radiation and chemotherapy in human reproduction, it is important to review the process of spermatogenesis and oogenesis.

Spermatogenesis

Development of the undifferentiated gonadal anlage into a testis occurs under the influence of a testis-determining factor (or factors) located on the sex-determining region (SRY) at the short-arm level of the Y chromosome (3–5). Finding a 46,XY phenotypic female with an intact *SRY* gene suggests that other genes located outside of this region may be important in sex determination (6).

During the sixth week of gestation, the primordial cells migrate from the yolk sac region into the mesonephric or gonadal ridges, where they undergo mitosis and are surrounded by coelomic epithelial cells (primordial Sertoli cells) to form seminiferous or sex cords (7). Initially under the influence of human chorionic gonadotropin (hCG) and later pituitary follicle-stimulating hormone (FSH) and luteinizing hormone (LH), both germ cells and Sertoli cells undergo active mitotic division during gestational weeks 8 to 14. The Sertoli cells produce, among other substances, müllerian-inhibitory substance, which plays a crucial role in the process of male and female internal genital differentiation. After the fourteenth gestational week, the germ and Sertoli cells continue dividing, but at a reduced pace, until puberty (8).

During the eighth gestational week, fetal Leydig cells begin to develop from mesenchymal cells of the gonadal ridge (9). Leydig cells multiply rapidly and secrete increasing amounts of testosterone, first under the influence of maternal hCG and later that of fetal LH secretion (10). Testosterone is converted to dihydrotestosterone (DHT) by the enzyme 5α-reductase. DHT is responsible for the induction of internal and external genitalia from the mesonephric ducts and urogenital sinus, respectively. After gestational week 17, the Leydig cells involute until puberty (11).

Despite low secretion of gonadotropins during fetal life and the neonatal, infancy, and prepuberal periods, Sertoli and germ cell numbers increase significantly and finally mature into spermatogonia. The number of cells that develop during this period of time is crucial to determining the size and maximum capacity of testicular function and sperm production (12).

At puberty, the hypothalamus and the pituitary mature, secreting gonadotropin-releasing hormone (Gn-RH) and stimulating the secretion of FSH and LH. This provides the proper input to the establishment of spermatogenesis and testosterone secretion (13). The adult testis is composed of seminiferous tubules, in which spermatogenesis occurs. The seminiferous tubules represent 90% of the testicular volume. The interstitium, where Leydig cells are located, is in close proximity to the seminiferous tubules. Locally, they deliver a high testosterone concentration that is important to maintaining spermatogenesis (14).

Spermatogenesis has been divided into three functional phases: proliferative, meiotic, and spermiogenetic. During the *proliferative phase*, some spermatogonia divide to replenish the stem cell pool (stem cell renewal), and others undergo mitotic divisions and differentiation and become spermatocytes. During the *meiotic phase*, the spermatocytes divide, giving rise to spermatids with a haploid number of chromosomes. During *spermiogenesis*, the spermatids mature to reach the stage of spermatozoa (15,16) (Fig. 1).

Spermatogonia are located in the basal compartment of the seminiferous tubules, separated from other germ cells by Sertoli cell tight junctions. There are three types of spermatogonia: A_d, A_p, and B. A_d (dark) spermatogonia are characterized by the darkness of the chromatin in their nucleus. They are the spermatogonial stem cells. Mitotic activity is low, and therefore they are *resistant* to external insults such as chemotherapeutic agents and radiation. A_d spermatogonia replenish the spermatogonia population by mitotic divisions. Complete damage to the A_d spermatogonia by radiation, chemotherapy, or vascular trauma results in irreversible azoospermia. After mitotic divisions, A_d spermatogonia give rise to A_p (pale) spermatogonia, characterized by the pale-staining chromatin in their nucleus. After mitotic divisions, the A_p spermatogonia differentiate into B spermatogonia. During these three phases, the spermatogonia maintain the diploid chromosome component of 46. B spermatogonia are the *most radiosensitive* germ cells. They are commonly affected by external radiation of the testis (17).

B spermatogonia undergo another mitotic division to produce preleptotene or resting primary spermatocytes that enter the prolonged phase of spermatogenesis. This phase lasts approximately 24 days. The spermatogonia do not separate completely during mitotic division. Groups of germ cells remain in contact with each other via cytoplasmic bridges and undergo further changes in a synchronous

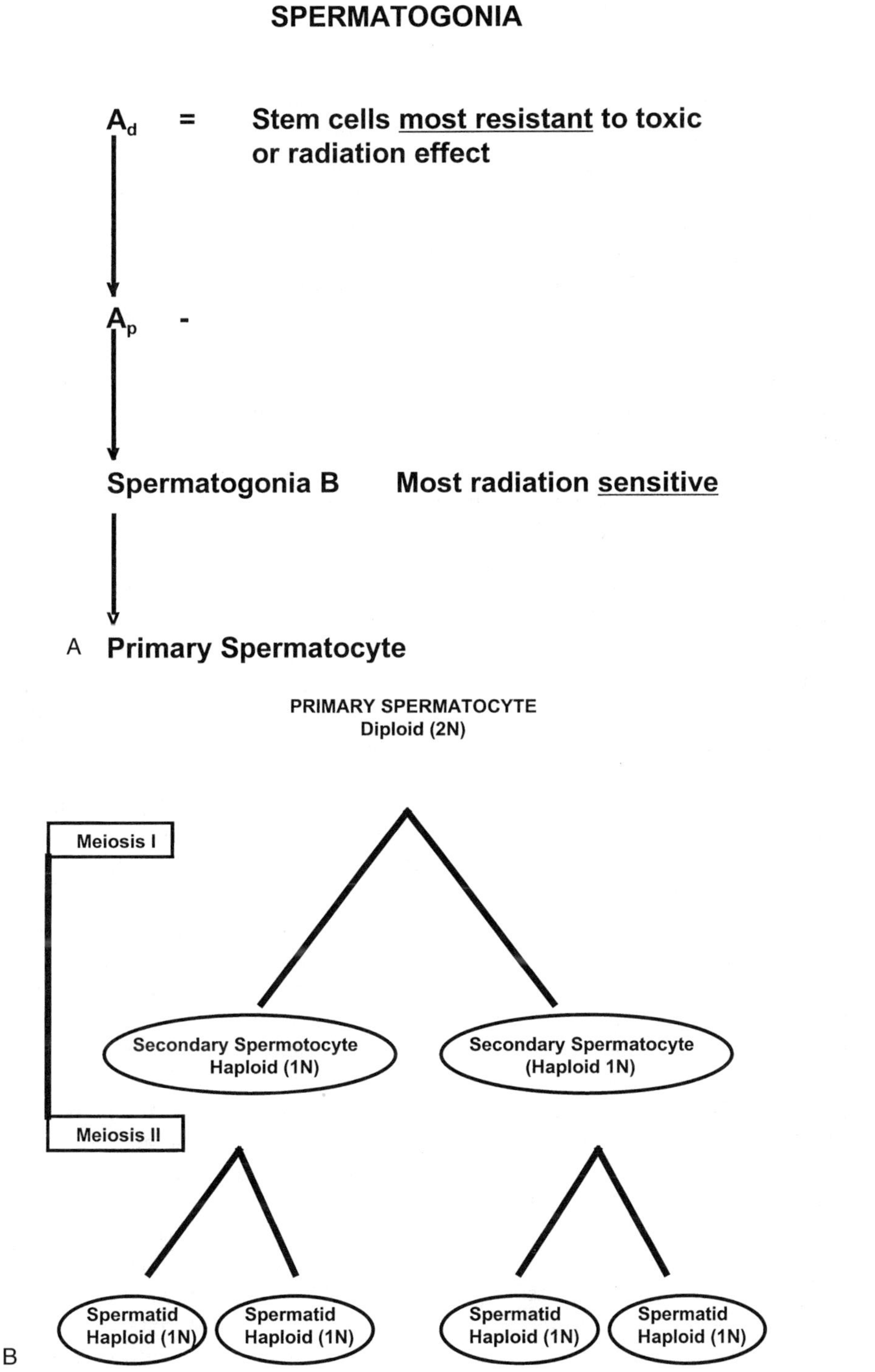

FIG. 1. A: Sensitivity of male germ cells to radiation. **B:** Spermatogenesis: meiosis I and II.

fashion. Preleptotene spermatocytes are smaller than B spermatogonia and have less chromatin. Active deoxyribonucleic acid (DNA) synthesis occurs during the preleptotene stage, and the amount of DNA duplicates. Therefore, preleptotene spermatocytes contain a diploid complement of chromosomes (46 chromosomes or 2*N*, where *N* is haploid chromosome number). Since each chromosome is composed of a pair of identical sister chromatids, the total DNA content in these germ cells is twice the diploid content (4*N*). Preleptotene spermatocytes are the final germ cells to undergo DNA synthesis during spermatogenesis (see Fig. 1).

On completion of DNA synthesis and sister chromatid formation, preleptotene spermatocytes enter prophase (prophase I) of the first meiotic division (meiosis I). During this phase, changes occur in the characteristics of the nucleus, which increases in size, and spermatocytes go through the stages of leptotene I, zygotene I, pachytene I, diplotene I, and diakinesis I.

In the leptotene stage, the chromosomes condense, but are unpaired and appear as finely filamentous and beaded chromatin threads in the nucleus (18). In pachytene spermatocytes, chromosomes are fully paired and remain so for 2 weeks. During this interval, exchange of genetic material occurs through crossing-over between chromatids of homologous chromosomes. This genetic recombination results in germ cell chromosomes that contain a unique combination of genetic material. Pachytene spermatocytes are characterized by their large ovoid nucleus containing short, thick chromatin material and prominent spheric nucleoli.

After the prolonged prophase I, the remaining stages of meiosis I proceed rapidly. Diakinesis I is followed by metaphase I. In metaphase I, the nuclear membrane breaks down and spindles appear. The spermatocytes go through anaphase and telophase I until the cell divides to give origin to two secondary spermatocytes, each containing one haploid number of chromosomes (23 chromosomes or 1*N*). Secondary spermatocytes are smaller than primary spermatocytes. The secondary spermatocyte stage lasts only 8 hours.

During meiosis II, secondary spermatocytes undergo similar changes to those during meiosis I, with the exception that the number of chromosomes of the secondary spermatocytes is haploid (23), each containing two sister chromatids. The final result is two spermatids, each containing a haploid number of chromosomes.

Chromosome abnormalities are the result of a disruption of the meiosis or mitosis processes. Aneuploidy due to an extra or missing chromosome is the most common and clinically significant chromosome abnormality, since it is associated with physical and/or mental abnormalities. Trisomy 21, or Down syndrome, is due to paternal meiotic nondisjunction in about 5% to 20% of cases. Klinefelter syndrome (47,XXY) is the result of errors in meiosis I and is related to abnormal spermatogenesis in 50% of cases. Turner syndrome (45,XO), in which one of the X chromosomes is missing, is due to paternal meiotic nondisjunction in 80% of cases (19).

Spermiogenesis is the final stage of spermatogenesis. It is the complex process by which spermatids are transformed into mature spermatozoa capable of fertilizing an oocyte. During this stage, spermatids develop the flagellum (tail) and the acrosome, with condensing of the chromosomes and nucleoproteins to form the spermatozoon head. At this stage, the spermatozoa are released into the seminiferous tubules, a process called *spermiation*. Newly formed spermatozoa migrate through the epididymis and the vas deferens and are stored within the seminal vesicles until the time of ejaculation (20).

The duration of spermatogenesis from the formation of A_p spermatogonia to the release of S_d spermatids is approximately 74 ± 4 days. Transit through the epididymis takes about 12 additional days (21). Therefore, any insult to the testis resulting in arrested development will not be manifested in the ejaculate until 3 months later.

A spermiogram is normal according to the following criteria:

Volume	2 to 5 mL
Count	>20 million/mL
Motility	>50%
Morphology	>50%

Any decrease in volume, sperm count, motility, or morphology may render a man subfertile but not sterile. A man is considered sterile when the sperm count shows azoospermia.

Oogenesis

The primordial germ cells originate from the endoderm of the yolk sac near the caudal end of the embryo. By the third week of preg-

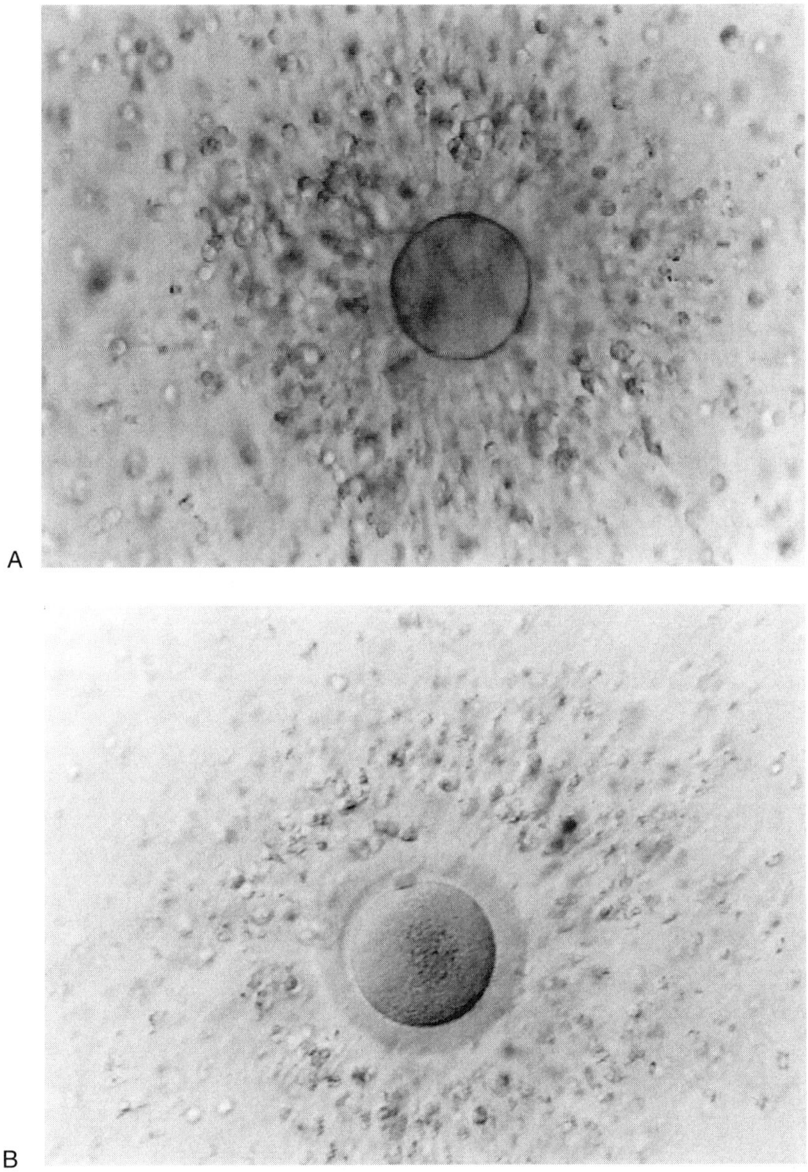

FIG. 2. A: Oocyte with expanded corona radiata. **B:** Close-up of metaphase II oocyte. Notice the polar body present at 12 o'clock.

nancy, the germ cells start to migrate toward the genital ridge by ameboid movements (22,23). This process is completed by the fifth gestational week. At this stage, germ cells are called *oogonia.* Between gestational weeks 5 and 7, the primordial gonadal structure constitutes no more than a bulge on the medial aspect of the urogenital ridge. This protuberance is created by proliferation of coelomic germinal epithelium, the underlying mesenchyma, and oogonia. The number of oogonia is estimated to be approximately 10,000 by the end of week 7. At this point, the gonads are in the undifferentiated stage. The absence of testicular development beyond gestational week 7 is considered presumptive evidence of ovarian formation. During the eighth gestational week, oogonia undergo persistent mitosis, and their number is estimated at about 600,000. At this point, oogonia are subject to simultaneously undergo mitosis, meiosis, and atresia. By gestational week 20, total germ cells are estimated to be 7 million, of which two-thirds are intrameiotic primary oocytes and the remainder oogonia. The process of mitosis ends by gestational week 30 (7 months of fetal life). Thereafter, the number of cells decreases in an organized fashion to approximately 2 million at birth and 400,000 to 500,000 at puberty. The mechanism by which germ cells are commanded into atresia is still unknown. The code used by the ovary to store and release the monthly cohort of follicles, from which only 400 to 500 will be ovulated during the reproductive years, is unknown as well (24).

The first primordial follicle can be identified within the ovary by gestational week 16. Nevertheless, some oogonia initiate the characteristic nuclear changes of prophase I of meiotic division (25). Once an oocyte enters the prophase I stage, it will remain in this dormant stage until the time of ovulation, probably because of the inhibitory action of the meiosis-inhibiting factor (MIF).

The process of oocyte maturation is different from spermatogenesis. The oocyte remains in prophase I of meiosis until the LH surge preceding ovulation occurs. At this point, MIF levels decrease, and the oocyte resumes meiosis to complete the first metaphase stage and formation of the first polar body (Fig. 2). The primary oocyte is converted into a secondary oocyte after ovulation only if it is penetrated by

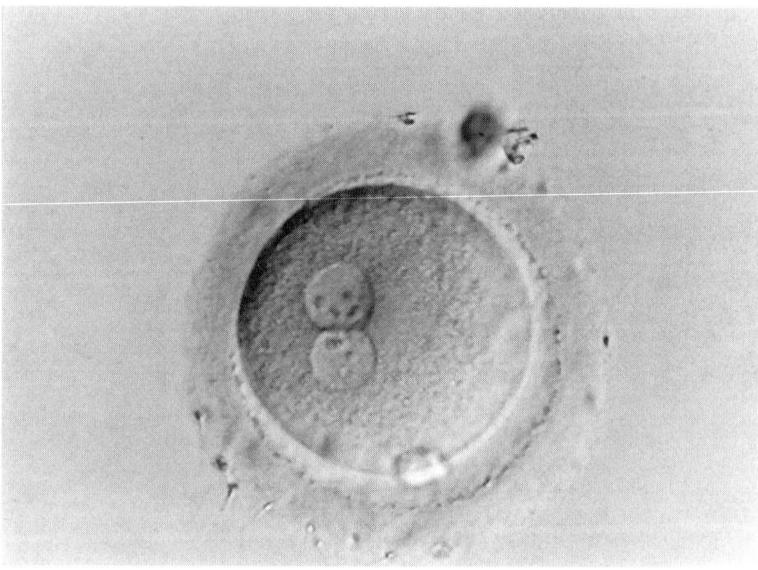

FIG. 3. Fertilized oocyte, two-pronuclei stage; second meiotic division. Notice the polar body at 3 and 6 o'clock.

a spermatozoon. It then undergoes a second meiotic division, during which the second polar body is extruded (Fig. 3). The ovum finally acquires its haploid component moments before fertilization takes place.

EFFECTS OF ONCOLOGY TREATMENT ON REPRODUCTION

In the United States, cancer is the second leading cause of death. Today, one of every three people living in the United States will eventually battle a life-threatening malignancy. With the exception of uterine and stomach cancers, the incidences of most malignancies have remained unchanged or have increased. Nevertheless, with advances in radiotherapy and chemotherapy, life expectancy has improved for certain malignancies, namely, lymphomas, leukemia, dysgerminomas, and seminomas, among others (26–29).

Physicians, nurses, and counselors play a critical role in the diagnosis, physical and psychologic assessment, and supportive care of cancer patients. As patients move through the different modalities of treatment, it is important to discuss the immediate and delayed effects of surgery, chemotherapy, and radiotherapy (30–33). In general, patients receive adequate information about local effects, nausea/vomiting, and other types of discomforts associated with treatment, as well as about prognosis based on recurrence and life expectancy; however, quite often sexuality and reproduction are only tangentially addressed.

Chemotherapy

The principle of chemotherapy is to attain maximal therapeutic cytotoxic effects without extreme toxicity to normal tissues. Unfortunately, in many instances, it is not feasible to obtain a therapeutic effect without temporally or permanently altering the functions of other cells, tissues, organs, and/or systems (27, 34–36).

Cancer is believed to arise when cell growth escapes normal growth-control mechanisms. The cell cycle has four stages:

G_1	Initial resting phase
S	Synthetic phase during which the DNA duplicates
G_2	Second resting (premeiotic) phase
M	Cell division, during which mitosis takes place

Phase G_0 indicates nonproliferating cells (cell death or loss) (27–30). Normally, there is an equilibrium between the number of cells in division and the number of cells dying. This generally occurs in every system, although in some cell systems the repair mechanism is slow or nonexistent, as with oogonia in women.

Chemotherapy effects depend on the cell-cycle time (Fig. 4). Basically, chemotherapeutic drugs are grouped according to their chemistry or mode of action:

- Alkylating agents
- Antimetabolites
- Vinca alkaloids
- Antimitotic antibiotics
- Miscellaneous

Alkylating agents contain an alkyl group that forms a covalent bond specifically at the cross-link on the DNA helix, preventing DNA duplication. Furthermore, alkylating agents attach to free guanine bases of DNA, preventing their action as templates for new DNA formation.

Antimetabolites have similar chemical structures to essential metabolites required by the cell prior to cell division. Antimetabolites may be incorporated into new nuclear material or combined with enzymes to inhibit cell division. They include the following:

Folic acid antagonist	Methotrexate
Purine antagonist	6-Mercaptopurine (Purinethol)
	6-Thioguanine
Thymidylate synthetase inhibitor	5-Fluorouracil
DNA polymerase inhibitor	Cytarabine (Cytosar-U)

Vinca alkaloids derived from the periwinkle plant (*Vinca rosea*) are metaphase-arrest agents. They bind to tubules, blocking microtubule formation and interfering with spindle

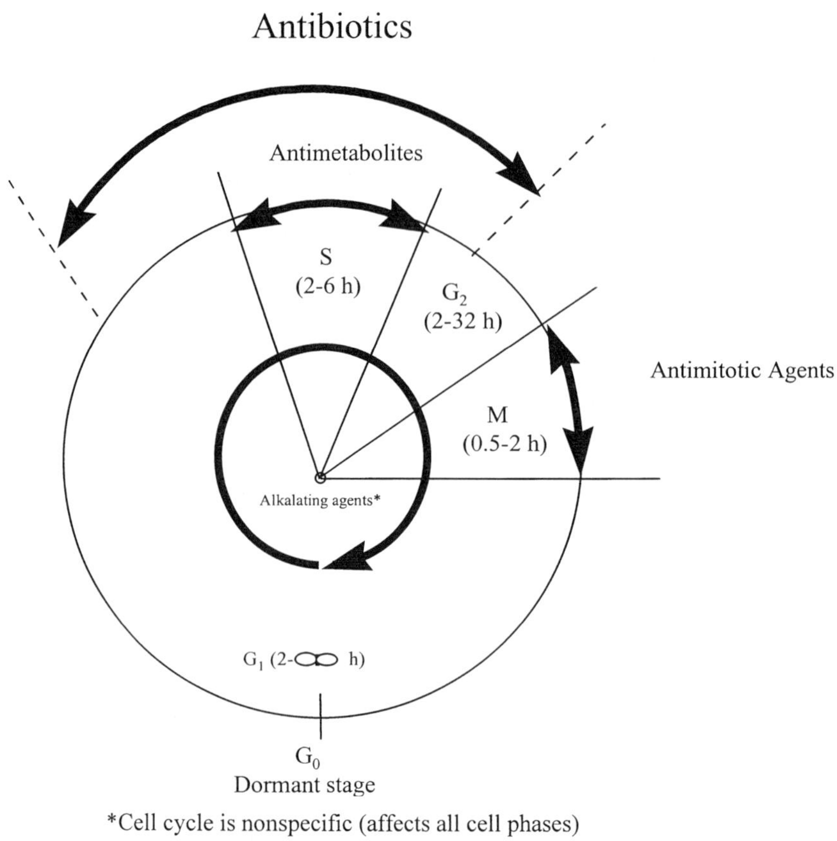

FIG. 4. Phases of the cell cycle, relative time intervals, and sites of action of the various classes of antineoplastic agents.

formation that is essential for the metaphase stage of mitosis.

Antimitotic antibiotics have many different modes of action, including increasing cell membrane permeability, inhibiting DNA and RNA synthesis, disrupting the DNA chain preventing mitosis, and blocking DNA replication.

Miscellaneous agents, belonging to none of the above categories, have different modes of action; they include the following:

- Paclitaxel (Taxol), a taxane that acts by spindle promotion
- Carboplatin (Paraplatin) and cisplatin (Platinol), nonclassical alkylating agents that block DNA replication
- Dacarbazine (DTIC-Dome), alkylating agent causes DNA breakage and strands crosslinking. Inhibits DNA and RNA synthesis.
- Procarbazine hydrochloride (Matulane), an analog of the monoamine oxidase inhibitors that works like an alkylating agent
- Etoposide (VePesid), a semisynthetic analog of podophyllotoxin, whose mode of action is not well understood but is thought to arrest DNA replication in the premitotic phase
- Hydroxyurea (Hydrea) analog of urea that inhibits RNA reductase and prevents DNA synthesis
- Chemotherapy is delivered intermittently—rather than at a constant dose—to exploit the fact that malignant cells have a less effective repair capacity than normal cells. The optimum dosing will achieve maximum tumor cell kill, with the next treatment cycle given when normal stem cells have had adequate time to recover from the previous treatment cycle. Furthermore, it

will give the immune system time to recover and maintain its function in tumor surveillance. Based on this principle, many chemotherapy agents induce azoospermia, oligospermia, or amenorrhea that is reversible over time.

Chemotherapeutic Agents

Chemotherapeutic agents and their effects on the reproductive system and pregnancy are listed on Table 1. Theoretically, the toxic effects of chemotherapy on the gonads could be minimized by suppression of their function using oral contraceptives in women or testosterone in men (37). In theory, similar effects could be obtained in both sexes by inducing pituitary suppression with Gn-RH analogs. Nevertheless, the published information is contradictory and limited. There are no prospective studies documenting hormonal protection of the gonads from chemotherapy.

Radiation Therapy

Radiation therapy is required as a single treatment, or more frequently as a coadjuvant treatment in cancer patients receiving chemotherapy. Radiation generates highly reactive free radical molecules that irreparably alter cells' DNA structure, therefore rendering cells incapable of proliferation. The rate of response to radiation depends on the cell cycle, the frequency with which the cell population turns over, oxygen concentration, and distance between the radiation source and the target tissue.

A unit dose of ionizing radiation causes similar degrees of DNA damage in most cell types. For most tumors, a dose of 200 centrigray (cGy) will reduce the number of reproductive cells by 50%. Therefore, several sessions of therapy are required before the tumor is destroyed. Because of a cumulative radiation effect or the tumor location, there is excessive damage to normal tissue. Testes and ovaries are highly radiosensitive. Different doses of radiation will produce the following:

50 to 150 cGy	Some gonadal dysfunction
200 to 500 cGy	Reversible gonadal dysfunction. Function is regained over time, depending on patient age and the amount of radiation given. It is estimated that recovery takes about 1 year for each 100 cGy administered
>600 cGy	Sterility

Gonadal dysfunction and infertility produced by irradiation are enhanced by the addition of chemotherapy, as well as by age in female patients. At 20 years of age or younger, there is a 30% chance of infertility; at 30 years and more than 40 years of age, there is an 80% and 100% chance, respectively.

Both the testes and the ovaries can be protected from radiation damage by orchiopexy or oophoropexy, with displacement of these organs to areas outside the proposed radiation field. Oophoropexy is accomplished by surgical mobilization of the ovaries, suspensory ligaments, and blood vessels outside the pelvic brim (38–41). Semen and oocytes can be cryopreserved. Animal studies suggest that cryopreservation with reimplantation of testicular and ovarian tissue may someday be possible.

Gonadal and Sexual Dysfunction

The magnitude of gonadal and sexual dysfunction in cancer patients is related to sex, age, diagnosis, and treatment.

Sex

The production of spermatozoa is a continuum process. Sertoli cells and spermatogonia are more susceptible to the action of different chemotherapeutic agents and radiation. In women, the ovaries contain primary oocytes that are arrested at the prophase I stage; as there is no DNA activity, oocytes have some protection from damage. This

TABLE 1. *Chemotherapeutic agents*

Name	Cell cycle action	Reproductive side effects	Pregnancy
Alkylating agents			
Busulfan (Myleran)	Nonspecific	Ovarian suppression Amenorrhea Menopause Testicular atrophy Azoospermia Impotence	Milk secretion unknown
Carboplatin, CBDCA (Paraplatin)	Nonspecific	Amenorrhea Menopause Gynecomastia Impotence Azoospermia	Milk secretion unknown
Carmustine, BCNU (BiCNU)	Nonspecific	—	Mutagenic Teratogenic
Chlorambucil (Leukeran)	Nonspecific	Amenorrhea Azoospermia	Milk secretion unknown
Cisplatin, *cis*-diamminedichloroplatinum, *cis*-DDP, CDDP, CACP (Platinol, Platinol-AQ)	Nonspecific	Gynecomastia Impotence Sterility	Contraindicated
Cyclophosphamide (Cytoxan, Endoxan, Neosar)	Nonspecific	Oligospermia (temporary) Azoospermia (temporary) Amenorrhea (1 yr) Ovarian fibroids Can produce sterility	Excreted in breast milk
Dacarbazine (DTIC-Dome)	Nonspecific	—	Teratogenic
Ifosfamide (IFEX)	Nonspecific	Oligomenorrhea Oligospermia Infertility	Excreted in milk
Lomustine, CCNU (CeeNU)	Nonspecific	Oligomenorrhea Oligospermia	Unknown
Mechlorethamine HCl, nitrogen mustard, NH2 (Mustargen)	Nonspecific	Oligomenorrhea Amenorrhea Menopause Impaired spermatogenesis Germinal aplasia Azoospermia	Unknown
Melphalan, L-phenylalanine mustard, L-PAM, L-sarcolysin (Alkeran)	Nonspecific	—	Contraindicated in pregnancy.
Pipobroman (Vercyte)	Nonspecific	—	—
Streptozocin, streptozotocin (Zanosar)	Nonspecific	Oligomenorrhea Oligospermia	Excreted in milk
Thiotepa, triethylenethiophosphoramide, TEPA (Thioplex)	Nonspecific	Amenorrhea (6–8 mos) Oligospermia Azoospermia (reversible and incomplete)	Excreted in milk
Uracil mustard	Nonspecific	Amenorrhea Oligospermia Azoospermia	—
Antimetabolites			
Cytarabine, cytosine arabinoside, ara-C (Cytosar-U, Cadastre-U)	S phase Inhibits cell development G_1 to S	—	Teratogenic

TABLE 1. *Continued.*

Name	Cell cycle action	Reproductive side effects	Pregnancy
Floxuridine, 5-fluorouracil deoxyribonucleoside, FUDR (Sterile FUDR)	S phase	—	Mutagenic Teratogenic
5-Fluorouracil, 5-FU, fluorouacil, (Adrucil, Efudex, Fluoroplex)	S phase	—	Mutagenic Teratogenic
6-Mercaptopurine, mercaptopurine, 6-MP (Purinethol)	S phase	Unknown	First trimester abortions Teratogenic
Methotrexate, MTX, amethopterin, methotrexate sodium (Folex, Mexate, Rheumatrex)	S phase	Oligomenorrhea Oligospermia	Abortion Teratogenic
Thioguanine, 6-thioguanine, 6-TG	S phase	Unknown	Abortion Teratogenic
Vinca alkaloids			
Vinblastine Sulfate (Velban, VLB)	Metaphase arrest M phase	Amenorrhea Azoospermia	Unknown milk secretion
Vincristine Sulfate Oncovin, VCR	Metaphase arrest M-S phase	Amenorrhea Azoospermia (permanent in postpubertal patients; unlikely if prepubertal administration)	Unknown if secreted in milk
Antimitotic alkaloids			
Bleomycin sulfate (Blenoxane)	G_2 and M phases	Unknown	Unknown
Dactinomycin, actinomycin D, DACT (Cosmegen)	Nonspecific G_1 phase	Unknown	Mutagenic Excreted in milk
Daunorubicin HCl, daunomycin HCl (Cerubidine)	Nonspecific	Unknown	Unknown
Doxorubicin HCl (Adriamycin)	Nonspecific	Unknown	Unknown
Mitomycin, mitomycin C (Mutamycin)	Nonspecific	Unknown	Unknown
Mitoxantrone HCl (Novantrone)	Nonspecific	Unknown	Mutagenic Teratogenic Unknown secretion in milk
Paclitaxel (Taxol)	Promotes microtubule formation	Unknown	Unknown
Plicamycin, mithramycin (Mithracin)	Nonspecific	Unknown	Unknown
Miscellaneous			
Asparaginase, L-asparaginase, L-ASP (Elspar)	G_1 specific	Unknown	Unknown
Etoposide, VP-16 (VePesid)	G_2-S_1		Mutagenic Genotoxic Excreted in milk
Interferon alfa-2a (Roferon-A)	Unknown	Unknown	Unknown
Procarbazine HCl, ibenzmethyzin (Matulane)	Nonspecific	Amenorrhea Azoospermia Gynecomastia Testicular atrophy	Mutagenic Teratogenic

mechanism explains why gonadal failure occurs in 80% of the men but only in 50% of women treated for Hodgkin's disease (26,35,37).

Age

Prepubertal boys and girls are more resistant to gonadal dysfunction. This is explained on the basis of the quiescent status of the testes and the increased number of oocytes in women. Once puberty is established, and with the initiation of spermatogenesis, the testes will be more vulnerable to toxic aggression (36,42,43). In women, the process of follicular atresia continues, and the number of oocytes available will be decreased over time.

Diagnosis

Diagnosis of gonadal failure in women is suspected by the symptoms of hot flashes, sweating, insomnia, and emotional instability. It is confirmed by pelvic examination showing vaginal dryness and atrophy of the vaginal epithelium and by determination of elevated serum FSH and LH levels and decreased estradiol (E_2) levels. In men, gonadal failure is diagnosed by complaints of decreased libido, impotence, depression, and muscular weakness. The diagnosis is confirmed by testicular atrophy and by elevated serum levels of FSH and LH, low serum testosterone levels, and azoospermia.

Treatment

One problem to determine is whether gonadal failure is transitory or permanent. It is important to evaluate each case and to consider the diagnosis, as well as treatment. Before cancer treatment begins, cancer patients should have appropriate counseling on issues of fertility and sexuality.

Sexual Dysfunction

Sexual dysfunction occurs frequently in cancer patients. It is caused by physical, hormonal, and emotional changes.

Physical Dysfunction

Obviously, some changes are the result of mutilating procedures that render patients unable to function physically. Patients with gynecologic cancer may require radical vulvectomy or vaginectomy, or men may require penectomy. Impotence is a common complaint in patients who undergo radical prostatectomy, as well as ejaculatory dysfunction in patients with bilateral retroperitoneal lymphadenectomy. Some of these patients develop retrograde ejaculation, in which most of the semen goes to the bladder (44,45).

Hormonal Dysfunction

Patients may develop premature menopause with atrophy of the introitus and vaginal dryness that make intercourse difficult or uncomfortable. Furthermore, their libido is decreased. In men, impotence and decreased libido due to low testosterone levels are the principal components of sexual dysfunction.

Emotional Dysfunction

Depression is one of the most constant symptoms in patients with a cancer diagnosis. They are concerned about their health, treatment, and survival, in addition to all the economic and familial problems that may arise. Feelings of rejection or undesirability from one's partner occur, especially when there are mutilation or major bodily changes in the genital region.

ASSISTED REPRODUCTIVE TECHNOLOGIES

IVF in humans was developed by Stepto and Edwards (1) in England. After the first successful pregnancy in 1978, IVF became the focus of interest for the treatment of infertility in patients with absence of or irreparable damage to the fallopian tubes. During the last 20 years, the technique has expanded its indications and allowed the development of other techniques such as gamete intrafallopian tube transfer (GIFT), zygote intrafallopian tube transfer (ZIFT), tubal embryo transfer (TET), and sperm microinjection techniques such as partial zona dissection (PZD), subzonal sperm injection (SUZI) and intracytoplasmic sperm injection (ICSI).

IVF Indications

According to the clinic-specific report in ARTs published by the Society for Assisted Reproductive Technologies (SART), the American Society for Reproductive Medicine (ASRM), and the Centers for Disease Control and Prevention, there were 59,142 cases involving ARTs in the United States during 1995 (46). The indications associated with these cases included the following:

Tubal-factor infertility	32%
Endometriosis	16%
Male-factor infertility	20%
Ovarian-factor infertility	9%
Unexplained infertility	14%
Other	9%

Tubal-factor Infertility

Tubal factors and pelvic adhesions account for approximately 30% of cases. Historically, prior to IVF, adoption was the only option for patients with bilateral salpingectomy secondary to ectopic pregnancies or severe pelvic inflammatory disease, as well as for patients with failed tuboplasty or frozen pelvis. Today, ARTs not only overcome infertility in these patients, but IVF results are superior to those of other microsurgical techniques, rendering these latter techniques obsolete (47).

Endometriosis

Severe pelvic endometriosis is accepted as a cause of infertility. Endometriosis in general is treated medically by suppression of ovulation using progestins, danazol (Danocrine), and Gn-RH analogs. In many instances, surgery (laparotomy or operative laparoscopy) is the standard of treatment to remove endometriomas and correct any pelvic adhesions that may interfere with normal functioning of the fallopian tubes. IVF is indicated in patients whose pregnancy is not achieved after medical or surgical treatment (48,49).

Male-factor Infertility

Pure male-factor infertility occurs in approximately 20% of cases and is associated with other factors in about 20%. Normal semen parameters require a sperm concentration greater than 20 million/mL, sperm motility greater than 50%, and normal morphology in excess of 50%, according to the World Health Organization (WHO) criteria, or more than 14% using the parameters of strict morphology described by Kruger et al. (50). Male infertility is considered when pregnancy is not established after 1 year of unprotected intercourse and when several separate semen analyses performed over a period of time show abnormalities such as oligospermia (low count), asthenospermia (low motility), teratospermia (abnormal forms), necrospermia (dead spermatozoa), and/or hypozoospermia (low volume). Characteristically, more than one parameter is altered in the semen analysis.

Other Factors

Other factors may interfere with sperm function. Antisperm antibodies may be associated with a history of testicular trauma, vasectomy reversal, testicular biopsy, and infections. Azoospermia (absence of sperm) could be primarily related to congenital absence of the vas deferens, spermatogenesis arrest, or obstruction due to infection or elective sterilization or secondary to chemotherapy, radiation therapy, or prostatectomy. In other instances, it could be related to ejaculatory dysfunction, such as retrograde ejaculation.

A history of exposure *in utero* to diethylstilbestrol (DES) is another factor related to infertility (51). Women whose mothers took DES during pregnancy are born with uterine anomalies consisting of hood cervix, a T-shaped uterus on hysterosalpingogram (HSG), irregular fimbriae, and ovulatory dysfunction. Chronic cervicitis and poor cervical mucus may cause infertility. DES patients have an increased risk for clear cell adenocarcinoma of the cervix and vagina. They also have increased risk for ectopic pregnancy, pregnancy loss during the first and second trimesters, and premature delivery due to cervical incompetence. In men, DES exposure accounts for oligospermia.

Idiopathic Infertility

Idiopathic infertility, commonly referred to as unexplained infertility or normal infertile couple, accounts for 20% of the infertile population. A complete infertility evaluation shows a normal postcoital test, normal HSG, normal ovulation, normal luteal phase, and normal laparoscopy. The prognosis in these patients is poor, and only 5% eventually achieve a pregnancy during the 5 years following the initial diagnosis. Nowadays, these patients are treated empirically with ovulation induction associated with intrauterine insemination (IUI); otherwise, they are candidates for IVF.

Patient Selection

It is generally accepted that IVF patients should enjoy good health and have no contraindications to pregnancy. They should be psychologically prepared to undergo all the stress related to the procedures, and should have the support of their partners. Other important factors involved in the selection of patients include age, ovarian reserve (functional ovaries), normal or adequate endometrial cavity, and functional spermatozoa that can be used for microinsemination (ICSI).

Age

Patient age is the singularly most important determinant factor for the success of IVF. It is well known that fertility declines after 36 years of age, but the decline is more pronounced after age 40 (52). Furthermore, spontaneous miscarriage rates increase with age and have been greater than 50% in patients older than 40 years because of an increased incidence of chromosome abnormalities. In the 1995 ARTs report, the live-birth rate per embryo transfer in patients younger than age 35 years was 30.6%, which is quite different from the 11.6% rate reported for patients older than 40 (46) (Table 2).

Ovarian Reserve

Ovarian reserve, the potential cohort of follicles available in any given menstrual cycle, is also an important determining factor in IVF success. In general, it is related to chronologic age. However, there are patients older than 40 who respond well to ovarian stimulation, as well as younger women who have a poor ovarian response. In these cases, one refers to the *biologic* age of the patient, which is extremely important for a select group of patients. Ovarian reserve can be evaluated by early serum determinations of FSH and E_2 and a baseline pelvic ultrasound on the second menstrual

TABLE 2. *1995 National pregnancy rates and the live-birth rates according to patient age*

	Age			
IVF cycles	<35	35–39	>40	Total
Numbers of cycles	21,019	16,728	8,159	45,906
Pregnancy/cycle (%)	29.7	23.4	13.2	24.4
Live birth/cycle (%)	25.3	18.2	8.0	19.6
Live birth/oocyte retrieval	28.0	21.5	10.2	22.0
Live birth/embryo transfer	30.6	23.6	11.6	25.1

IVF, *in vitro* fertilization.
Modified from ref. 46, with permission.

cycle day (53). An elevated FSH level (greater than 13 mIU/mL) and an extremely low E_2 level (less than 20 pg/mL) associated with inactive ovaries by ultrasound are indicative of a poor ovarian reserve. However, in my experience, there are cycles in which the FSH baseline level is within the normal range (less than 10 mIU/mL), the E_2 level is greater than 80 pg/mL, and pelvic ultrasound shows a follicle that is already greater than 12 mm in diameter. In this case, the prognosis is not good because of early follicular selection, in which an early elevation of FSH has recruited the dominant follicle even before menstrual bleeding occurs (54). The low FSH levels are secondary to down-regulation induced by early E_2 secretion from the follicular granulosa cells. A cancer survivor who received chemotherapy or subdiaphragmatic radiation should undergo assessment of ovarian reserve before enrollment in an IVF program.

Endometrial Cavity

A woman under evaluation for an IVF program should have an HSG performed within the previous 2 years to evaluate the size of the endometrial cavity and rule out endometrial polyps, submucous fibroids, or intrauterine synechiae. Furthermore, it is important to rule out the presence of hydrosalpinx (55). Several reports have proven the toxic effect of hydrosalpinx fluid on the embryo, decreasing IVF success (56–58). If a patient is interested in GIFT, ZIFT, or TET, it is important to be sure that at least one fallopian tube is normal and patent. An endometrial biopsy should demonstrate that there is no progesterone deficiency, or should reveal the need for extra progesterone or hCG support during the luteal phase.

Semen Analysis

A semen analysis must be performed to evaluate the concentration, motility, morphology, and other characteristics of the sperm (59,60). Sperm wash and Percoll gradient separations are important to define the needs for conventional insemination or to see whether ICSI is required. In severe oligospermia or azoospermia, men require a urologic evaluation to rule out a varicocele, testicular tumor, or other pathology such as obstruction or congenital absence of the vas deferens (61,62). Furthermore, the urologist will decide whether the man is a candidate for microscopic epididymal sperm aspiration (MESA) or testicular sperm aspiration (TESA) (63).

Finally, cervical and semen cultures for *Ureaplasma urealyticum, Chlamydia,* gonococci, and other microorganisms are important before initiation of the IVF cycle (64,65).

In Vitro Fertilization

Several steps are required in IVF:

- Ovarian stimulation
- Follicular aspiration
- Oocyte classification
- Sperm preparation
- Oocyte insemination
- Embryo culture
- Embryo transfer

Ovarian Stimulation

The first IVF pregnancy followed the fertilization of a single oocyte obtained during a spontaneous menstrual cycle (1). Nevertheless, the experiences gained in the United States and Australia between 1979 and 1981 proved that monitoring natural ovulation was feasible and much improved but the procedure was cumbersome and inefficient, and ovarian stimulation became the gold standard in IVF programs (66). During the last few years, there have been a few publications in which the authors claimed a successful delivery rate of 12% per cycle during the natural menstrual cycle in a selected group of patients (67).

IVF success is related not only to patient age but also to the number of embryos transferred, among others factors (52,68). The number of embryos obtained in any given IVF cycle depends on the number of oocytes obtained after ovulation induction and follicular aspiration. There are several protocols for ovarian stimulation—all based in the physiologic principle of follicular recruitment, selection, and dominance described by Hodgen (69).

Clomiphene Citrate

Today, clomiphene citrate (CC) is infrequently used in IVF. The CC-only protocol consists of 5- to 7-day treatment using doses of 100 to 150 mg per day, starting on the second menstrual cycle day. The ovarian response is monitored by pelvic ultrasound and determinations of serum E_2 and LH levels. Once the follicle reaches 18 mm in diameter, LH needs to be measured every 3 to 4 hours to detect a premature LH surge (70–72). Oocyte retrieval needs to be carried out 24 to 26 hours after the LH surge. The advantages of this protocol are its low cost and the nonexistent risk of ovarian hyperstimulation syndrome (OHSS). The major disadvantages include a low oocyte yield (one or three per cycle), a frequent and unexpected LH surge that leads to oocyte retrieval at any time of the day, a cancellation rate of 50%, and a low pregnancy rate (73).

Clomiphene Citrate and Human Menopausal Gonadotropins

The association of CC with human menopausal gonadotropins (hMG) has the advantage of increasing the number of recruited follicles. The dose of CC (100 to 150 mg per day) is similar to that of the CC-only protocol; hMG is administered concurrently or for 2 to 7 days after CC at a dose of 150 IU per day. Frequent ultrasound and daily determinations of E_2 and LH are required, as well as frequent determinations of LH once the follicular diameter reaches 15 mm. The follicular size is smaller with this protocol. The follicle completes its development at a diameter of 17 to 18 mm; therefore, 10,000 IU of hCG needs to be administered intramuscularly to complete the oocyte maturation. Oocyte aspiration should be carried out 35 hours after the hCG injection. Disadvantages of this protocol are premature luteinization, spontaneous LH surge, and a 25% to 50% cancellation rate.

Human Menopausal Gonadotropins

Administration of hMG for ovarian stimulation has been one of the breakthrough steps in IVF (74,75). Use of hMG has evolved with the introduction of new technologies and the generation of pure FSH gonadotropins that can be used subcutaneously; furthermore, recombinant FSH and LH gonadotropins are currently available:

Preparation	FSH	LH	Trade name
hMG (menotropins)	75 IU	75 IU	Humegon, Repronex
Pure FSH (urofollitropin)	75 IU	<1 IU	Metrodin
Ultrapure FSH (urofollitropin)	75 IU	<0.1 IU	Fertinex
Recombinant FSH (follitropin -alpha and -beta)	75 IU	0	Gonal-F, Follistim
Recombinant LH	0	75 IU	Not available in United States

Gonadotropin doses vary between 150 and 450 IU per day. In general, gonadotropins are started on the second or third menstrual cycle day. The response is monitored by daily serum E_2 determinations and later by pelvic ultrasound. Frequent LH determinations are required to determine an LH surge. Once the follicular diameter reaches 17 to 18 mm, gonadotropins are discontinued and 10,000 IU of hCG is administered that evening. Oocyte retrieval is carried out 35 hours later. Ovulation induction seems to be more predictable with the use of gonadotropins. Nevertheless, spontaneous LH surges occur in about 25% of cycles and account for one reason to cancel the ovulation induction cycle (76,77).

Regardless of the use of gonadotropins, there is a group of patients (poor responders) in whom only two to three follicles develop and/or the oocytes are of poor quality. The possibility for a successful pregnancy is seriously compromised. In general, patients with poor response to gonadotropin stimulation have a rather poor ovarian reserve manifested by elevated baseline FSH levels on the second or third menstrual cycle day, as well as early follicle recruitment. Some patients respond with premature luteinization due to elevated tonic LH levels that are responsible for premature elevation of progesterone, compromising oocyte quality (78–81). Analysis of each ovarian stimulation cycle is important to modify future stimulations and increase patient response.

Gonadotropin-releasing Hormone Analogs

Initially, Gn-RH analogs were used in patients with premature luteinization, spontaneous LH surge, and a less than acceptable or ideal ovarian stimulation response (82–84). Gn-RH analogs can be used in two protocols: flare-up and luteal-phase protocols.

In the *flare-up protocol,* advantage is taken of the agonistic effect that induces a temporary elevation of FSH during the first 4 days (85,86). This elevation helps in the follicular recruitment process. After 5 days of Gn-RH analog administration, the pituitary undergoes down-regulation that will prevent premature luteinization and spontaneous LH surge. Administration of gonadotropins must be initiated on the fifth menstrual cycle day. In the *luteal-phase protocol*, a Gn-RH analog is started on menstrual cycle day 17 or 21. By the time of menstrual cycle onset, the phenomenon of down-regulation is in effect, so the gonadotropin administration will be started on the second day of bleeding (86).

The adjunctive use of Gn-RH analogs in ovarian stimulation leads to an overall improvement in IVF. It accounts for the increase in the number, quality, and synchronization of the oocytes recovered per cycle, which is reflected by the improvement in the fertilization rate, number and quality of embryos, and increased pregnancy rate (87–89). More embryos than the number used in a fresh embryo transfer are available, giving the opportunity to cryopreserve the excess embryos for a future transfer (90).

Potential risks and disadvantage of Gn-RH analog use include an increased amount of gonadotropin doses, increased costs due to increased days of therapy, and the risk of OHSS due to excessively high E_2 levels (91).

Follicular Development

Regardless of the ovulation-induction agent used, ovarian follicles are subject to the phases of follicular recruitment, selection, dominance, and maturation. In the general menstrual cycle, only one out of several hundred available follicles is recruited and selected to undergo full development and ovulation with the chance to be fertilized. Using ovulation-induction agents, the number of follicles recruited is increased, depending on patient age, ovarian reserve, and the type of ovarian stimulation. Generally, follicular development is monitored by ultrasound and by serum E_2 determination. The diameter of the preovulatory follicle varies according to the ovarian stimulation as follows:

Natural menstrual cycle	18 to 24 mm
CC	23 to 25 mm
hMG	17 to 20 mm
FSH	15 to 18 mm

Therefore, it is important to be familiar with the above diameters so that hCG can be administered at the appropriate time to prevent premature luteinization (92–94).

Follicular Aspiration

Oocyte aspiration is undertaken 35 to 36 hours after hCG administration. Originally, all aspirations were done through *laparoscopy* (74,95,96). This requires general anesthesia, a skillful laparoscopist, and major discomfort for the patient, in addition to the risks involved in the laparoscopic procedure itself. Furthermore, there are patients with severe pelvic adhesions that render the ovaries inaccessible and make it impossible to attain an oocyte aspiration (97).

Ultrasound-guided oocyte aspiration is another method currently utilized. Follicular aspirations under ultrasound guidance were first done transabdominally through the urethra and later transvaginally. Transvaginal ultrasound-guided oocyte aspiration is the dominant method used by most IVF programs. For transvaginal oocyte aspiration, the patient is placed in the dorsal lithotomy position, the bladder is catheterized, and the vaginal wall is prepared with povidone-iodine. A 5- to 7-MHz ultrasound probe is inserted into the vagina to localize the ovaries and the follicles. Then, a 17-gauge needle is passed through the vaginal fornix into the ovaries. The follicular fluid is aspirated, and the fluid is delivered to the IVF laboratory, which ideally should be adjacent to the operating room (98–102).

Ultrasound-guided oocyte aspiration has the advantage of not requiring general anesthesia; conscious (twilight) sedation is sufficient. The risk of bowel injury is almost nil, allowing oocyte retrieval in patients with a frozen pelvis in whom laparoscopic retrieval is not possible. Furthermore, one avoids the use of carbon dioxide pneumoperitoneum that may alter the pH of the follicular fluid. The major risk is damage to the pelvic vessels and pelvic infection, which can be avoided if the procedure is carefully carried out under aseptic conditions.

Oocyte Classification

Classification of the oocyte is a crucial step for IVF success. The follicular fluid is scanned under either a dissecting or an inverted microscope, and oocytes are graded by the appearance of the corona–cumulus complex. The presence of a polar body (metaphase II stage) and/or germinal vesicle (prophase stage) is a determining factor for the preincubation time prior to insemination. Other oocyte classifications are *atretic* and *fractured zona,* constituting less than 15% of oocytes obtained (103) (Fig. 5; see also Fig. 2B).

A

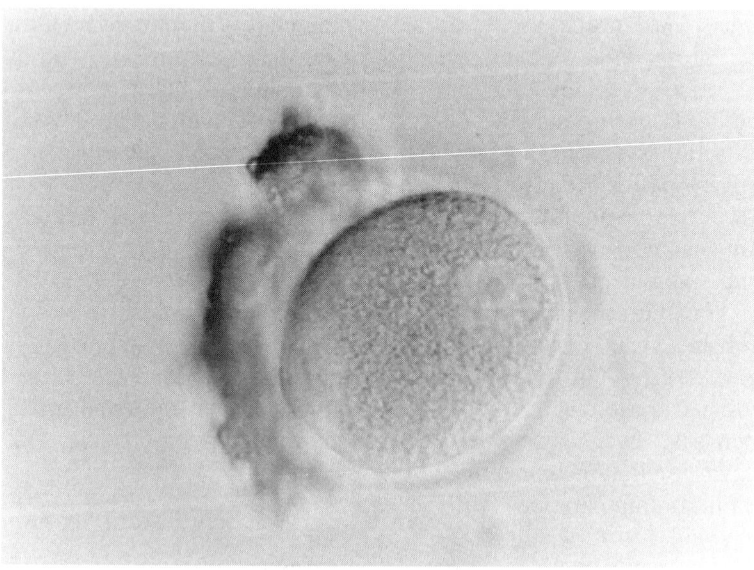

FIG. 5. A: Germinal vesicle.

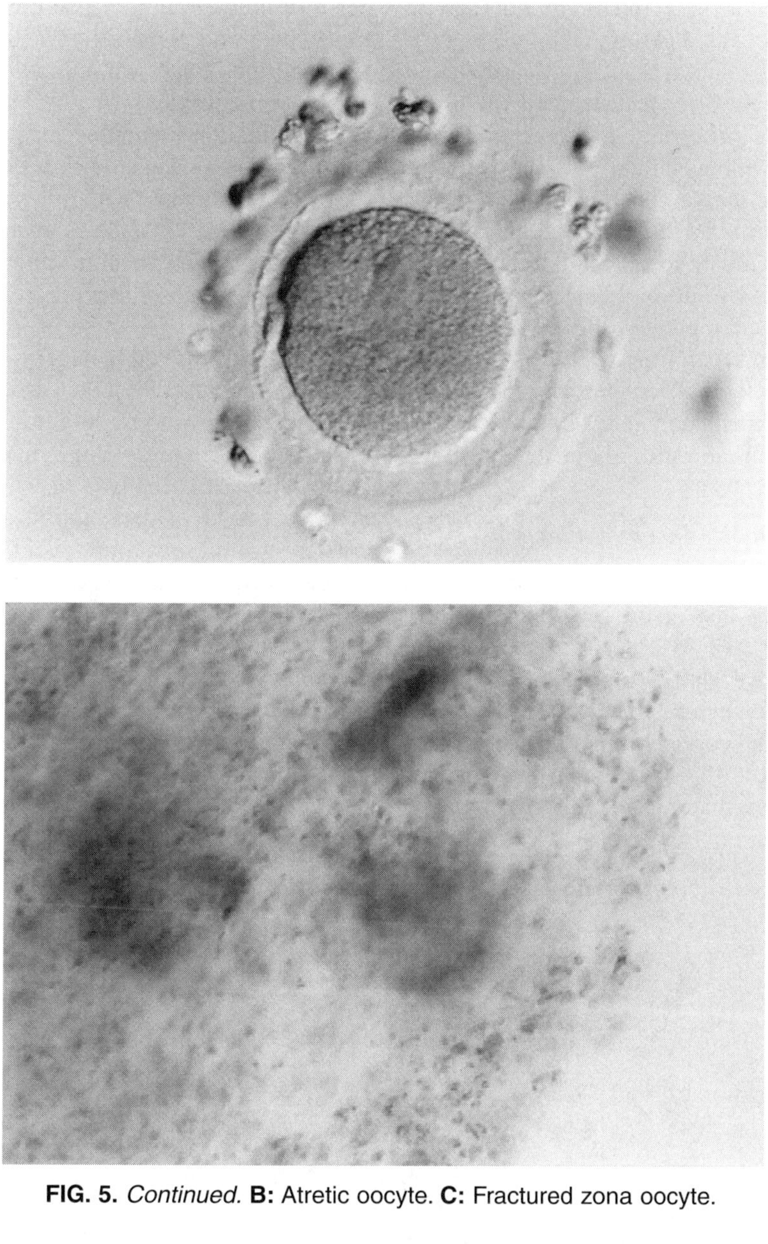

B

C

FIG. 5. *Continued.* **B:** Atretic oocyte. **C:** Fractured zona oocyte.

Sperm Preparation

The semen sample is produced just before or a few hours after oocyte aspiration. Frozen sperm can be used as well, provided that the sperm count is sufficient and motility is good before cryopreservation of the semen. The semen specimen should be collected in a sterile plastic container by masturbation or by coitus using a Silastic condom without a spermicide (104). If there is an ejaculatory dysfunction, such as retrograde ejaculation, the patient must take a urine-alkalizing agent (sodium bicarbonate) in advance. A urine sample should be collected immediately following ejaculation (105). The semen sample is allowed to liquefy at room temperature for about 30 minutes. The seminal plasma is washed by the addition of a medium containing 7.5% to 10% heat-inactivated serum, followed by centrifugation. The supernatant is discarded, and the sperm pellet is resuspended in fresh medium. This procedure is repeated twice. Spermatozoa enhancement is achieved by a swim-up technique consisting of adding layers of medium over the sperm pellet and allowing it to incubate for 30 to 60 minutes. The active sperm swim up to the surface, and this fraction is then pipetted off. Another technique is sperm separation using Percoll gradient centrifugation. The spermatozoa recovered are then incubated at 37°C in 5% carbon dioxide concentration for about 1 hour (106).

Oocyte Insemination

Metaphase II oocytes are inseminated in a Falcon culture disk using a suitable culture medium, such as Earl's balanced salt solution or human tubal fluid, supplemented with a protein source such as maternal serum, heat-inactivated fetal cord serum, or human plasma protein fraction. In conventional IVF insemination, approximately 50,000 spermatozoa per milliliter of culture medium are required to obtain good fertilization (104). In oligospermia, the concentration could be adjusted to 500,000 sperm artificially by using a microinsemination technique, in which oocytes and sperm are incubated in a droplet of culture medium covered with mineral oil to avoid evaporation (106). Culture dishes are incubated at 37°C in an atmosphere containing 5% carbon dioxide and a relative humidity of 98% (103). After 18 hours of incubation, the oocytes are examined to confirm the presence of two pronuclei (2PN), the earliest indication of fertilization, and to rule out the presence of three or more pronuclei indicative of polyspermia (Fig. 6; see also Fig. 3). Polyspermia is indicative of a dysfunction at the oocyte cortical-granule reaction level that should be triggered off at the time of fertilization by a single spermatozoon (106). Normal fertilization varies between 75% and 90% for metaphase II oocytes. For immature oocytes, it is reduced to 50% to 60%. In severe male-factor infertility, the fertilization rate is low unless microinsemination techniques are used.

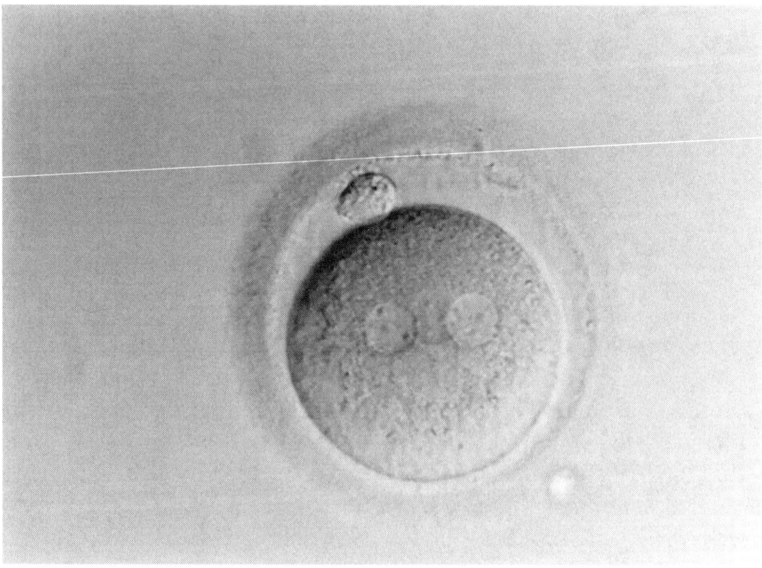

FIG. 6. Three pronuclei indicative of polyspermia.

Embryo Culture

The 2PN embryos are transferred to a growth culture medium containing a 15% concentration of serum supplementation. Incubation is continued until the transfer day, traditionally on the second or third day after oocyte aspiration. Normal embryos should cleave to the two-cell stage by 24 to 29 hours after insemination and reach the four- to eight-cell stage between 48 and 72 hours (103). Today, there is a tendency to delay the transfer for an additional 2 days, or until the embryo reaches the blastocyst stage (107) (Fig. 7).

Embryo quality is important and correlates well with the pregnancy rate. Embryo quality

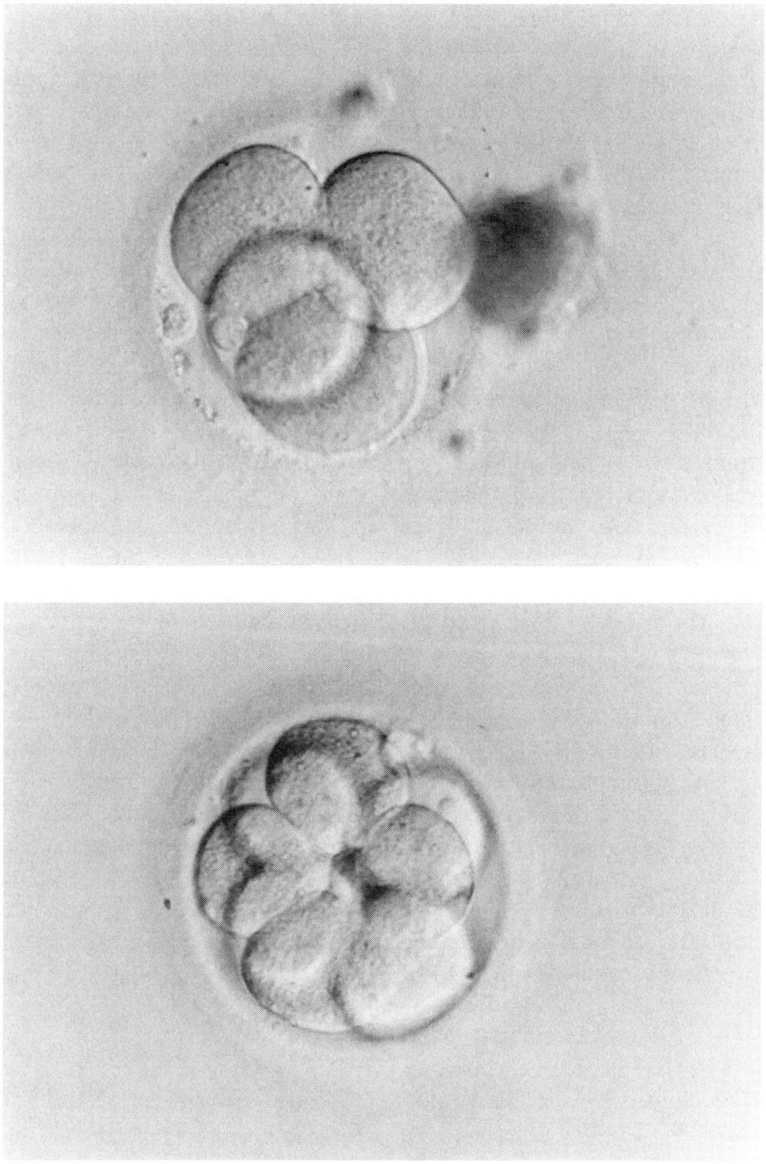

A

B

FIG. 7. A: Four-cell-stage embryo (two with single nuclei). **B:** Eight-cell-stage embryo.

is based on the cleavage rate, the number of blastomeres, their size and synchronization, and the presence of fragments in and granularity of the ooplasma. Furthermore, it is important to determine the thickness of the zona pellucida because thinning of the zona may be required prior to embryo transfer (assisted hatching) (108).

Embryo Transfer

Embryo transfer can be performed at the 2PN stage or at the four- to eight-cell stage 48 or 72 hours after insemination, unless the embryos are delayed until the blastocyst stage, which should occur by the fifth day postinsemination. The number of embryos to be transferred depends on patient age, the quality of the embryos, and the experience and success of the IVF program (109,110). Multiple pregnancy is one problem that results from an increased number of transferred embryos and also depends on patient age. At the Johns Hopkins Hospital IVF program, only three embryos are transferred to patients younger than age 30 years, four embryos to patients between age 31 and 39 years, and six embryos to patients older than 40 years.

The embryo transfer technique does not require anesthesia. The patient is placed in the dorsal lithotomy position. A sterile bivalve speculum is placed into the vagina. The cervix is cleansed with culture medium to remove excess cervical mucus. The embryos are loaded into an embryo transfer catheter using only 30 to 50 μL of culture medium to avoid reflux into the endocervical canal. In general, the transfer is an easy nonsurgical procedure. Sometimes, due to the position of the uterus and curvature of the endocervical/endometrial cavity, a cervical tenaculum needs to be placed in the cervix for traction and correction of the angle of the endocervical canal. The transfer must be a gentle technique. Bleeding must be avoided because blood clots may interfere with the implantation. Following the embryo transfer, the patient rests for 30 to 60 minutes.

In Vitro Fertilization–Related Techniques

Other techniques designed as alternatives to IVF include the following:

- Gamete intrafallopian transfer (GIFT)
- Zygote intrafallopian transfer (ZIFT)
- Tubal embryo transfer (TET)
- Intrauterine insemination (IUI)

Gamete Intrafallopian Transfer

GIFT was described by Ash et al. (111) in 1984. This technique is more appealing to patients with moral and/or religious objections to IVF because it is considered more natural. Indications for GIFT are similar to those for IVF, but normalcy of at least one fallopian tube is required.

The GIFT procedure shares the same type of ovarian stimulation, follicular aspiration, oocyte classification, and sperm preparation as in IVF, except that the sperm must be provided and prepared (washed) in advance. Once oocytes are retrieved, the patient undergoes laparoscopy for gamete transfer. The fimbriae are picked up with an atraumatic forceps, and gametes are delivered to the ampullary portion using a special catheter previously loaded with the oocytes and 150,000 sperm. The GIFT technique ensures that the oocytes and sperm are delivered to the natural place where fertilization normally takes place. Once fertilization occurs, the embryos arrive at the endometrial cavity through their normal mechanism. GIFT initially showed a greater success rate than IVF in many centers; however, in good, large IVF centers, there is no significant difference between the two procedures (112,113). In 1995 in the United States, 3,672 GIFT procedures were performed, with a 26.8% success rate (46).

Zygote Intrafallopian Transfer and Tubal Embryo Transfer

One disadvantage of GIFT is the lack of knowledge about fertilization; in another words, if GIFT does not produce a pregnancy, it is impossible to determine whether it was related to lack of fertilization or lack of embryo implantation. Therefore, ZIFT (114,115) and TET (116) were developed as alternatives to GIFT.

The ZIFT and TET procedures are identical to those of IVF: ovulation induction, oocyte aspiration, sperm wash, and IVF. In ZIFT, embryos are transferred into the fallopian tubes at the 2PN stage. Twenty-four hours after oocyte aspiration, the patient is returned to the operating room for laparoscopy. In a similar technique to GIFT, embryos are transferred to the ampullary portion of the fallopian tube. The TET procedure is similar, except that the embryos have already cleaved and are transferred at any time from the two- to eight-cell stage. For both ZIFT and TET, lack of success (i.e, failure to become pregnant) is due to failure of embryo implantation because fertilization and cleavage have already taken place. There is a great deal of controversy about the effectiveness of ZIFT and TET compared with IVF (116). Again, in well established IVF programs, the difference in results seems to be nil.

Intrauterine Insemination

Intrauterine insemination was proposed as a means of increasing the number of sperm that reaches the fallopian tube. In the 1950s, a procedure involving injection of raw semen into the endometrial cavity resulted in severe allergic reactions because raw semen contains proteins and other substances that normally do not enter the endometrial cavity, being filtered by the cervical mucus (117,118). Therefore, the technique was of limited use until the mid-1970s and became more popular with the introduction of sperm-washing techniques associated with IVF (119,120).

Indications for IUI

Male factor	Oligospermia
	Teratospermia
	Hypospermia
	Asthenospermia
Cervical factor	Hostile cervical mucus
	Chronic cervicitis
	DES exposure
	Cervical cone
Luteal-phase deficiency	Endometriosis without tubal damage
	Idiopathic infertility
	CC ovulation induction
	Dryness of the cervix

In male-factor infertility, IUI is indicated only if there is a minimum total motile sperm of 1.5 million recovered after sperm wash using the swim-up technique or Percoll gradient separation. Pregnancies are the exception with concentrations of less than 1 million sperm; therefore, these patients have a better prognosis using IVF or donor sperm (119).

Consensus has not been reached about ovulation timing—and its importance—before IUI. Some authors recommend that IUI should be performed on 2 consecutive days, while others recommend that one well timed IUI is enough to succeed with a pregnancy (121).

Ovulation for IUI can be detected in a spontaneous menstrual cycle by LH determination using a urinary LH predictor kit or by monitoring the follicular development by ultrasound and serum LH determinations once the follicle reaches 18 mm in diameter (122). The LH surge precedes ovulation by 28 to 29 hours (123). Therefore, the IUI should be scheduled around that time. The fecundity rate varies from 0.08 to 0.12 per month, which is different from the 0.22 rate of the general population (124).

Ovulation induction with CC has been used to increase the number of follicles available and the fecundity rate (125). CC is started on menstrual cycle day 2 or 5 at a dose of 50 to 100 mg per day for 5 days. Regrettably, there is a tendency to perform the IUI on menstrual cycle day 13 or 14, without any follicle monitoring. In my experience, it is well established that when CC is administered to normal-ovulatory patients just for the purpose of IUI, ovulation may occur at any time between menstrual cycle days 12 and 23. Therefore, it is important to monitor patients closely, with ultrasound on menstrual cycle day 12 to determine the diameter of the follicle and schedule future tests accordingly. The follicle may be ovulated at any time after its diameter reaches 18 mm, but usually after reaching 24 mm. Serum LH determinations should be done once the follicle reaches 18 mm. When the LH surge is detected, the IUI can be done 30 to 32 hours later. If the LH level remains low regardless of the full follicular size (24 mm), then 10,000 IU of hCG should be given intramuscularly to induce ovulation and prevent luteinized unruptured follicle syndrome. The IUI should be carried out 40 to 44 hours following the hCG injection.

Ovarian stimulation with hMG has been used to increase the fecundity rate in IUI patients, especially those who have not succeeded with a pregnancy after several cycles of CC ovulation induction with IUI. In general, mild ovulation induction is carried out using 150 IU of hMG or pure FSH starting on menstrual cycle day 2 or 3, followed by follicle monitoring as previously described. The IUI will be performed between 40 and 44 hours after the hCG injection (124). The use of gonadotropins in IUI carries the risk of multiple pregnancy and OHSS.

The IUI technique consists of inserting a bivalve speculum into the vagina. The cervical mucus is cleansed with a cotton swab, and the sperm is delivered into the endometrial cavity by the insertion of a plastic catheter already loaded with a 0.5-mL volume containing the sperm wash. The patient remains in the recumbent position for 15 minutes.

Variations of IUI include selective tube insemination and transperitoneal insemination (126). *Selective tube insemination* is performed by selective catheterization of the ostium either by ultrasound guidance or free hand (127). *Transperitoneal insemination* is performed by injection of sperm into the peritoneum through the posterior vaginal fornix (128). Although there have been a few reports of the success of these procedures, one should question their usefulness because sperm could be detected in the peritoneal fluid within 10 minutes after the IUI.

Eighty-five percent of pregnancies occur during the first four IUIs (129). If a patient has not conceived by then, diagnostic laparoscopy is indicated before further inseminations. If artificial insemination has been done using donor sperm, a new donor is recommended. If the female evaluation is normal, then IVF is the next step in treating the infertility.

In Vitro Fertilization by Microinjection

To obtain a good fertilization rate through IVF, a sperm concentration of about 1 million after sperm washing is required; otherwise, the fertilization rate decreases significantly, or fertilization does not occur. Several microinjection techniques have been developed during the past decade (130–132):

Partial zona dissection (PZD)
Subzonal injection (SUZI)
Intracytoplasmic sperm injection (ICSI)

Partial Zona Dissection

PZD consists of creating a small rent mechanically or by digestion of the zona pellucida with a low-PH Tyrode's solution. This facilitates sperm fertilization of the oocyte when the post-sperm-wash concentration is between 500,000 and 1 million sperm. The disadvantages of PZD are a high rate of polyspermia (50%), a fertilization rate of only 25%, and an overall pregnancy rate of less than 5% per retrieval (130).

Subzonal Injection

SUZI is indicated when the post-sperm-wash concentration is between 300,000 and 500,000. The procedure consists of suspending the oocyte in a hyperosmolar sucrose solution to create a bigger perivitelline space. Three to five sperm are injected into this space using a microneedle. Polyspermia is high (50%), and oocyte damage occurs in 3% to 10% of cases. The fertilization rate per oocyte is around 20%, and the pregnancy rate is only 3%. Both PZD and SUZI have been replaced by ICSI (131).

Intracytoplasmic Sperm Injection

Palermo et al. (132) were the first to succeed with ICSI. They were able to inject a single sperm into the oocyte's cytoplasm to obtain fertilization and a viable pregnancy. ICSI requires a special microscope, armed with joysticks, that allows stabilization of the oocyte and injection of the sperm. The sperm must be immobilized and loaded within the injector needle by suction, tail first. The technique requires only a single live sperm per oocyte, making it possible for men with severe male-factor infertility to become biologic parents. ICSI has been expanded to patients with azoospermia due to acquired epididymal obstruction and to those with congenital absence of the vas deferens, in which the sperm can be obtained by microaspiration of the epididymis (MESA) (133,134) or testicular biopsy (TESA) (135). Furthermore, ICSI is the solution for patients with a history of antisperm antibodies or failed vasovasostomy (136,137). The fertilization rate per oocyte fluctuates between 70% and 90% and the pregnancy rate between 25% to 35% per cycle (138,139). ICSI allows fertilization in approximately 95% of all severe male-factor-infertility patients. The risk of congenital malformation after ICSI does not seem to be greater than the risk with conventional IVF (139).

CRYOPRESERVATION IN ASSISTED REPRODUCTIVE TECHNOLOGIES

Cryopreservation is the process by which cells can be stored at low temperatures for future use. The successful cryopreservation of cells is affected by the rate of freezing and the composition of the solution in which the cells are frozen. As the cells approach the freezing temperature, water outside the cell freezes first, removing liquid solvent from the extracellular broth, resulting in increased extracellular osmolarity. Water then leaves the cells to follow the osmotic gradient, concentrating the intracellular components sufficiently to eliminate supercooling. This phenomenon occurs when cells are cooled too rapidly, in which case the cells do not lose water fast enough to avoid intracellular freezing and are thereby damaged. Because of the osmotic difference, more water leaves the cells, resulting in shrinkage.

Cryopreservation is cell-specific because cells may differ both in the amount of intracellular water and the permeability of the cell membrane. For example, spermatozoa, due to their small volume, large surface, and small amount of intracellular water, require a different freezing technique from that used with oocytes or any other cells.

Sperm Cryopreservation

In 1953, it was demonstrated that thawed semen was capable of fertilizing and inducing normal embryonic development in humans (140). This success came almost two centuries after Spallanzani reported the effects of cryopreservation on human semen in 1776. Semen cryopreservation has been widely used by veterinarians, who were the first to establish sperm banks for commercial purposes (141).

Human sperm banks were established during World War II as a way for women to have legitimate children after their husband's death. These sperm banks proliferated when artificial insemination with fresh donor semen became unacceptable for the treatment of severe male infertility because of the risk of transmission of venereal and other pathogens, such as human immunodeficiency virus (HIV), hepatitis B virus, cytomegalovirus, and so on. Then, screening tests for donors and a 6-month quarantine for semen became mandatory (142). These actions resulted in an increased need for sperm cryopreservation and the creation of sperm banks.

Fewer than 15% of spermatozoa survive freezing and thawing without the addition of a cryoprotectant. Several cryoprotectants, such as glycerol and dimethyl sulfoxide, have been used to prevent damage to the plasma membrane, acrosomal leakage, and breakdown. These traumas sustained by spermatozoa account for a decreased fertilization capability and a 50% decrease in sperm motility after thawing (143,144). Therefore, sperm cryopreservation for the purpose of cervical insemination was not useful in patients with oligospermia or asthenospermia, unless multiple samples were pulled together or other ARTs were used, including IUI, IVF, and in extreme cases ICSI.

The freezing–thawing process has been improved by the use of various media called extenders. Extenders assist glycerol during cryopreservation by optimizing the osmotic pressure and pH, by providing an energy source, to prevent the undesirable use by sperm of their own intracellular phospholipid, by preventing bacterial contamination when an antibiotic is included, and by permitting dilution of semen while offsetting the deleterious effect on survival produced by high dilution (145). These extenders, such as TRIS (hydroxymethyl) aminomethane or N-TRIS methylaminoethane sulfonic acid (TES), may improve motile sperm recovery by their ability to bind heavy metals such as copper, zinc, or gold, which can decrease human sperm motility. The life expectancy of stored and properly cryopreserved semen is considered unlimited.

Oocyte Cryopreservation

Oocyte cryopreservation has been one of the goals of ARTs. Unfortunately, the size of the oocyte and its high water concentration have been major obstacles to ensuring the viability of cryopreserved oocytes. Chen (146) reported the first successful pregnancy after fertilization of a cryopreserved oocyte. Van Uem et al. (147) reported the second pregnancy.

Oocyte cryopreservation would eliminate the ethical, moral, religious, and legal issues created by embryo cryopreservation; it would also limit the number of oocytes to be inseminated, eliminate some of the risks of multiple pregnancy and its consequences, and optimize the benefits of ovarian stimulation. Today, cryopreservation of oocytes benefits the treatment of cancer patients who require radiotherapy or chemotherapy, without the need for the transfer of fresh embryos that could delay cancer treatment. Another relative indication concerns patients who postpone their reproductive function until they achieve professional career goals. Oocyte cryopreservation at a younger age could decrease or almost eliminate the risk of chromosome abnormalities related to maternal age, as well as the risk of poor ovarian response observed with advanced age.

To date, cryopreservation of metaphase II oocytes is still under development due to low cryosurvival and poor fertilization rates. However, fertilization has improved by means of ICSI, which indicates that during the process of oocyte cryopreservation there is damage to the zona pellucida and/or dysfunction at the cortical-granule reaction mechanism. Another concern with oocyte cryopreservation is the potential damage to the meiotic spindle with subsequent chromosome aberrations.

Still under development is cryopreservation of immature oocytes and ovarian tissue.

Embryo Cryopreservation

Embryo cryopreservation has been used by veterinarians for many years. Trounson and Mohr (148) reported the feasibility of human embryo cryopreservation in 1983. Cryopreservation may be accomplished at different stages after oocyte insemination: at the 2PN, zyngamy, four- or eight-cell, or blastocyst stages. Depending on the number of blastomeres, the freezing technique may require special cryoprotectants and different cooling techniques (149–152).

Cryopreservation at the 2PN stage has been the most frequently used and has the advantage in some programs of avoiding the moral/religious dilemma of human cryopreservation. The procedure has proven to be successful. It is done the day following oocyte insemination, once the decision has been made about the number of embryos that will be allowed to continue cleaving for a fresh embryo transfer. There is no problem in selecting which embryos will be cryopreserved and which will be transferred fresh because 2PN-stage embryos are alike and the selection is done at random. The survival rate after thawing varies between 60% and 80% and the pregnancy rate between 15% and 30% (152).

Cryopreservation at the four- to eight-cell stage is becoming more acceptable because it allows the embryos to cleave for 24 to 48 hours. Early embryonic arrest is detected. It also provides the opportunity to better select the embryos to be transferred fresh, and increases the possibility of a successful pregnancy. At the same time, it allows adjustment of the number of embryos to be transferred according to patient age and embryo quality. A disadvantage is that embryos of poor quality will be cryopreserved, with a decreased possibility for survival with thawing. During the freezing–thawing process some blastomeres will die, but in general an embryo may survive up to a 50% blastomere attrition (152).

Cryopreservation of blastocysts has been one of the best improvements in embryo cryopreservation (153). One drawback in IVF has been the relatively low embryo-implantation rate, a phenomenon poorly understood at present. One hypothesis explaining the poor implantation rate concerns the low number of embryos capable of reaching the blastocyst stage within the endometrial cavity. Nowadays, a special culture medium allows the embryo to cleave up to the blastocyst stage in the IVF laboratory. Therefore, fresh transfer of up to three blastocysts is feasible, with cryopreservation of the rest for future use (154). Approximately 50% of blastocysts implant, which represents an improvement in the IVF pregnancy rate. At the same time, it allows the transfer of a small number of embryos, decreasing the incidence of multiple pregnancies.

Cryopreservation of Testicular Tissue

The development of ICSI has been one of the major accomplishments in the history of assisted human reproduction. ICSI permits the treatment of infertility in patients otherwise considered sterile. It is well known that patients with a diagnosis of Sertoli-only cell syndrome or Klinefelter syndrome may still have a few sperm within the seminiferous tubules that could be removed by TESA and isolated under the microscope. Some sperm could be used to perform ICSI, and the rest cryopreserved for future use. TESA could be used in patients with leukemia, lymphomas, or any other cancer before treatment with radiation or chemotherapeutic agents renders the patient sterile (155–157). The same applies to patients who require castration as a treatment for testicular tumor.

GAMETE DONATION

Donor Sperm

Sperm donation has traditionally been the treatment for male infertility associated with azoospermia, oligospermia, or teratospermia, alone or in combination. It has also been used for men with uncorrectable sexual dysfunction of psychologic or traumatic origin. It has been used when other forms of therapy have failed and as a sperm backup in patients with obstructive azoospermia or Sertoli-only cell syndrome undergoing TESA, MESA for IVF, and ICSI. There is an increasing demand for donor sperm among single women who decline to have a heterosexual relationship.

Preferably, the source of the sperm should be anonymous, although there are patients who request that a nonconsanguineous relative be the donor, such as a father- or brother-in-law or a close friend. Regardless of the semen source, fresh inseminations are banned; all donors must comply with the regulations formulated by the ASRM, the SART, and by the tissue bank (142). Therefore, prior to the semen sample collection, a donor should have a complete history and physical examination, including a complete family history for inheritable problems (Tay-Sachs disease, sickle cell anemia, thalassemia, and so on) and screening for HIV disease, hepatitis B and C, gonorrhea, syphilis, cytomegalovirus infection, and other transmittable diseases. A psychologic evaluation of the donor should be performed by a certified psychologist or psychiatrist. The semen sample is cryopreserved and quarantined for at least 6 months, at which time the donor should be rescreened. If tests remain negative, then the semen sample is ready for donation. Although there is no consensus about the age of a donor, he should be younger than age 45 years because there is some risk of genetic problems related to age.

The selection of a sperm donor should be based on the phenotype and race of the infertile couple. Sperm sex selection is still under investigation. There are reports describing particular methods for separating the X- or the Y-bearing spermatozoon based on its motility and DNA component; nevertheless, there is no 100% guarantee.

Delivery of the frozen donor sperm is performed as follows: The prospective couple should be screened for HIV and hepatitis for medicolegal reasons. The recipient should have at least one patent fallopian tube, normal secretory endometrial biopsy, and endometriosis or pelvic adhesions should be ruled out. Ovulation could be monitored during a natural or ovulation-induction cycle (see "Intrauterine Insemination" above).

The success of artificial insemination by donor sperm (AID) is based on recipient age and the association of any other infertility-producing factors. If a woman is normal and the indication for AID is related to azoospermia, the fecundity rate is approximately 15% to 20% per cycle. If the indications are oligoovulation and/or are associated with other factors, then the success rate is estimated between 10% and 15%. The majority of pregnancies (85%) are achieved within the first four cycles of AID. If a pregnancy has not been achieved by that time, further evaluation is in order, including diagnostic laparoscopy and repeat HSG. If no other infertility-producing factor is detected, a new sperm donor is recommended.

Donor Oocyte

With the advent of IVF and ovulation induction with Gn-RH analogs, as well as the aspiration of more oocytes than will be inseminated, the possibility of creating oocyte donation arose (158–163). Donor oocyte is indicated in patients with or without ovarian function as follows:

Without ovarian function	Premature menopause
	Premature ovarian failure (before age 40, due to radiation therapy or chemotherapy)
	Bilateral oophorectomy (infection, cancer, other surgeries)
	Gonadal dysgenesis (Turner syndrome, pure gonadal dysgenesis)
	Physiologic menopause
	Desire to prolong reproductive age
With ovarian function	Genetic disease carriers (Tay-Sachs disease, cystic fibrosis, hemophilia, and so on)
	Carriers of chromosome abnormalities (fragile X)
	Poor ovarian reserve

The source of an oocyte should preferably be anonymous. Early on, donor oocyte sources were IVF patients currently undergoing ovarian stimulation. Regrettably, due to absent or poor insurance coverage, today's IVF patients are reluctant to donate any oocytes and opt for a larger number of embryos to be cryopreserved for future transfer. Therefore, the majority of donor oocytes are from patients recruited for this purpose, sometimes involving a patient's relative or close friend.

The oocyte donor should undergo the same screening process as the sperm donor: a complete history and physician examination, including a family history of inheritable problems, and screenings for HIV, hepatitis B and C, and other transmittable diseases. as well as a psychologic evaluation. Because freezing oocytes is not available or is in the development process, oocyte quarantine is not required at present. The recipient and her husband should have the same screenings for medicolegal reasons.

Selection of the oocyte donor should be based on the patient's phenotype, race, and age. Ideally, the oocyte donor should be between 21 and 30 years of age, although up to age 35 is acceptable. Age greater than 35 is not recommended because of the increased risk of chromosome abnormalities and a poor response to ovarian stimulation. Furthermore, it is preferable that the oocyte donor has been pregnant in the past, is monogamous, and uses mechanical contraception during the cycle of ovarian stimulation.

The complexity of the oocyte donor program lies in preparation of the recipient patient's endometrium and in ovarian stimulation of the oocyte donor. The endometrium is artificially stimulated by the administration of increasing doses of estradiol valerate or the use of transdermal estradiol patches. If the patient's ovarian function is still active, downregulation of pituitary gonadotropins is required using a Gn-RH analog from days 17 or 21 of the preceding menstrual cycle; the Gn-RH analog can be discontinued on the first day of estradiol administration. Maturation of the endometrium is started when the oocyte donor begins ovulation induction (first day of gonadotropins administration). If the recipient has a diagnosis of ovarian failure, there is no need for Gn-RH analog administration. On the day of donor oocyte aspiration, the recipient patient should be started on micronized progesterone (Prometrium), 200 mg every 6 hours vaginally (164).

Before the initiation of any therapy, both the oocyte donor and the recipient must sign a detailed consent form. The consent form should include a full explanation of the procedure including the protocols, frequent blood and ultrasound tests, oocyte aspiration technique, risk of anesthesia, oocyte aspiration, and potential side effects of gonadotropin use, such as OHSS, ovarian torsion, and ovarian rupture. The risk of an undesirable pregnancy and the importance of using sexual abstinence or mechanical contraception should also be included. It must be clear that the oocytes retrieved and the embryos resulting from the insemination will be the property of the recipient couple. Furthermore, the oocyte donor must be informed of any state legislation about parenthood, adoption, and custodial rights (165).

The success of the donor oocyte program is related to donor age, number of embryos transferred, and synchronization of the recipient to have a fresh embryo transfer. In general, the donor oocyte program is more successful than IVF using a patient's own oocytes. Success rates vary between 50% and 60% if the donor is younger than age 30 and a maximum of three embryos are transferred fresh into the well synchronized endometrium. If the oocyte donor's age is between 31 and 35 years, the pregnancy rate will be reduced to 30% to 35%. Multiple pregnancy occurs in 50% of recipients; therefore, one should consider limiting the number of embryos to be transferred and cryopreserve the remaining embryos for future transfer(s).

Donation of gametes must be voluntary. It is not legal to sell or buy gametes. However, the donors can be compensated for their time and inconvenience (165).

EMBRYO DONATION

The primary goal for embryo cryopreservation is to store supernumerary embryos for future transfer. This technique has brought great benefits to IVF patients by decreasing the frequency of ovarian stimulation and helping decrease the number of multiple pregnancies. Nevertheless, an increasing number of cryopreserved embryos have been donated to IVF programs as a result of unforeseeable circumstances such as delivery of multiple pregnancies following previous embryo transfer, divorce, and death of one or both parents. Sometimes, embryos are abandoned and become the property of an IVF program. In the consent form, duly signed by an infertile couple, ownership of the embryos should be clearly stipulated, as well as contingencies in case the couple relinquishes the desire of having additional children. One contingency is embryo donation to an anonymous couple or to someone designated by the couple (166,167).

Donor embryo is equivalent to the earliest adoption, except that the embryo recipient must undergo endometrial preparation as previously described. A donor embryo program requires the same screening process for transmittable diseases as for IVF and other ARTs. The recipient must be aware of the limited embryo implantation and pregnancy rates, which are determined by donor age at the time of ovarian stimulation and the quality and number of cryopreserved–thawed embryos. Furthermore, once implantation takes place, chorionic villus sampling or amniocentesis is indicated, but only depending on donor age.

Embryos cannot be sold as commodities, and expenses should be limited to screening, endometrial stimulation, embryo culture, and embryo transfer fees. An administrative fee is acceptable; however, no payment should be made to the donor or to the IVF program (163). A detailed consent form must be signed by the recipient couple assuming all risks and responsibilities of pregnancy, delivery, and child support if embryo transfer is successful. The IVF program and all team members are released from any legal responsibility. In most states, the legal mother is the one who delivers the baby, and the legal father is the husband or partner at the time of delivery.

SUMMARY

The most significant advances in ARTs, such as IVF and ICSI and the cryopreservation of embryos and gametes, make reproduction possible for oncology patients. Further research is necessary to decrease the risk of toxic effects from chemotherapy and radiation therapy on gametes. Cancer patients should receive appropriate counseling before, during, and after cancer treatment about issues of reproduction and sexuality.

REFERENCES

1. Steptoe PC, Edwards RG. Birth after preimplantation of a human embryo. *Lancet* 1978;2:366.
2. Hook EB, Cross PK, Schresnema Chess DM. Chromosomal abnormality rate at amniocentesis and in live-born infants. *JAMA* 1983;249:2034.
3. McLaren A. Sex determinations in mammals. *Trends Genet* 1988;4:153.
4. Welshons WJ, Russell LB. The Y chromosome as a bearer of male determining factors in the mouse. *Proc Natl Acad Sci U S A* 1959;45:560.
5. Besta P, Hawkins JR, Sinclair AH, et al. Genetic evidence equating SRY and the testis-determining factor. *Nature* 1990;348:448.
6. Jager RJ, Anvret M, Hall K, Schern G. A human XY female with a frame shift mutation in the candidate testis-determining gene SRY: nonsense and missense mutations in XY sex reversal. *Hum Genet* 1992;88:471.
7. Gier HT, Marion GB. Development of the mammalian testis and genital ducts. *Biol Reprod* 1969;1:1.
8. Winter JSD, Faiman C, Reges F. Sexual endocrinology of fetal and perinatal life. In: Austin CR, Edwards RG, eds. *Mechanisms of sex differentiation in animals and man.* London: Academic Press, 1981:205.
9. Cunha GR, Shannon JR, Neubauer BL, et al. Mesenchymal-epithelial interaction in sex differentiation. *Hum Genet* 1981;58:68.
10. Wilson JD, Griffin JE, George FW, Leshin M. The role of gonadal steroids in sexual differentiation. *Recent Prog Horm Res* 1981;37:1.
11. Fairman C, Winter JSD, Reyes FI. Patterns of gonadotropins and gonadal steroids throughout life. *Clin Obstet Gynecol* 1976;3:467.
12. Trans D, Meusy-Dessola N, Josso N. Anti-mullerian hormone is a functional marker of fetal Sertoli cell. *Nature* 1977;269:411.
13. Forest MC, dePeretti E, Bertrand J. Hypothalamic-pituitary-gonodal relationship in man from birth to puberty. *Clin Endocrinol (Oxf)* 1976;5:551.
14. Maisumoto AM. The testis and male sexual function. In: Wyngarrden JB, Smith LH, Bennett JC, eds. *Cecil textbook of medicine*. Philadelphia: WB Saunders, 1991;2:1333.
15. Kerr JB. Functional cytology of the human testis. *Baillieres Clin Endocrinol Metab* 1992;6:235.
16. Russell LD, Ettlin RA, Sinha Hikim AP, Clegg ED. Mammalian spermatogenesis. In: Russell LD, Ettlin RA, Sinha Hikim AP, Clegg ED, eds. *Histological and histopathlogical evaluation of the testis.* Clearwater, FL: Cache River Press, 1990:1.
17. Rowley MJ, Leach DR, Warner GA. Effect of graded doses of ionizing radiation on the human testis. *Radiat Res* 1974;59:665.
18. Clermont Y. The cycle of the seminiferous epithelium in man. *Am J Anat* 1963;112:35.
19. Thompson MW, McKinnes RR, Willard HF. The sex chromosomes and their abnormalities. In: Thompson MW, McKinnes RR, Willard HF, eds. *Thompson and Thompson genetics in medicine*, 5th ed. Philadelphia: WB Saunders, 1991:231.
20. deKaetser DM, Kerr JB. The cytology of the testis. In: Knobil E, Neill J, et al., eds. *The physiology of reproduction.* New York: Raven Press, 1988;2:837.
21. Heller CG, Clermont Y. Spermatogenesis in man: an estimate of its duration. *Science* 1963;140:184.
22. Bigers J, Schultz A, eds. *Oogenesis.* Baltimore: University Park Press, 1973.
23. Franchi L, Mandl A, Zakerman S. The development of the ovary and the process of oogenesis. In: Zuckerman

S, ed. *The ovary,* vol. 1. New York: Academic Press, 1963:1.
24. Baker TG. A quantitative and cytological study of germ cells in human primordial oocytes. *Proc R Soc London (Biol)* 1963;158:417–433.
25. Baker TG, Franchi L. The fine structure of oogonia and oocytes in human ovaries. *J Cell Sci* 1967;2:213.
26. Solt I, Weyl M, Arush B, Lightman A, Kuten A. Fertility status of long-term survivors of childhood lymphomas. Presented at Anti-cancer Treatment VI International Congress 1996, Feb 6–9, Paris, France.
27. Simmonds PD, Mead GM, Sweetenhan A, et al. PACE BOM chemotherapy: a 12-week regimen for advanced Hodgkin's disease. *Ann Oncol* 1997;8:259.
28. Novakovic B, Fears TR, Horowitz ME, Wexler LH. Genetic epidemiology in survivors of Ewing's sarcoma family tumors. *J Pediatr Hematol Oncol* 1997;19:220.
29. *Ovarian cancer: screening, treatment, and follow-up.* National Institutes of Health Consensus Development Conference Statement 1994, April 5–7. 12(3):1, Bethesda, Maryland.
30. Pont J, Albrech W. Fertility after chemotherapy for testicular germ cell cancer. *Fertil Steril* 1997;68:1.
31. Stephenson WT, Poirier SM, Rubin L, Einhorn L. Evaluation of reproductive capacity in germ cell tumor patients following treatment with cisplatin, etoposide and bleomycin. *J Clin Oncol* 1995;13:2278.
32. Hansen PV, Glavind K, Panduro J, Pedersen M. Paternity with testicular germ cell cancer: pre-treatment and post-treatment findings. *Eur J Cancer* 1991;27:1385.
33. Heindenreich A, Vorreuther R, Neubauer S, Engelman UH. Paternity in patients with bilateral testicular germ cell tumors. *Eur Urol* 1997;31:246.
34. Rosenshein NB, Grumbine FC, Woodruff JD, Ettinger DS. Pregnancy following chemotherapy for an ovarian immature embryonal teratoma. *Gynecol Oncol* 1979; 8:234.
35. Sutcliffe SB. Cytotoxic chemotherapy and gonadal function in patients with Hodgkin's disease. *JAMA* 1979;242:1898.
36. Lampe H, Horwich A, Noman A, Nicholls J, Dearnaley DP. Fertility after chemotherapy for testicular germ cell cancers. *J Clin Oncol* 1997;15:239.
37. Dein RA, Mennuti MT, Lovach P, Gabbe SG. The reproductive potential of young men and women with Hodgkin's disease: review. *Obstet Gynecol Surv* 1984; 39:474.
38. Husseinzadeth N, Nahhas WA, Velkley DE, Whitney CW. The preservation of ovarian function in young women undergoing pelvic radiation therapy. *Gynecol Oncol* 1984;18:373.
39. Baker TG. Radiosensitivity of mammalian oocytes with particular reference to the human female: review. *Am J Obstet Gynecol* 1971;110:746.
40. Gomes PJ, Rustin GJ. Attempted preservation of one gonad in patients with bilateral germ cell tumors. *Clin Oncol* 1996;8:397.
41. Gonzalez-Lira G, Escudero-De Los Rios P, Salazar-Martinez E, Lazcano-Ponce EC. Conservative surgery for ovarian cancer and effect on fertility. *Int J Gynaecol Obstet* 1997;56:155.
42. Ash P. The influence of radiation on fertility in man. *Br J Radiology* 1980;53:271.
43. Arai Y, Kawakita M, Okada Y, Yoshida O. Sexuality and fertility in long-term survivors of testicular cancer. *J Clin Oncol* 1997;15:1444.
44. Turlington WT, Wright BD, Powell JL. Impact of the LEEP electrosurgical excision procedure on future fertility. *J Reprod Med* 1996;41:815.
45. Steele GS, Richie JP. Current role of retroperitoneal lymph node dissection in testicular cancer. *Rev Oncol* 1997;11:717.
46. Society for Assisted Reproductive Technology and the American Society for Reproductive Medicine. Assisted Reproductive Technology in the United States and Canada: 1995 Results generated from the American Society for Reproductive Medicine, Society for Assisted Reproductive Technology Registry. *Fertil Steril* 1998;69:389–398.
47. Jones GS. Update in *in vitro* fertilization. *Endocrinol Rev* 1984;5:62.
48. Garcia JE, Tran T, Smith RD, Padilla SL. Relationship of endometriosis staging and *in vitro* fertilization outcome. *Hum Reprod* 1991;6(suppl 1):74(abst).
49. Feldberg D, Davis O, Grifo J, et al. Severity of endometriosis does not impact on pregnancy success after *in vitro* fertilization. Presented at the 7th IVF World Congress, June/July 1991, Paris, France.
50. Kruger TF, Acosta AA, Simmons KF, et al. Predictive value of abnormal sperm morphology in *in vitro* fertilization. *Fertil Steril* 1988;49:112.
51. Muasher SJ, Garcia JE, Jones HW Jr. Experience with diethylstilbestrol-exposed infertile women in a program of *in vitro* fertilization. *Fertil Steril* 1984;42:20.
52. Romeu A, Muasher SJ, Acosta AA, et al. Results of *in vitro* fertilization attempts in women 40 years of age and older: the Norfolk experience. *Fertil Steril* 1987; 47:130.
53. Scott RT, Muasher SJ, Oehninger S, Robinson S, Rosenwaks Z. Follicle-stimulating hormone level on cycle day 3 are predictive of *in vitro* fertilization outcome. *Fertil Steril* 1989;51:651.
54. Coulam CB, Adamson SC, Annegers JF. Incidence of premature ovarian failure. *Obstet Gynecol* 1986;67:604.
55. Sachdev R, Kemman E, Bohrer MK, El-Danosouri I. Detrimental effect of hydrosalpinx fluid on the development and blastulation of mouse embryos in *in vitro* fertilization. *Fertil Steril* 1997;68:531.
56. Strandell A, Waldenstrom U, Nilson L, Hamberger L. Hydrosalpinx reduces *in vitro* fertilization/embryo transfer pregnancy rates. *Hum Reprod* 1994;9:861.
57. Vandromme J, Chasse E, Lejune B, Van Rysselberger M, Delvigne A, Leroy F. Hydrosalpinges in *in vitro* fertilization: an unfavorable prognostic feature. *Hum Reprod* 1995;10:576.
58. Rawe VF, Liu J, Shaffer S, Compton MG, Garcia JE, Katz E. Effect of human hydrosalpinx fluid on murine embryo development and implantation. *Fertil Steril* 1997;8:668.
59. David G, Jouanette P, Martin-Boyce A, Spira A. Schwartz D. Sperm count in fertile and infertile men. *Fertil Steril* 1979;31:453.
60. Overstreet JW, Davis RO, Katz DF. Semen evaluation. *Infertil Reprod Med Clin North Am* 1992;3:329.
61. Jimenez C, Grizard G, Pouly JL, Boucher D. Birth after combination of cryopreservation of sperm recovered from urine and intracytoplasmic sperm injection in a case of complete retrograde ejaculation. *Fertil Steril* 1997;68:542.
62. Palermo G, Joris H, Desdre MP, Camus M, Devroey P, Van Steirteghem AC. Sperm characteristics and outcome of human assisted fertilization by subzonal in-

semination and intracytoplasmic sperm injection. *Fertil Steril* 1993;59:826.
63. Madgar I, Hourvitz A, Levron J, et al. Outcome of *in vitro* fertilization and intracytoplasmic sperm injection of epididymal and testicular sperm extracted from patients with obstructive and non-obstructive azoospermia. *Fertil Steril* 1998;69:1080.
64. Tjiam KH, Zeilmaker GH, Alberda AT, et al. Prevalence of antibodies to *Chlamydia trachomatis, Neisseria gonorrhoeae* and *Mycoplasma hominis* in infertile women. *Genitourin Med* 1985;61:175.
65. Moller BR, Taylor-Robinson D, Furr PM, et al. Serological evidence that *Chlamydia* and *Mycoplasma* are involved in infertility in women. *J Reprod Fertil* 1985; 73:237.
66. Garcia JE, Jones GS, Wright G Jr. Prediction of the time of ovulation. *Fertil Steril* 1981;36:308.
67. Paulson RJ, Sauer MV, Francis MM, Macaso TM, Lobo RD. *In vitro* fertilization in unstimulated cycle: the University of Southern California experience. *Fertil Steril* 1992;57:290.
68. Wilkes CA, Rosenwaks Z, Jones DL, Jones HW Jr. Pregnancy related to infertility, diagnosis, number of attempts and age in a program of *in vitro* fertilization. *Obstet Gynecol* 1985;66:350.
69. Hodgen GD. The dominant ovarian follicle. *Fertil Steril* 1982;38:281.
70. Trounson AO. Pregnancies in humans by fertilization *in vitro* and embryo transfer in controlled ovulatory cycle. *Science* 1981;212:681.
71. O'Herlily C, Pepperell RJ, Robinson HP. Ultrasound timing of human chorionic gonadotropin administration in clomiphene-stimulated cycles. *Obstet Gynecol* 1982;59:40.
72. Quigly MM: Selection of agents for enhanced follicular recruitment in an *in vitro* fertilization and embryo replacement treatment program. *Ann N Y Acad Sci* 1985;442:96.
73. Stanger JD, Yovitch JL. Reduced *in vitro* fertilization of human oocytes from patients with raised basal luteinizing hormone levels during follicular phase. *Br J Obstet Gynaecol* 1985;92:385.
74. Steptoe PC, Edwards RC. Laparoscopic recovery of preovulatory human oocyte after priming of ovaries with gonadotropins. *Lancet* 1970;1:683.
75. Diezfalvzy E, Haslin J. Clinical-pharmacological studies on human menopause gonadotropin. *Hum Reprod* 1988;3:21.
76. Garcia JE, Jones GS, Acosta AA, Wright G Jr. Human menopausal gonadotropin/human chorionic gonadotropin in follicular maturation for oocyte aspiration: phase I, 1981. *Fertil Steril* 1981;39:167.
77. Garcia JE, Jones GS, Acosta AA, Wright G Jr. Human menopausal gonadotropin/human chorionic gonadotropin follicular maturation for oocyte aspiration: phase II 1981. *Fertil Steril* 1981;39:174.
78. Howles CM, Macnamee MC, Edwards RG, Goswamy R, Steptoe PC. Effect of high tonic levels of luteinizing hormone in outcome of *in vitro* fertilization. *Lancet* 1986;2:521.
79. Punnomen R, Ashom R, Vilja P, Heinonen PK, Kujansuu E, Tuohimoa P. Spontaneous luteinizing hormone surge and cleavage of *in vitro* fertilized embryos. *Fertil Steril* 1988;49:479.
80. Regan L, Owen EJ, Jacobs HS. Hypersecretion of LH, infertility and miscarriages. *Lancet* 1990;336:1141.
81. Seegar Jones GE, Acosta AA, Garcia JE, Rosenwaks Z. Specific effects of FSH and LH on follicular development and oocyte retrieval as determined by a program for *in vitro* fertilization. *Ann N Y Acad Sci* 1985; 442:119.
82. Devroey P, van Steirteghem A, Mannaerts B, Bennink HC. Successful *in vitro* fertilization and embryo transfer after treatment with recombinant human FSH. *Lancet* 1992;339:1171.
83. Rutherford AS, Suback-Sharpe SJ, Dawsib KJ, Margova RA, Franks S, Winston RML. Improvement of *in vitro* fertilization after treatment with buserelin, an agonist of luteinizing hormone-releasing hormone. *BMJ* 1988;296:1765.
84. Macnamee MC, Howles MC, Edwards RG, Taylor PJ, Elder KT. Short-term luteinizing hormone-releasing hormone agonist treatment: prospective trial of a novel ovarian hyperstimulation regime for *in vitro* fertilization. *Fertil Steril* 1989;52:264.
85. Padilla SL, Smith RD, Garcia JE. The Lupron screening test: tailoring the use of leuprolide acetate in ovarian stimulation for *in vitro* fertilization. *Fertil Steril* 1991;53:79.
86. Garcia JE, Damewood M, Katz E. Follicular-phase luprolide acetate and human menopause gonadotropins in *in vitro* fertilization: intimacies of the flareup protocol in a major IVF program. Presented at the 51st Annual Meeting of the American Society for Reproductive Medicine, Oct 7–12, 1995, Seattle, Washington.
87. Kenigsberg D, Littman BA, Williams RF, Hodgen GD. Medical hypophysectomy. II. Variability of ovarian response to gonadotherapy. *Fertil Steril* 1984;42:116.
88. Bentick B, Shaw RW, Iffland CA, Burford G, Bernard A. A randomized comparative study of purified follicle-stimulating hormone and human menopausal gonadotropin after pituitary desensitization with buserelin for superovulation and *in vitro* fertilization. *Fertil Steril* 1988;50:79.
89. Schoot DC, Coeling-Bennink HJT, Mannaerts BMJL, Lamberts SWJ, Bouchard P, Fauser BCJM. Human recombinant follicle-stimulating hormone induces growth of preovulatory follicles without concomitant increase in androgen and estrogen biosynthesis in a woman with isolated gonadotropin deficiency. *J Clin Endocrinol Metab* 1992;74:1471.
90. Out HJ, Mannaerts BMJL, Driessen SGAJ, Coelingh-Bennink HJH. A prospective, randomized, assessor-blind multicenter study comparing recombinant and urinary follicle-stimulating hormone (Puregon vs. Metrodin) in *in vitro* fertilization. *Hum Reprod* 1995; 10:2534–2540.
91. Navot D, Rosenwaks Z, Anderson F, Hodgen GD. Gonadotropin-releasing hormone agonist-induced ovarian hyperstimulation: low-dose side effects in women and monkeys. *Fertil Steril* 1991;55:1069.
92. Hackeloer BJ, Fleming R, Robinson HP, Adams AH, Coutts JR. Correlation of ultrasonic and endocrinologic assessment of human follicular development. *Am J Obstet Gynecol* 1979;135:122.
93. Bryce RL, Sluter B, Sinosich MJ, Stiel JN, Picker RH. The value of ultrasound, gonadotropin and estradiol measurements for precise ovulation prediction. *Fertil Steril* 1982;37:42.
94. Mantzavinos T, Garcia JE, Jones HW Jr. Ultrasound measurement of ovarian follicles stimulated by human

gonadotropins for oocyte recovery and *in vitro* fertilization. *Fertil Steril* 1983;40:461.
95. Steptoe PC. Laparoscopy and ovulation 1968. *Lancet* 1968;2:913.
96. Steptoe PC, Edwards RG. Reimplantation of a human embryo with subsequent tubal pregnancy. *Lancet* 1976; 1:880.
97. Feitchinger W, Kemeter P. Laparoscopic or ultrasonically guided follicular aspiration for *in vitro* fertilization. *J In Vitro Fertil Embryo Transfer* 1984;1:244.
98. Wikland M, Nilsson L, Hansson R. Collection of human oocytes by the use of sonography. *Fertil Steril* 1983;39: 603–608.
99. Lenz S, Lauritsen JG, Kjellow M. Collection of human oocytes for *in vitro* fertilization by ultrasonically guided follicular puncture. *Lancet* 1981;1:1163.
100. Gleitcher N, Friberg J, Fullan N. Egg retrieval for *in vitro* fertilization by sonographically controlled vaginal culdocentesis. *Lancet* 1983;2:508.
101. Dellenbach P, Nisand I, Moreau I. Transvaginal sonographically controlled ovarian punch for egg retrieval. *Lancet* 1984;1:1467.
102. Seifer DB, Collins RL, Paushter DM, George CR, Quigley MM. Follicular aspiration: a comparison of an ultrasound endovaginal transducer with fixed needle guide and other retrieval methods. *Fertil Steril* 1988; 49:462.
103. Veeck LL, ed. *Atlas of the human oocyte and early conceptus*. Baltimore: Williams & Wilkins, 1987.
104. Windt ML, Menkveld R, Kruger TF. Sperm separation. In: Acosta AA, Swanson, RJ, Ackerman SB, Kruger TF, Van Zyl JA, Menkveld R. eds. *Human spermatozoa in assisted reproduction*. Baltimore: Williams & Wilkins, 1990:85.
105. Braude PR, Ross LD, Bolton YN, Ockenden K. Retrograde ejaculation: a systematic approach to non-invasive recovery of spermatozoa from post-ejaculatory urine for artificial insemination. *Br J Obstet Gynaecol* 1987;94:76.
106. Kruger TF, Menkveld R, Scott RT, Jeyendran RS, Zaneveld LJD Windt ML. Spermatozoa motile fraction separation. In: Acosta AA, Swanson, RJ, Ackerman SB, Kruger TF, Van Zyl JA, Menkveld R. eds. *Human spermatozoa in assisted reproduction*. Baltimore: Williams & Wilkins, 1990:181.
107. Gardner DK, Vella P, Lane M, Wagley L, Schlenker T, Schoolcraft WB. Culture and transfer of human blastocysts increases implantation rates and reduces the need for multiple embryo transfers. *Fertil Steril* 1998; 69:84–88.
108. Cohen J, Alikani M, Trowbridge J Rosenwaks Z. Implantation enhancement by selected hatching using zona drilling of human embryos with poor prognosis. *Hum Reprod* 1992;7:685.
109. Jones HW, Acosta AA, Garcia JE, Veeck LL. On the transfer of conceptuses from oocytes fertilized *in vitro*. *Fertil Steril* 1983;39:241.
110. Jones HW Jr. Embryo transfer. *Ann N Y Acad Sci* 1985;442:375.
111. Ash RH, Ellworth LR, Balmaceda JP, Wong PC. Pregnancy after translaparoscopic gamete intrafallopian transfer. *Lancet* 1984;2:1034.
112. Toth T, Oehninger S, Toner J, Brzyski R, Acosta A, Muasher S. Embryo transfer to the uterus or the fallopian tube after *in vitro* fertilization yields similar results. *Fertil Steril* 1992;57:1110.
113. Leong MKH, Leung CKM, Marriot VM. Comparative study of combined GIFT and IVF-ET with GIFT alone. *Hum Reprod* 1988;9:877.
114. Devroey P, Braeckmans P, Smith J. Pregnancy after translaparoscopic zygote intrafallopian transfer in a patient with sperm antibodies. *Lancet* 1986;1:1329.
115. Yovich JL, Blakledge DG, Richardson PA, Matson PL, Turner SR, Draoer R. Pregnancies following pronuclear stage tubal transfer. *Fertil Steril* 1987;48:851.
116. Tournaye H, Camus M, Khan I, Staessen C, Van Steirthgham AC, Devroey P. *In vitro* fertilization, gamete or zygote intra-fallopian transfer for the treatment of male infertility. *Hum Reprod* 1991;6:263.
117. Hanson FM, Rock J. Artificial insemination with husband's sperm. *Fertil Steril* 1951;2:162.
118. Mastrioanni L Jr, Laberge JL, Rock J. Appraisal of the efficacy of artificial insemination with husband's sperm and evaluation of insemination technique. *Fertil Steril* 1957;8:260.
119. Serhal PF, Katz M. Intrauterine insemination. *Lancet* 1987;1:52.
120. Urry RL, Middleton RG, McGavin S. A simple and effective technique for increasing pregnancy rate in couples with retrograde ejaculation. *Fertil Steril* 1986;14: 1124.
121. Dodson W, Haney A. Controlled ovarian hyperstimulation and intra-uterine insemination for treatment of infertility. *Fertil Steril* 1991;55:457.
122. Mill M, Eddowes H, Cahill D, et al. A prospective controlled study of *in-vitro* fertilization, gamete intra-fallopian transfer and intrauterine insemination combined with superovulation. *Hum Reprod* 1992;7:490.
123. Garcia JE, Jones GS, Wright GL Jr. Prediction of the time of ovulation. *Fertil Steril* 1981;36:308.
124. Guzick DS, Sullivan MW, Adamson GD, et al. Efficacy of treatment for unexplained infertility. *Fertil Steril* 1998;70:207.
125. Dodson WC, Whitesides DB, Hughes CL. Superovulation with intrauterine insemination in the treatment of infertility: a possible alternative to gamete intrafallopian transfer and *in vitro* fertilization. *Fertil Steril* 1987; 48:441.
126. Weathersbee PS, Werlin LB, Stone SC. Peritoneal recovery of sperm after intrauterine insemination. *Fertil Steril* 1984;42:322.
127. Jansen RPS, Anderson JC, Radomic I, Smith J. Pregnancies after ultrasound-guided fallopian insemination with cryostored donor semen. *Fertil Steril* 1988;49: 920.
128. Forrler (Menard) A, Dellenbach P, Nisand I, et al. Direct intraperitoneal insemination in unexplained and cervical infertility. *Lancet* 1986;1:916.
129. Garcia JE, Bayati J, Padilla SL, Smith R. Fertility Update Presented at the Greater Baltimore Medical Center's Fertility Center Seminar, April, 1989, Baltimore, Maryland.
130. Cohen J, Malter H, Wright G, et al. Partial zona dissection of human oocytes when failure of the zona pellucida is anticipated. *Hum Reprod* 1989;4:435.
131. Fishel S, Jackson P, Antinori S, Johnson J, Grossi S. Subzonal insemination for the alleviation of infertility. *Fertil Steril* 1990;54:828.
132. Palermo G, Joris H, Devroey P, Van Steirthghem AC. Pregnancies after intracytoplasmic injection of a single spermatozoon into an oocyte. *Lancet* 1992;40:17.
133. Silber SJ, Ash RH, Balmaceda JP, Borrero C, Ord T.

Pregnancy with sperm aspiration from the proximal head of the epididymis: a new treatment for congenital absence of the vas deferens. *Fertil Steril* 1988;50:525.

134. Madgar I, Hourvitz A, Levron J, et al. Outcome of *in vitro* fertilization and intracytoplasmic injection of epididymal and testicular sperm extracted from patients with obstructive and nonobstructive azoospermia. *Fertil Steril* 1998;69:1080.
135. Silber SJ, Ord T, Balmaceda JP, Patrizio P, Ash RH. Congenital absence of the vas deferens: the fertilizing capacity of human epididymal sperm. *N Engl J Med* 1990;323:1788.
136. Devroey P, Liu J, Nagy Z, et al. Pregnancies after testicular sperm extraction and intracytoplasmic sperm injection in non-obstructive azoospermia. *Hum Reprod* 1995;10:1457.
137. Craft I, Tsirigotis M, Shrivastav P. Value of percutaneous epididymal sperm aspiration. *Fertil Steril* 1995; 63:208–209.
138. Van Steirteghem AC, Nagy Z, Joris H, Liu J, Staessen C, Devroey P. High fertilization and implantation rate after intracytoplasmic sperm injection. *Hum Reprod* 1993;6:1061.
139. Van Steirteghem AC, Liu J, Joris H, et al. Higher success rate by intracytoplasmic sperm injection than by subzonal insemination: report of a second series of 300 consecutive treatment cycles. *Hum Reprod* 1993; 8:1055.
140. Bunge RG, Sherman JK. Fertilizing capacity of frozen human spermatozoa. *Nature* 1953;172:767.
141. Phillips PH. The presentation of bull semen. *J Biol Chem* 1939;130:415.
142. American Fertility Society. New guidelines for the use of semen donor insemination. *Fertil Steril* 1986;46:955.
143. Matheson CW, Carlburg L, Gemzell C. Frozen human semen for artificial insemination. *Am J Obstet Gynecol* 1969;104:495.
144. Taylor PJ, Wilson J, Laycock R, Weger S. A comparison of freezing and thawing methods for the cryopreservation of human semen. *Fertil Steril* 1982;37:100.
145. Mahony MC, Mahmood M, Scott R, DeVilliers A, Erasmus E. Role of spermatozoa cyropreservation in assisted reproduction. In: Acosta AA, Swanson, RJ, Ackerman SB, Kruger TF, Van Zyl JA, Menkveld R. eds. *Human spermatozoa in assisted reproduction*. Baltimore: Williams & Wilkins, 1990:310.
146. Chen C. Pregnancy after human oocyte cryopreservation. *Lancet* 1986;1:884.
147. Van Uem JFHM, Siebzehubl ER, Schuh B, Koch R, Trotnow S. Birth after cryopreservation of unfertilized oocytes. *Lancet* 1987;2:752.
148. Trounson AO, Mohr L. Human pregnancy following cryopreservation, thawing and transfer of an eight-cell embryo. *Nature* 1983;305:707.
149. Trounson A. Preservation of human eggs and embryos. *Fertil Steril* 1986;46:1.
150. Quinn P, Kerin JFP. Experience with the cryopreservation of human embryo using the mouse as a model to establish successful techniques. *J In Vitro Fertil Embryo Transfer* 1986;3:40.
151. Freeman L, Trounson A, Kirby C. Cryopreservation of human embryos: progress on the clinical use of the technique in human *in vitro* fertilization. *J In Vitro Fertil Embryo Transfer* 1986;3:53.
152. Veeck LL. Cryopreservation of embryos/egg. In: Adashi E, Rock JA, Rosenwaks Z, eds. *Reproductive endocrinology, surgery, and technology*, vol. 2. Philadelphia: Lippincott–Raven Publishers, 1995:2354.
153. Menezo Y, Nicollet B, Andre D. Freezing co-cultured human blastocysts. *Fertil Steril* 1992;58:977.
154. Hartshorne GM, Elder K, Crow J, Dyson H, Edwards RG. The influence of *in vitro* development upon post-thaw survival and implantation of cryopreserved human blastocysts. *Hum Reprod* 1991;6:136.
155. Sanger WG, Armitage JO, Schmidt MA. Feasibility of semen cryopreservation in patients with malignant disease. *JAMA* 1980;244:789.
156. David OK, Bedford JM, Berkeley AS, Graf MJ, Rosenwaks Z. Pregnancy achieved through *in vitro* fertilization with cryopreserved sperm from a man with Hodgkin's lymphoma. *Fertil Steril* 1990;53:377.
157. Rowland GF, Cohen J, Steptoe PG, Hewitt J. Pregnancy following *in vitro* fertilization using cryopreserved semen from a man with testicular carcinoma. *Urology* 1985;26:33–36.
158. Rosenwaks Z, Veeck LL, Liu H-G. Pregnancy following transfer of *in vitro* fertilized donor oocytes. *Fertil Steril* 1986;45:417.
159. Yovich JL, Blackledge DG, Richardson PA, et al. *Prost* for ovum donation. *Lancet* 1987;1:1209–1210.
160. Formight L, Formigli G, Roccio C. Donation of fertilized uterine ova to infertile women. *Fertil Steril* 1987; 47:162.
161. Asch R, Balmaceda JP, Ord T, Borrero G, Cefalu E, Rajos F. Oocyte donation and gamete intrafallopian transfer in premature ovarian failure. *Fertil Steril* 1988;49:263.
162. Sauer MV, Paulson RS, Lobo RA. A preliminary report on oocyte donation extending reproductive potential to women over 40. *N Engl J Med* 199;323: 1157.
163. Sauer MV, Paulson RJ, Lobo RA. Pregnancy after age 50: application of oocyte donation to women after natural menopause. *Lancet* 1993;341:321.
164. Navot D, Jaufer N, Kopolovic J, et al. Artificially induced endometrial cycles and establishment of pregnancies in the absence of ovaries. *N Engl J Med* 1986; 314:806.
165. American Fertility Society. American Law and assisted reproductive technologies. *Fertil Steril* 1994; 62(suppl 1):85.
166. Trounson A, Leeton J, Besanko M, Wood C, Conti A. Pregnancy established in an infertile patient after transfer of a donated embryo fertilized *in vitro*. *BMJ* 1983;286:835.
167. Lutzen P, Trounson A, Leeton J, Findlay J, Wood C, Remou P. The establishment and maintenance of pregnancy using *in vitro* fertilization and embryo donation in a patient with primary ovarian failure. *Nature* 1984; 307:174.

5

Childbearing After Cancer Treatment

Michael E. Lantz

Department of Obstetrics and Gynecology, Johns Hopkins Bayview Medical Center, Baltimore, Maryland 21224; and Johns Hopkins University School of Medicine, Baltimore, Maryland 21287

Becoming pregnant is an affirmation of life—that something is growing inside of you that is not killing you, but is healthy and strong (1).

—Nora Frenkiel, J.D., breast cancer survivor since 1987 and mother of 7-year-old Emma and 1-year-old Bartholamue

The desire to bear children and to experience motherhood does not end with the diagnosis of cancer. The prospect of pregnancy after cancer treatment can represent a sense of normalcy and expectation. More and more women are reaching reproductive age after treatment of childhood or adolescent malignancy (2,3). Furthermore, women experiencing cancer during their reproductive years can now expect better long-term survival and hope for successful pregnancy.

Patients diagnosed with cancer during pregnancy or wishing to become pregnant after cancer therapy represent a special group of women who will require intense counseling and a multidisciplinary approach to their care. It is imperative that obstetricians, oncologists, and counselors work together to provide these patients with accurate and up-to-date information when available. This chapter reviews the current literature on general issues related to pregnancy management during cancer therapy and to pregnancy outcome after cancer.

LIMITATIONS OF AVAILABLE DATA

Study of the effects of cytotoxic chemotherapy and radiation therapy on pregnancy outcome is limited by several factors. Most reports involve single cases or case series describing a limited number of patients. These studies have utilized retrospective cohorts of cancer survivors and controls, with data collected from medical record reviews and patient interviews. These study techniques lend themselves to ascertainment and/or recall bias in favor of poorer outcomes among cancer survivors. Because these cohorts of cancer survivors were often treated in childhood or during adolescence, long-term follow-up is necessary to acquire outcome data on pregnancy. It is likely that assessment of their offspring is incomplete.

Pregnancy data have now become available on cancer survivors treated during the 1940s through 1970s. The pregnancy outcomes of these patients may differ from those cancer survivors contemplating pregnancy today because of the likelihood that the latter patients have received newer, more refined cancer treatments. Evaluation of pregnancy outcomes in cancer patients being treated today will require several decades.

Due to the relative paucity of patients having children after cancer treatment, outcome data have often been drawn from patient cohorts having several different types of cancers and therefore several different types of cancer treatments. Doses and types of radiotherapy and combined chemotherapy differ greatly depending on the cancer being treated. This makes the determination of attributable risk from any single therapy difficult.

The study of birth defects due to cancer treatments has relied heavily on data obtained from animal experiments. Experience has shown that caution must be used in the application of animal data on congenital anomalies to humans. Acetylsalicylic acid is highly teratogenic in rodents but not in humans (4), while the thalidomide epidemic may have been prevented if experiments had been conducted in animals other than mice or rats (5). Furthermore, many concerns about the teratogenicity of certain drugs come from animal experiments in which extremely large doses of the agents were administered. It is important to note that large doses of even benign agents may be teratogenic in experimental animals (6).

Interpretation of the available data must take these limitations into consideration, particularly during counseling of cancer patients on pregnancy management and outcome.

RADIATION THERAPY DURING PREGNANCY—GENERAL CONSIDERATIONS

Radiotherapy is a common treatment modality for several cancers encountered in women of reproductive age. These include lymphomas, cancers of the breast, leukemias, and cancer of the thyroid. The treatment of a cancer patient with radiation during pregnancy should be aimed at optimizing the benefit to the patient while minimizing the possible detrimental effects on the fetus.

The effect of radiotherapy on the fetus depends on both gestational age at the time of exposure and total radiation dose. The effects of ionizing radiation on development include embryonic death, congenital malformations, intrauterine growth restriction, and central nervous system disturbances (7) (Table 1). During the first 1 to 2 weeks after conception, there appears to be an all-or-nothing effect of radiation exposure on the embryo. Radiation exposure during this period may result in embryonic death but not in congenital anomalies or growth restriction (8). The lethality of radiation to the human embryo is difficult to quantitate, because these early losses may go unrecognized clinically and there is a high background loss rate (up to 60%) in early pregnancy. Data from experimental mice show a loss rate of 10% to 15% when mice are exposed to 0.5 Gy of gamma radiation during the preimplantation period (9).

The greatest susceptibility to the fetus for the development of congenital malformations, regardless of the type of exposure, is during the period of organogenesis (Table 2). For most organ systems in humans, this encompasses the second through eighth weeks after conception (10). The exception is the

TABLE 1. *Relationship between the time of fetal exposure to radiotherapy by gestational period and the effects on the fetus*

	Preimplantation period	Organogenesis period (wk)		Fetal period (wk)	
Fetal effects	0–9 Days	2–8	8–15	15–25	≥25
Lethality	+++	+	–	–	–
Malformations	+++	±	±	–	±
Mental retardation	–	+++	–	++	–
Growth retardation	+	+	–	+	+
Carcinogenicity	+	+	–	+	+

–, no observed effect; ±, almost no observed effect; +, demonstrated effect; ++, readily apparent effect; +++, occurs at a high incidence.

From Kusama T. Fetal exposure to radiation and its effects. *Maternal Health* 1996;37:9; with permission

TABLE 2. *Simple malformations in offspring of cancer survivors and in offspring of sibling controls, and rate per 10,000 live births*

	Offspring with malformations (rate per 10,000 live births)	
Malformations	Survivors	Controls
Anencephaly	0 (0)	2 (1)
Spina bifida	9 (2)	9 (4)
Hydrocephalus	9 (2)	0 (0)
Transposition of the great vessels	0 (0)	4 (2)
Septal defects	55 (12)	46 (21)
Patent ductus arteriosus	23 (5)	13 (6)
Cleft lip without cleft palate	14 (3)	7 (3)
Cleft lip with or without cleft palate	9 (2)	9 (4)
Tracheoesophageal fistula	5 (1)	0 (0)
Rectal atresia/stenosis	5 (1)	2 (1)
Hypospadias	23 (5)	18 (8)
Clubfoot	73 (16)	106 (48)
Limb-reduction deformity	5 (1)	20 (9)
Hip dislocation	55 (12)	66 (30)
Renal agenesis	0 (0)	4 (2)

None of the findings achieved statistical significance.
From ref. 59, with permission.

central nervous system, which is known to undergo rapid and marked structural changes throughout the first half of gestation and retains its sensitivity to ionizing radiation up to approximately 25 weeks (11).

Several factors influence the total radiation dose received by the fetus during radiation therapy (12):

- Body area to be radiated
- Field size
- Distance of the fetus from the treatment field
- Total radiation prescribed for tumor control

The change in uterine size and the relative position of the growing fetus must be taken into account when radiotherapy during pregnancy is planned. Stovall et al. (13) estimated fetal doses of radiation during treatment for several different cancers and the reduction achieved with different shielding techniques. They suggested that for most patients receiving radiation therapy during pregnancy, a reduction in the fetal dose of approximately 50% can be achieved with proper shielding techniques.

Microcephaly, usually combined with mental retardation, and eye malformations are the most commonly reported malformations observed in humans exposed to high doses of radiation *in utero*. During the first half of the 20th century, radiation therapy was used to treat several gynecologic conditions including menorrhagia, leiomyomas, and carcinoma of the uterine corpus and cervix. As of 1929, Goldstein and Murphy (14,15) had collected data on 106 women reported to have received radiation therapy during pregnancy. Thirty-eight (51%) of 74 children born at full-term were said to have serious health and development problems, with 42% of affected children having microcephaly and mental retardation. Eye abnormalities within this cohort included microphthalmia, cataracts, strabismus, retinal degeneration, and optic atrophy.

Further information on the effects of ionizing radiation during pregnancy has come from observational data obtained after the atomic bombings of Hiroshima and Nagasaki in 1945. Eleven years after the bombings, Miller (16) reported on 169 exposed children in Hiroshima examined prior to 9 years of age. Almost 20% of the children had head circumferences at least 2 standard deviations (SD) below the mean, and 9% were considered mentally retarded. A later report on the same children evaluated the incidence of microcephaly and mental retardation in relation to the maximum dose of maternal radiation sustained and the gestational age at the time of exposure (17). Almost 50% of the children whose mothers received an estimated radiation dose of at least 1.5 Gy had head circumferences 2 or more SD below the mean and were mentally retarded. The highest percentage of children with small head size and mental retardation were at a gestational age of 15 weeks or less at the time of exposure. No mental retardation was observed in children exposed in the third trimester.

A larger cohort of 1613 Hiroshima and Nagasaki children *in utero* at the time of the atomic bombings has been reported on by the Atomic Bomb Casualty Commission (18). Among the Hiroshima children, those who had received at least 0.5 Gy *in utero* were at a substantially increased risk of being mentally retarded, compared to nonexposed controls. Relative risk values for mental retardation were consistently greater than 10 for doses greater than 0.5 Gy in Hiroshima and 2.0 Gy in Nagasaki. The lower threshold seen in Hiroshima was thought to be secondary to differences in the quality of radiation (neutron versus gamma) between the two bombs. The gestational age of those with mental retardation spanned from 6 to 27 weeks, with the highest concentration exposed prior to 15 weeks.

Dekaban (11) presented outcome data on 22 pregnant women treated for various indications with moderate to high doses of pelvic radiation between 4 and 20 weeks' gestation. Care was taken to quantitate accurately the radiation dose to the midpelvic region. The average dose to this area was 2.5 Gy. The following were the most common abnormalities identified in children who received long-term follow-up:

- Intrauterine growth restriction and stunted growth (95%)
- Microcephaly (95%)
- Mental retardation (86%)
- Microphthalmos (59%)
- Pigmentary degeneration of the retina (27%)
- Genital and skeletal malformations (27%)
- Cataracts (14%)

In summary, radiation exposure during pregnancy can have significant detrimental effects on the fetus. Atomic bomb exposure thresholds for congenital malformations may not apply to radiotherapy for cancer treatment, since the latter is usually fractionated and given over a 4- to 6-week period. Therapeutic radiation to a pregnant woman will result in fetal doses far greater than the commonly used threshold of 0.05 Gy for occupational exposure during pregnancy (19). If possible, radiation treatment during pregnancy should be delayed until the midsecond trimester (after 15 weeks) to minimize fetal risks. Aggressive efforts at shielding the abdomen and pelvis should be made. Medical and radiation oncologists should provide the patient with a pretreatment estimate of the fetal radiation dose and counsel accordingly using the available data.

PREGNANCY AFTER ABDOMINAL RADIATION

Abdominal irradiation remains a mainstay in the treatment of cancers encountered in children and in women of reproductive age. Cancer survivors who have received abdominal radiation appear to be at increased risk for spontaneous abortion, fetal death, preterm birth, and low birthweight. These adverse outcomes may be due to decreased uterine blood supply from radiation fibrosis, as well as disruption in normal uterine function secondary to radiation.

Cancers commonly treated with abdominal irradiation include Wilms' tumor, Hodgkin's disease, and non-Hodgkin's lymphomas. A possible association of poor pregnancy outcome in women having received abdominal radiation in childhood was described by Green et al. (20) in a group of patients treated for Wilms' tumor. Among 33 offspring of women treated with abdominal irradiation, 10 (30%) weighed less than 2500 g at birth. Twenty-one percent of these deliveries were reported to occur prior to 38 weeks' gestation. In contrast, term deliveries were reported for all 10 offspring of women with Wilms' tumor who did not receive abdominal irradiation and for 94% of the 16 offspring of the wives of male Wilms' tumor patients.

Li et al. (21) reported on the pregnancy experience of 99 women after treatment of Wilms' tumor in childhood. They compared outcome data from those treated with abdominal irradiation to those not treated with radiation and to the wives of male patients treated at several pediatric centers in the United States. An adverse outcome was reported in 30% of the 114 pregnancies that occurred in women treated with abdominal irradiation, compared to 3% of the 77 pregnancies in nonirradiated women and the wives of irradiated male patients. There was an increase among the irradiated female patients in fetal deaths, low-birthweight infants, and preterm deliveries. When compared to white women in the United States, the group treated with abdominal radiation had a relative risk of 7.9 for perinatal mortality and a relative risk of 4.0 for the delivery of an infant weighing less than 2500 g. A large survey of pregnancy outcomes among childhood cancer survivors who received abdominal irradiation in Great Britain between 1940 and 1977 showed an increased risk of spontaneous abortion and a mean birthweight of 300 g less in exposed patients compared to nonexposed (22).

Several theories have been put forth to explain the adverse pregnancy outcomes in pediatric patients receiving abdominal irradiation, particularly for Wilms' tumor. Functional impairment of visceral organs and fibrosis of the abdominal musculature are known complications of radiotherapy in patients treated for Wilms' tumor (23,24). It is also possible that vascular damage to uterine blood flow may occur after radiation therapy (25), resulting in uteroplacental insufficiency. Patients considering pregnancy who were treated with abdominal radiation in childhood should be made aware of the possible effects that this therapy may have on childbearing.

Data to support an adverse pregnancy outcome after abdominal irradiation for the treatment of Hodgkin's disease and non-Hodgkin's lymphoma are less convincing. Holmes and Holmes (26) studied the pregnancy outcome in a cohort of patients who had received radiotherapy, chemotherapy, or both for Hodgkin's disease. Eighteen female patients received irradiation only. These patients went on to have 37 pregnancies. When compared to sibling controls, there was no difference in fetal wastage or abnormal offspring. A later study evaluated 103 women younger than age 40 years treated for Hodgkin's disease with total lymphoid irradiation, combination chemotherapy, or both (27). Twenty women became pregnant after therapy, resulting in a total of 28 pregnancies. There were no spontaneous abortions in any of the pregnancies and no birth defects among 24 live-born children.

It is possible that the few studies addressing this issue do not have sufficient power to detect a difference in pregnancy outcome among reproductive-age women who receive abdominal irradiation. It could also be theorized that the radiation effects seen in adults after childhood treatment may take years to develop and therefore do not have the same detrimental effects on pregnancy.

In summary, abdominal irradiation during childhood, particularly for the treatment of Wilms' tumor, appears to be associated with more adverse pregnancy outcomes, including an increased risk of spontaneous abortion, low birthweight, and higher perinatal mortality.

CHEMOTHERAPY DURING PREGNANCY—GENERAL CONSIDERATIONS

Since most cytotoxic agents used to treat cancer in humans have their greatest effect on rapidly dividing cells, the fetus would theoretically be highly susceptible to these agents when exposed *in utero*. In fact, methotrexate has successfully been used as an abortifacient and is now a common treatment in the management of ectopic pregnancy (28).

Most chemotherapeutic agents possess certain characteristics including a low molecular weight, high lipid solubility, and loose binding to plasma proteins, allowing them to readily cross the placenta and enter the fetal circulation (29). Several studies have shown that cytotoxic chemotherapy, given during specific points of gestation, can cause congenital malformations in animals (30–32). For these reasons, concern has been raised about the possible detrimental effects of single or multiagent chemotherapy administration during human pregnancy.

Several case reports and small case series have confirmed the teratogenicity of chemotherapy in humans when these agents are administered during the first trimester, particularly from the third to the eighth week of development. This represents the period of organogenesis and the maximum susceptibility of the fetus for the development of congenital malformations (33). It has been estimated that 10% to 20% of fetuses exposed to cytotoxic chemotherapy in the first trimester will be born with major congenital malformations, compared to 3% of the general population (34). In an extensive literature review of first-trimester chemotherapy exposure, Doll et al. (29) found a rate of fetal malformations of 14% in fetuses exposed to alkylating agents, 19% in fetuses exposed to antimetabolites, and 7% in fetuses exposed to vinblastine sulfate (Velban).

A list of suspected congenital malformations caused by first-trimester exposure to commonly used chemotherapeutic agents is shown in Table 3. However, these data are based mainly on case reports and small case series and should be interpreted cautiously. Determination of a causal effect for each agent is made difficult because most fetuses born with congenital anomalies received multiagent chemotherapy and many received radiation. It is also quite possible that the number of patients described is too small to reflect the true risk of malformations associated with the various chemotherapeutic agents.

Treatment with chemotherapeutic agents in the second and third trimesters does not result in fetal malformations but is associated with the delivery of low-birthweight infants and perinatal myelosuppression. Nicholson (35) reported on a cohort of women exposed to cytotoxic chemotherapy during pregnancy in whom 40% of exposed fetuses were low birthweight. Other factors such as underlying maternal disease and nutrition may contribute to the degree of prematurity and growth restric-

TABLE 3. *Possible anomalies associated with first-trimester exposure to commonly used chemotherapeutic agents*

Chemotherapeutic agent	Possible associated anomalies
Antimetabolites	
Methotrexate (Folex, Mexate, Rheumatrex)	Limb deformities, oligodactyly, cranial defects, hypertelorism
Alkylating agents	
Cyclophosphamide (Cytoxan, Endoxan, Neosar)	Facial anomalies, absent or hypoplastic digits, imperforate anus
Chlorambucil (Leukeran)	Unilateral renal agenesis, cardiovascular anomalies
Busulfan (Myleran)	Liver anomalies, pyloric stenosis, renal anomalies, facial anomalies
Antibiotics	
Bleomycin sulfate (Blenoxane)	None identified
Dactinomycin (Cosmegen)	None identified
Doxorubicin HCl (Adriamycin)	Imperforate anus, rectovaginal fistula[a]
Plant alkaloids	
Vinblastine sulfate (Velban)	Atrial septal defect
Vincristine sulfate (Oncovin, Vincasar PFS)	None identified
Taxanes	
Pacditaxel (Taxol)	None identified
Other	
Cisplatin (Platinol)	None identified
Prednisone	Cataracts
Procarbazine HCl (Matulane)	Limb deformities, oligodactyly, renal anomalies, cardiovascular anomalies

[a]Based on a single infant who also received cyclophosphamide and unshielded radiation.

tion seen in patients exposed to chemotherapy during pregnancy.

Myelosuppression has been shown to occur with the use of multiple chemotherapeutic agents later in pregnancy. Reynoso et al. (36) reported on women treated for acute leukemia with multiagent chemotherapy during pregnancy and found that over 30% of the infants were pancytopenic at birth.

The decision to initiate chemotherapy during pregnancy must weigh the benefit to the mother against the potential risk to the fetus. Gestational age at the time of diagnosis, type of malignancy, maternal prognosis, and recommended chemotherapeutic regimen should all be taken into consideration when this decision is made.

Several congenital malformations may occur after chemotherapy in the first trimester. The development of major anomalies, however, is not inevitable. A few general recommendations can be made. Antimetabolites, such as methotrexate, should be avoided during the first trimester. A therapeutic equivalent can almost always be substituted for methotrexate in the curative treatment of cancers encountered in reproductive-age women. Combination chemotherapy can be initiated in the second and third trimesters without increasing the risk for congenital malformations. Nonetheless, the most suitable regimen with the least risk of teratogenicity should still be used. Patients should be counseled about the possible adverse effects on pregnancy outcome with treatment after the first trimester. When possible, the timing of delivery should coincide with the period when maternal myelosuppression is at its lowest. Women should be monitored closely in both the antepartum and peripartum periods for signs and symptoms of infection.

Women who are unknowingly exposed to chemotherapeutic agents in the first trimester or who chose to initiate therapy early in gestation should be counseled with the available data on the risk of congenital malformations. Those unwilling to accept the possible untoward effects of these agents should be offered pregnancy termination. Management of these patients should involve a multidisciplinary approach including a high-risk obstetrician, oncologist, pediatrician, and religious, social, and psychiatric support, when necessary.

PREGNANCY AFTER BONE MARROW TRANSPLANTATION

Bone marrow transplantation after high-dose chemotherapy or total body irradiation is often a curative therapy for several cancers encountered in childhood, adolescence, and reproductive-age women. These would include hematologic cancers, lymphomas, and breast cancer. The number of long-term survivors following bone marrow transplantation has steadily increased (37,38), and as of 1998 there have been more than 250 offspring born to patients having received a bone marrow transplant (39). Until recently, data on pregnancy outcomes after bone marrow transplantation have been limited to case reports (40–42), with no comparative data for patients receiving different transplant-preparative regimens. Sanders et al. (43) recently evaluated pregnancy outcomes among 76 patients receiving bone marrow transplants at a single institution from 1971 to 1992. Forty-one female patients and partners of 35 male patients had 146 pregnancies after transplantation. The rates of clinically recognized spontaneous abortion and preterm delivery were significantly higher among the female patients who received total body irradiation with or without cyclophosphamide (37% and 63%, respectively), compared to those who had received only cyclophosphamide (7% and 18%, respectively). There was no increase over the background rate in congenital anomalies among the female patients who had received either cyclophosphamide with or without total body irradiation–preparative therapy. In addition, there was no increase in adverse pregnancy outcomes in the partners of male patients who had received preparative therapy followed by bone marrow transplantation.

The available data suggest that preparative high-dose chemotherapy with or without total body irradiation followed by bone marrow transplantation does not result in an increased rate of congenital malformations among survivors giving birth. It appears that total body irradiation may predispose these patients to higher rates of spontaneous abortion and preterm delivery, compared to those patients receiving only high-dose chemotherapy. However, choosing chemotherapy alone as a preparative therapy based on its benefits to pregnancy outcome may not outweigh the treatment benefits achieved with the addition of total body irradiation.

CANCER IN THE OFFSPRING OF CANCER SURVIVORS

Improvements in high-dose multiagent chemotherapy, radiotherapy, and other treatments have resulted in an overall survival of greater than 70% for childhood and adolescent cancers (44). The high doses of such therapies required to treat these cancers has led to concern regarding the future fertility of these patients and the possible adverse effects that these therapies may have on their unborn children. Several observational studies have now addressed the hypothesis that treatment of childhood and adolescent cancer patients may lead to an increase in cancer among their offspring.

In 1985, Mulvihill and Bryne (45) reported on over 700 survivors of childhood and adult cancers, mostly Hodgkin's disease and gestational trophoblastic neoplasia. Among 1194 offspring, there were no cancers. The same authors later presented retrospective data on a cohort of 2283 cancer survivors and 3604 controls (46). They found a rate of cancer of 0.3% in the offspring of cancer survivors, compared to 0.23% in the offspring of controls. This difference was not statistically significant. The observed cancer cases were not significantly different from those expected in the general population. Importantly, this study reported a power of 79% to detect a threefold excess of cancer to 11 years of age.

Hawkins et al. (47) presented a similar study on the offspring of patients successfully treated for childhood cancer in Great Britain prior to 1978. Excluding bilateral retinoblastoma, which is known to be inherited as an autosomal trait, 1199 offspring were born to 629 survivors of childhood malignancies. There was one case each of acute monocytic leukemia and acute lymphoblastic leukemia, a higher than expected frequency when compared to the general population. However, these two offspring and the cancer found in their parents followed a previously known aggregation of cancers. The offspring in this cohort were followed to an average of 6 years of age.

The largest trial to date was a collaborative study from five Scandinavian countries, in which the risk of cancer was assessed among 5847 offspring of 14,652 survivors of childhood or adolescent cancers diagnosed in the 1940s and 1950s (48). The median age at the end of follow-up was 14 years. When cancers known or likely to be hereditary were excluded, there was no evidence of a significantly increased risk of cancer in the offspring of childhood cancer survivors.

Further supporting evidence comes from two decades of data collected on the offspring of survivors of the Hiroshima and Nagasaki atomic bombings. Using death certificates and tumor registries maintained in these cities, the Radiation Effects Research Foundation collected data on 31,150 live-born children, one or both of whose parents received greater than 0.01 Sv of radiation at the time of the atomic bombings, and on 41,066 controls whose parents were not exposed (49). Malignant tumors were ascertained in 0.14% of the children of exposed parents compared to 0.12% in the controls. Linear regression analysis revealed no increase in malignancies in the children of exposed parents.

The available data suggest that the children of patients receiving cancer therapy in childhood or adolescence do not have an increased risk for the development of cancer. It should be noted that follow-up in the offspring of cancer survivors has been limited for the most part to childhood and adolescence. The possibility of an increased risk of adult cancers among these offspring has yet to be addressed.

CONGENITAL ANOMALIES AND GENETIC DISEASE IN THE OFFSPRING OF CANCER SURVIVORS

Much concern has been raised regarding the effects of radiation and chemotherapy on gonadal function and the risk of mutagenesis in germ cells. Studies in mammalian cell cultures have shown that ionizing radiation can cause cytologically visible chromosomal aberrations (50). Furthermore, chemotherapeutic agents used to treat cancer in humans are known to have damaging effects on deoxyribonucleic acid (DNA). Alkylating agents can cause base alterations, cisplatin (Platinol) induces interstrand and intrastrand DNA cross-links, etoposide (VePesid) results in protein-associated DNA cleavage, and bleomycin sulfate (Blenoxane) has been shown to cause DNA single-strand or double-strand breaks (51).

Several studies have addressed the concern that radiation and chemotherapy may lead to an increase in congenital malformations and genetic disease among the offspring of cancer survivors previously treated with these agents. Much of the data has been derived from patient questionnaires or surveys of practitioners caring for long-term cancer survivors. While the concern for ascertainment bias is evident, the vast majority of the data suggests no increased risk to these offspring.

The survivors of the Hiroshima and Nagasaki atomic bombings have provided a large sample size and long-term prospective data on the possible effects of ionizing radiation on the well-being of offspring. Established in 1948, a systematic survey was undertaken in Japan to evaluate differences in sex ratio, congenital defects, viability at birth, birthweight, and survival during the neonatal period among the children of men and women exposed and not exposed to the one-time dose of ionizing radiation. Over a 6-year period, sufficient data were available for analysis in nearly 70,000 newborn infants born to parents in Hiroshima and Nagasaki. From these data, no statistically significant effect of ionizing radiation has emerged with regard to major or minor congenital malformations (52), the frequency of balanced structural rearrangements of chromosomes or sex chromosome aneuploidy (53), or growth and development (54).

Early reports on pregnancy outcomes of cancer survivors were limited to small case series or case reports. Over the past 15 years, more extensive data have become available on the subsequent risk of congenital malformations and genetic disease among the offspring of patients treated for cancer. These cohorts include patients treated with multiagent chemotherapy, radiotherapy, or both, making an assessment of the attributable risk from any one agent more difficult.

Two separate studies from 1984 presented pregnancy-outcome data among patients treated with cytotoxic chemotherapy for gestational trophoblastic disease (55,56). There was no increase in the incidence of congenital malformations among live-born offspring in 596 subsequent pregnancies.

Green et al. (57) performed a study on the outcome of pregnancies reported by 306 men and women diagnosed with pediatric cancer between 1960 and 1984 at Roswell Park Cancer Institute. Pregnancies of at least 20 weeks' gestation were reported in 60 male and female respondents who had chemotherapy as part of their treatment regimen. The 60 former patients had a total of 100 live-born and two stillborn children. The type of chemotherapy and the cumulative dose for these patients were determined. The rates of congenital malformations were 8.1% and 7.9%, respectively, among the live-born children of the female patients and the live-born children of the wives of the male patients. However, in 20 women who had received dactinomycin (Cosmegen) as part of their treatment regimen, two had structural congenital heart defects. This 10% incidence was significantly higher than that among the children in a multicenter survey of congenital malformations. There was no association found between the number or the cumulative dose of chemotherapeutic agents used and the incidence of congenital anomalies.

Dodds et al. (58) conducted a case–control study using a computerized record linkage that identified congenital anomalies in the first year of life among a large population in Canada. No significant associations were found between congenital malformations in the offspring and type of cancer treatment in either parent. More recently, Byrne et al. (59) conducted an interview study of long-term survivors of pediatric cancers treated with chemotherapy, radiotherapy, or both before 1976. Genetic disease (defined as a birth defect, a cytogenetic abnormality, or a single-gene defect) occurred in 3.4% of 2198 offspring of survivors compared to 3.1% of 4544 offspring of controls. This did not represent a statistically significant difference. Although data were not provided, the authors stated that no congenital heart defects were identified in mothers who received dactinomycin.

In summary, the overall data are reassuring and do not support an increased risk of congenital malformations or genetic disease in the offspring of long-term survivors of cancer treatment. The exception may be a possible association between dactinomycin exposure in mothers and structural congenital heart defects in their future children. Until further data are available, this subset of cancer patients should probably undergo fetal echocardiography in the second trimester of pregnancy.

SUMMARY

Patients who have a good prognosis for cancer survival or have achieved long-term survival should not be discouraged from bearing children solely based on a history of prior cancer treatment. Although the data are limited, congenital malformations and nonhereditary cancers do not appear to be increased in the offspring of patients who received radiation or chemotherapy.

Patients who have undergone cancer treatment often have several concerns related to the prospects of bearing children. There is concern that their infants may be abnormal or deformed as a result of the treatment that they received. Several patients reported their understanding, based on physician counseling, that it would be impossible for them to have children (60). For this reason, patients who become pregnant during or after cancer therapy may opt for pregnancy termination.

Cancer survivors contemplating pregnancy should be counseled on the theoretical risk of germ cell mutations and the implications this may have in their offspring. However, the available observational data in humans should be used to reassure patients that there does not appear to be an increased risk of congenital malformations or nonhereditary cancers in their offspring. If a patient does become pregnant, liberal use of targeted ultrasound and prenatal diagnosis may help reduce anxiety. Cancer survivors who underwent abdominal irradiation in childhood or adolescence should be warned about the possible increased risk of fetal wastage and low birthweight that may occur if they become pregnant.

Parents whose children undergo cancer treatment in childhood or adolescence should be provided with accurate records regarding the type of treatment and dosage received. This will permit more accurate counseling when these patients reach reproductive age.

REFERENCES

1. Frenkiel N. A question of life. *The New York Times Magazine* May 3, 1992:36.
2. Miller GA, Ries LAG, Hankey BF, Kosary CL, Edwards BK, eds. *Cancer statistics review, 1973–1989.* NIH publication no. 92-2789. National Cancer Institute, 1992.
3. Byrne J, Kessler LJ, Devesa SS. The prevalence of cancer among adults in the United States, 1987. *Cancer* 1992;69:2154.
4. Warkany J, Takacs E. Experimental production of congenital malformations in rats by salicylate poisoning. *Am J Pathol* 1959;35:315.
5. Shepard TH. Counseling pregnant women exposed to potentially harmful agents during pregnancy. *Clin Obstet Gynecol* 1983;26:478.
6. Nishimura H, Miyamoto S. Teratogenic effects of sodium chloride in mice. *Acta Anal Nippon* 1969;74:121.
7. Brent RL. The effects of embryonic and fetal exposure to x-ray, microwaves, and ultrasound. *Clin Obstet Gynecol* 1983;26:484.

8. Rush R, Grupp E. Response of very early mouse embryo to low levels of ionizing radiation. *J Exp Zool* 1959;141:571.
9. Devi PU, Basker R. Influence of gestational age at exposure on the prenatal effects of gamma-radiation. *Int J Radiat Biol* 1996;70:45.
10. Congenital malformations and inherited disorders. In: Cunningham FG, MacDonald PC, Gant NF, eds. *Williams obstetrics*, 18th ed. Norwalk, CT: Appleton & Lange, 1989:561.
11. Dekaban AS. Abnormalities in children exposed to x-irradiation during various stages of gestation: tentative timetable of radiation injury to the human fetus. *J Nucl Med* 1968;9:471.
12. Nakagawa K, Aoki Y, Kusama T, Ban N, Nakagawa S, Sasaki Y. Radiotherapy during pregnancy: effects on fetuses and neonates. *Clin Ther* 1997;19:770.
13. Stovall M, Blackwell CR, Cundiff J, et al. Fetal dose from radiotherapy with photon beams: report of AAPM radiation therapy committee task group no. 36. *Med Phys* 1995;22:63.
14. Goldstein L, Murphy DP. Microcephalic idiocy following radium therapy for uterine cancer during pregnancy. *Am J Obstet Gynecol* 1929;18:189.
15. Goldstein L, Murphy DP. Etiology of ill health in children born after maternal pelvic irradiation. II. Defective children born after postconceptional maternal irradiation. *Am J Roentgenol* 1929;22:322.
16. Miller RW. Delayed effects occurring within the first decade after exposure of young individuals to the Hiroshima atomic bomb. *Pediatrics* 1956;18:1.
17. Wood JW, Johnson KG, Omori Y. *In utero* exposure to the Hiroshima atomic bomb: an evaluation of head size and mental retardation twenty years later. *Pediatrics* 1967;39:385.
18. Blot WJ, Miller RW. Mental retardation following *in utero* exposure to the atomic bombs of Hiroshima and Nagasaki. *Radiology* 1973;106:617.
19. Brent RL. Radiation teratogenesis. *Teratology* 1980;21:281.
20. Green DM, Fine WE, Li FP. Offspring of patients treated for unilateral Wilms' tumor in childhood. *Cancer* 1982;49:2285.
21. Li FP, Gimbrere K, Gelber RD, et al. Outcome of pregnancy in survivors of Wilms' tumor. *JAMA* 1987;257:216.
22. Hawkins MM, Smith RA. Pregnancy outcomes in childhood cancer survivors: probable effects of abdominal irradiation. *Int J Cancer* 1989;43:399.
23. Green DM, Jaffe N. Wilms' tumor: model of a curable pediatric malignant solid tumor. *Cancer Treat Rev* 1978;5:143.
24. Riseborough EJ, Grabias SL, Burton RI, et al. Skeletal alterations following irradiation for Wilms' tumor. *J Bone Joint Surg Am* 1976;58:526.
25. Hopewell JW. The importance of vascular damage in the development of late radiation effects in normal tissues. In: Meyn RE, Withers HR, eds. *Radiation biology in cancer research.* New York: Raven Press, 1980:449.
26. Holmes GE, Holmes FF. Pregnancy outcome of patients treated for Hodgkin's disease: a controlled study. *Cancer* 1978;41:1317.
27. Horning SJ, Hoppe RT, Kaplan HS, Rosenberg SA. Female reproductive potential after treatment for Hodgkin's disease. *N Engl J Med* 1981;304:1377.
28. Stovall TG, Ling FW. Single-dose methotrexate: an expanded clinical trial. *Am J Obstet Gynecol* 1993;168:1759.
29. Doll DC, Ringenberg QS, Yarbro JW. Antineoplastic agents and pregnancy. *Semin Oncol* 1989;16:337.
30. Murphy ML, Karnovsky DA. Effect of azaserine and other growth-inhibiting agents on fetal development of the rat. *Cancer* 1956;9:955.
31. Gulluni CM, Santoro DL. Teratogenic effects of L-asparaginase on anuran amphibians. *Rev Biol* 1977;70:283.
32. Sieber SM, Whang-Peng J, Botkin C, Knutsen T. Teratogenic and cytogenetic effects of some plant-derived antitumor agents in mice. *Teratology* 1978;18:31.
33. Sorosky JI, Sood AK, Buekers TE. The use of chemotherapeutic agents during pregnancy. *Obstet Gynecol Clin North Am* 1997;24:591.
34. Gililland J, Weinstein L. The effects of cancer chemotherapeutic agents on the developing fetus. *Obstet Gynecol Surv* 1983;38:6.
35. Nicholson HO. Cytotoxic drugs in pregnancy. *J Obstet Gynaecol Br Commonwlth* 1968;75:307.
36. Reynoso EE, Shepherd FA, Mesner HA, et al. Acute leukemia during pregnancy: the Toronto Leukemia Study Group experience with long-term follow-up of children exposed *in utero* to chemotherapeutic agents. *J Clin Oncol* 1987;5:1098.
37. Kernan NA, Bartsch G, Ash RC, et al. Analysis of 462 transplantations from unrelated donors facilitated by the National Marrow Donor Program. *N Engl J Med* 1993;328:593.
38. Peters WP, Shpall EJ, Jones RB, et al. High-dose combination alkylating agents with bone marrow support as initial treatment for metastatic breast cancer. *J Clin Oncol* 1988;6:1368.
39. Gulati SC, Van Poznak CV. Pregnancy after bone marrow transplantation. *J Clin Oncol* 1998;16:1978.
40. Card RT, Holmes IH, Sugarman RG, Stord R, Thomas ED. Successful pregnancy after high dose chemotherapy and marrow transplantation for treatment of aplastic anemia. *Exp Hematol* 1980;8:57.
41. Jacobs P, Dubovsky DW. Bone marrow transplantation followed by normal pregnancy. *Am J Hematol* 1981;11:209.
42. Russel JA, Hanley DA. Full-term pregnancy after allogeneic transplantation for leukemia in a patient with oligomenorrhea. *Bone Marrow Transplant* 1989;4:579.
43. Sanders JE, Hawley J, Levy W, et al. Pregnancies following high-dose cyclophosphamide with or without high-dose busulfan or total-body irradiation and bone marrow transplantation. *Blood* 1996;87:3045.
44. Ries LAG, Miller BA, Hankey BF, Kosary CL, Harras A, Edwards BK, eds. *SEER cancer statistics review, 1973–1991:* tables and graphs. NIH publication no. 94-2789. National Cancer Institute, 1994.
45. Mulvihill JJ, Byrne J. Offspring of long-time survivors of childhood cancer. *Clin Oncol* 1985;4:333.
46. Mulvihill JJ, Connelly RR, Austin DF, et al. Cancer in offspring of long-term survivors of childhood and adolescent cancer. *Lancet* 1987;2:813.
47. Hawkins MM, Draper GJ, Smith RA. Cancer among 1,348 offspring of survivors of childhood cancer. *Int J Cancer* 1989;43:975.
48. Sankila R, Olsen JH, Anderson H. Risk of cancer among offspring of childhood-cancer survivors. *N Engl J Med* 1998;338:1339.

49. Yoshimoto Y, Neel JV, Schull WJ, et al. Malignant tumors during the first 2 decades of life in the offspring of atomic bomb survivors. *Am J Hum Genet* 1990;46: 1041.
50. Cox R, Masson WK. Do radiation-induced thioguanine-resistant mutants of cultured mammalian cells arise by HGPRT gene mutation or X-chromosome rearrangement? *Nature* 1978;276:629.
51. Epstein RJ. Drug-induced DNA damage and tumor chemosensitivity. *J Clin Oncol* 1990;8:2062.
52. Neel JV, Schull WJ, Awa AA, et al. The children of parents exposed to atomic bombs: estimates of the genetic doubling dose of radiation for humans. *Am J Hum Genet* 1990;46:1053.
53. Awa AA, Honda T, Neriishi S, et al. Cytogenetic studies of the offspring of atomic bomb survivors. In: Obe G, Basler A, eds. *Cytogenetics:* basic and applied aspects. Berlin: Springer-Verlag, 1987:163.
54. Furusho T, Otake M. A search for the genetic effects of atomic bomb radiation on the growth and development of the F1 generation. V. Stature of 6- to 11-year-old elementary school pupils in Hiroshima. *Radiation Effects Research Foundation Technical Report* 1985;1:9.
55. Goldstein DP, Berkowitz RS, Bernstein MR. Reproductive performance after molar pregnancy and gestational trophoblastic disease. *Clin Obstet Gynecol* 1984;27:221.
56. Rustin GJS, Booth M, Dent J, et al. Pregnancy after cytotoxic chemotherapy for gestational trophoblastic tumours. *BMJ* 1984;228:103.
57. Green DM, Zevon MA, Lowrie G, Seigelstein N, Hall B. Congenital anomalies in children of patients who received chemotherapy for cancer in childhood and adolescence. *N Engl J Med* 1991;325:141.
58. Dodds L, Marrett LD, Tomkins DJ, Green B, Sherman G. Case-control study of congenital anomalies in the children of cancer patients. *BMJ* 1993;307:164.
59. Byrne J, Rasmussen SA, Steinhorn SC, et al. Genetic disease in offspring of long-term survivors of childhood and adolescent cancers. *Am J Hum Genet* 1998;62:45.
60. Blatt J, Mulvihill JJ, Ziegler JL, Young RC, Poplack DG. Pregnancy outcome following cancer chemotherapy. *Am J Med* 1980;69:828.

6

Genitourinary Disease in Women with Cancer

Jennifer Cohen-Kogan and *Thomas C. Randall

*Division of General Internal Medicine and *Department of Obstetrics and Gynecology, Hospital of the University of Pennsylvania, Philadelphia, Pennsylvania 19104*

Women with cancer often suffer lower genitourinary (GU) problems. These problems range from those specific to particular malignancies (including the complications or treatments of malignancy) to those also seen in women without cancer. For example, women treated with the chemotherapeutic agents cyclophosphamide or ifosfamide (IFEX) are at risk for hemorrhagic cystitis, while women with hematologic malignancies often suffer recurrent candidal infections. It is important therefore that women who have cancer and lower GU complaints be approached and managed in a systematic and comprehensive fashion with consideration of both cancer- and noncancer-related diseases. This chapter provides an overview of common problems of the lower urogenital system and reviews problems specific to cancer patients, such as those induced by radiation and certain chemotherapeutic agents.

ANATOMY AND PHYSIOLOGY

In the evaluation of women with GU symptoms, it is helpful to be familiar with normal female anatomy and physiology. The female genital tract is composed of both squamous and columnar epithelium. These different types of epithelium are susceptible to different infectious agents. The vagina and ectocervix are composed of squamous epithelium that is more susceptible to infections with *Candida* species and *Trichomonas vaginalis*. The columnar epithelium of the endocervix, however, is more susceptible to *Neisseria gonorrhoeae* and *Chlamydia trachomatis*. Both squamous and columnar epithelium are susceptible to the herpes simplex virus (HSV).

The normal vaginal flora represents a mix of organisms, with hydrogen peroxide–producing lactobacilli being most prominent. These lactobacilli act in suppressing overgrowth of anaerobic bacteria such as *Bacteroides* species, *Gardnerella vaginalis,* viridans streptococci, *Staphylococcus epidermidis*, and *Candida* species.

GENITOURINARY SYMPTOMS

The different diseases of the female lower urogenital tract, such as vaginitis, vulvitis, cervicitis, and cystitis, share many overlapping signs and symptoms including dysuria, pruritus, irritation, dyspareunia, and vaginal discharge. Therefore, in the evaluation of a woman with GU symptoms, a detailed history and a thorough physical examination, including pelvic examination, are important for distinguishing among vaginitis, vulvitis, cervicitis, and urethritis. For example, women with cystitis more commonly present with symptoms of frequency, urgency, suprapubic pain, flank pain, hematuria, and fever. Women with vaginitis are more likely to report pruritus, vaginal odor, and dyspareunia with fewer symptoms of frequency and urgency. Finally, women with cervicitis are more likely to report a new sexual partner, a sexual partner with symptoms, subacute onset over several weeks, and accompanying symptoms such as odor and discharge (1).

Another common GU complaint is vaginal discharge. While this may represent underlying pathology, as will be discussed, it is important to remember that certain discharges are physiologic. A benign vaginal discharge is composed of sloughed epithelial cells, bacteria, and endocervical secretions. Characteristically, the pH is 3.8 to 4.5, although it can be elevated secondary to exposure to sperm, blood, or cervical mucus (2). Anything that increases the rate of vaginal desquamation, such as stress, can subsequently increase the amount of vaginal discharge (2). A normal vaginal discharge can also be differentiated from a pathologic discharge because the former characteristically pools in the posterior fornix, is usually odorless, and is not associated with other symptoms such as itching and burning (2).

PHYSICAL EXAMINATION

The first step in the examination of any patient with suspected GU disease is inspection and palpation of both the vulva and vestibule. Palpation should be performed using the tip of a cotton swab. After inspection and palpation, examination using a speculum should follow for further evaluation of the vaginal mucosa. The examiner should note the presence of any ulcerations, edema, erythema, petechiae, atrophy, or discharge. If vaginal secretions are present, their color, consistency, and volume should be noted. Finally, the cervix should be inspected, with attention to any discharge from the cervical os or any friability of the cervical mucosa.

The next step in the examination is the collection of a specimen to assess vaginal pH. Determining the pH can be accomplished by swabbing secretions from the middle third of the vagina and placing the secretions on hydrazine paper. Secretions should also be obtained for the preparation of a saline and 10% potassium hydroxide (KOH) wet mount that will be examined by light microscopy. A final swab can be obtained and added to 10% KOH for a whiff test (amine elaboration). If indicated, bacterial and/or fungal cultures should be taken. Finally, a urine specimen should be obtained for dipstick, microscopy, and culture, if clinically indicated.

MICROSCOPY

Microscopic evaluation of a vaginal discharge involves examination of a saline and KOH wet mount. The purpose of saline microscopic examination is to identify clue cells, yeast hyphae, and trichomonads. In addition, the ratio of polymorphonuclear (PMN) leukocytes to squamous cells should be noted. A normal ratio is less than 1 PMN per squamous cell. Higher ratios are considered abnormal. Next, the clinician can determine whether the vaginal epithelial cells show evidence of atrophic vaginitis secondary to estrogen deficiency. Finally, the examiner should take note of the background vaginal flora. As mentioned previously, the normal vaginal flora primarily is composed of lactobacilli that appear rod-like. These organisms are present in moderate quantity. A change from a predominance of lactobacilli to primarily coccobacillary forms may indicate infection with *T. vaginalis* or bacterial vaginosis (BV). Finally, the KOH slide should be evaluated to help identify the presence of yeast.

VAGINITIS

Vaginitis is a common problem seen in women of all ages and accounts for 5 to 10 million office visits per year (2). Vaginitis is rarely a cause of mortality; however, it is a source of considerable morbidity and therefore necessitates a careful evaluation and diagnosis. Women with vaginitis can present with a variety of symptoms, including vaginal discharge, vaginal pruritus, irritation, dyspareunia, and dysuria. Unfortunately, the presenting signs and symptoms of vaginitis are nonspecific and therefore play a limited role in the evaluation of patients. This can become frustrating for clinicians trying to differentiate among even the most common causes of vaginitis such as BV, trichomoniasis, and vulvovaginal candidiasis. It is important to appreciate that despite workup, as many as one-third to one-half of patients lack a final microbiologic diagnosis. In a prospective study of 123 symptomatic women, only 49% received a diagnosis of candidiasis, trichomoniasis, or BV (3). This study also found that itching was the only symptom that was more frequently seen in patients in whom a diagnosis was made. Further, there was no significant difference in the presenting symptoms of the three infections, and the absence of vaginal odor, seen more frequently in a yeast infection, was the only significantly different sign.

Differential Diagnosis

The differential diagnosis of vaginitis is extensive but can be separated into infectious and noninfectious causes (Table 1). The most common causes of infectious vaginitis are BV, vulvovaginal candidiasis, and trichomoniasis. Other, less common infectious etiologies include atrophic vaginitis complicated by a secondary infection, desquamative inflammatory vaginitis, streptococcal vaginitis, ulcerative vaginitis associated with *Staphylococcus aureus* and toxic shock syndrome, and a secondary anaerobic bacterial infection from a foreign body such as a forgotten tampon, diaphragm, or condom (4). Causes of noninfectious vaginitis include allergic, hypersensitivity, and contact dermatitis, vaginitis from chemicals or irritants, traumatic vaginitis, and atrophic vaginitis. Among cancer patients, both radiation and chemotherapy can cause vaginitis. A comparison of the typical findings for the different causes of vaginitis is presented in Table 2.

TABLE 1. *Differential diagnosis of vaginitis in the oncology patient*

Infectious vaginitis
Bacterial vaginosis
Vulvovaginal candidiasis
Trichomoniasis
Atrophic vaginitis with secondary bacterial infection
Foreign body with secondary infection
Desquamative inflammatory vaginitis
Streptococcal vaginitis (group A)
Ulcerative vaginitis associated with *Staphylococcus aureus* and toxic shock syndrome
Idiopathic vulvovaginal ulceration associated with human immunodeficiency virus infection
Noninfectious vaginitis
Chemical or irritant
Allergic, hypersensitivity, and contact dermatitis (lichen simplex)
Traumatic vaginitis
Erosive lichen planus
Collagen vascular disease
Pemphigus syndromes
Radiation-induced atrophy and/or fibrosis
Idiopathic

Modified from ref. 4, with permission.

Bacterial Vaginosis

BV is the most common cause of vaginitis in women of childbearing age (4). However, despite causing 40% to 50% of cases of infectious vaginitis, the pathophysiology of BV is complex and poorly understood. BV is characterized by a decrease in the prevalence and concentration of hydrogen peroxide–producing lactobacilli (5): Of unaffected women, 96% have hydrogen peroxide–producing strains of lactobacilli, compared with only 6% of women with BV (2). It is believed that this lack of hydrogen peroxide–producing lactobacilli causes bacterial overgrowth of other flora, including *G. vaginalis, Mobiluncus* species, *Mycoplasma hominis,* anaerobic gram-negative rods, *Bacteroides* species, and *Peptostreptococcus* species (6). The *G. vaginalis* carrier state is two to three logs higher in women with BV (2).

It is unclear whether BV is sexually transmitted. Male sexual contacts of women with BV have been found to carry similar organisms, and BV is often associated with other sexually transmitted diseases (STDs) (2,7). The prevalence of BV in virgins is low, whereas it can be diagnosed in sexually abused girls (8). However, some reject the

TABLE 2. *Differential diagnosis of vaginitis*

Variable	Normal	Candidiasis	Bacterial vaginosis	Trichomoniasis	Atrophic vaginitis
Symptoms	None	Pruritus, soreness, dyspareunia	Malodorous discharge; no dyspareunia	Malodorous discharge; dyspareunia	Dyspareunia; vaginal dryness
Signs	None	Vulvar erythema, edema, fissures	Adherent discharge	Purulent discharge, erythema	Vaginal thinning
pH	4–4.5	4–4.5	>4.5	5–6	>6
Amine test	Negative	Negative	+ (70%–80%)	Often positive	Negative
Saline microscopy PMN:EC ratio	<1	<1	<1	PMN+++	PMN+ to ++
Other	Rods dominate; squames	Pseudo-hyphae (40%)	Increased coccobacilli clue cells (>90%)	Motile trichomonads (60%)	Loss of rods; parabasal cells
KOH test	Negative	Pseudohyphae (70%)	Negative	Negative	Negative

EC, epithelial cells; KOH, potassium hydroxide; PMN, polymorphonuclear leukocytes.
Modified from ref. 4, with permission.

theory that BV is sexually transmitted because the diagnosis has been made in virginal adolescents and the treatment of sexual partners does not decrease the likelihood of recurrent disease (9,10).

Several risk factors associated with the development of BV have been identified. These risk factors include use of an intrauterine device (IUD), white race, prior pregnancy, sexual activity, prior history of STDs, tobacco use, a recent change in sexual partner, and douching (4,11). BV has been implicated in preterm labor and delivery of low-birth-weight infants, plasma-cell endometritis, postpartum fever, posthysterectomy vaginal cuff cellulitis, postcesarean section endometritis, and abnormal Papanicolaou (Pap) smears (2,12).

Clinical Presentation

The presentation of BV is variable. As many as 50% of women are asymptomatic, while others present with a fishy, amine-odored discharge that may be more prominent after unprotected intercourse. There is usually no inflammation, hence the term *vaginosis* rather than vaginitis. Dysuria and dyspareunia are less common.

Examination of the vaginal vault often reveals a mild to moderate amount of thin, off-white discharge that is homogeneous and adherent to the vaginal wall. The characteristic pH is greater than 4.5. A pH less than 4.5 is not consistent with the clinical diagnosis of BV. BV is characterized by a positive whiff test in which there is increased odor after the addition of 10% KOH to the discharge. Examination of the vaginal walls reveals an absence of inflammation.

Diagnosis

The Amsel criteria are used to diagnose BV (11). Using these criteria, the diagnosis is based on the presence of three of the following four clinical signs:

- Thin, homogeneous discharge
- pH greater than 4.5
- Amine odor
- Clue cells on wet-mount examination

The Amsel criteria have been further refined to increase the specificity of the diagnosis. According to these refined criteria, at least 20% of the epithelial cells on the wet mount must be clue cells (5).

Wet-mount examination of the vaginal discharge is extremely important for diagnosing BV. Wet-mount examination is used to identify the presence of clue cells, which are the single most reliable predictor of BV (5). Clue cells are squamous cells with frayed borders and represent vaginal epithelial cells with such a heavy coating of bacteria that the peripheral borders are obstructed (5) (Fig. 1). Identification of clue cells can be facilitated by using more saline in the wet-mount preparation, which helps to separate the epithelial cells from each other (2). Loss of coccobacilli, also characteristic of BV, may be noted on the wet mount. Finally, the wet mount may reveal numerous white cells; however, the absence of increased PMN leukocytes does not rule out the diagnosis of BV.

Gram stain also has been used to make the diagnosis of BV. The Spiegel and Nugent criteria are the two different Gram stain–based methods that have been described (13,14). The Spiegel criteria bases the diagnosis of BV on the presence of fewer than five lactobacillus morphotypes, five or more *Gardnerella* morphotypes, and five or more other morphotypes (gram-positive cocci, small gram-negative rods, curved gram-variable rods, or fusiforms) (13). The Nugent system, developed by the Vaginal Infection and Prematurity Study Group, has become the gold standard for diagnosis and grades the severity of BV on a 0 to 10 scale (Table 3). A score of 0 to 3 represents normal flora, 4 to 6 is indeterminate, and 7 to 10 is diagnostic of BV (14).

The sensitivity and specificity of the vaginal Gram stain using the Nugent criteria in the diagnosis of BV have been evaluated in comparison with the Amsel criteria. In one study, the sensitivity and specificity of the Gram stain compared with the Amsel criteria were 89% and 83%, respectively (15). When the Gram stain was used as the criterion for diagnosis, the sensitivity and specificity of the Amsel criteria were 70% and 94%, respectively. Yet despite the reliability of the Gram stain in the diagnosis of BV, clinicians do not take advantage of this underused tool.

Culture does not play a role in the diagnosis of BV because 50% to 60% of healthy asymptomatic women have a positive culture (4).

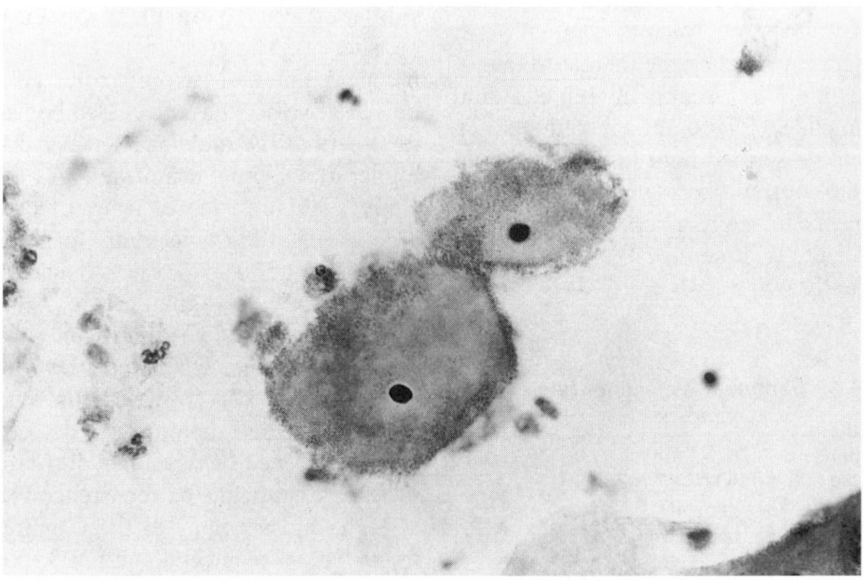

FIG. 1. Clue cells. These are mature squamous epithelial cells with adherent bacteria that are more prominent at the periphery. Note that there is no prominent background of inflammatory cells. (Courtesy of Cindy McGrath, M.D., and Prabody Gupta, M.D., University of Pennsylvania Health System, Philadelphia, PA.)

TABLE 3. *Nugent criteria for the diagnosis of bacterial vaginosis*

Score	*Lactobacillus* morphocytes	Gardnerella/Bacteroides morphotypes	Curved gram-variable rods
0	4+	0	
1	3+	1+	1+ or 2+
2	2+	2+	3+ or 4+
3	1+	3+	
4	0	4+	

Morphotypes: scored as the average number seen per oil-immersion field. Note that less weight is given to curved gram-variable rods. Total score = lactobacilli + G vaginous and *Bacteroides* + curved rods.

0, no morphotypes present; 1, <1 morphotype present; 2, 1–4 morphotypes present; 3, 5–30 morphotypes present; 4, 30 or more morphotypes present.

Modified from ref. 14, with permission.

Treatment

Several different treatment options are available for BV (Table 4). Therapy consists of metronidazole, 400 to 600 mg twice daily for 7 days. This leads to a 90% to 95% initial cure, although the cure rate decreases to only 80% at 1 month (16). Metronidazole can also be given as a single 2-g oral dose. The immediate cure rate of the single metronidazole dose is similar to the 7-day treatment regimen, although the former is associated with a higher incidence of recurrence (4). Advantages of the single-dose regimen are improved compliance and lower rates of vaginal yeast infection; however, given the increased rate of recurrence, the 7-day treatment course should be recommended for compliant patients (2). All patients prescribed metronidazole should be warned to abstain from alcohol to avoid a disulfiram-like reaction. Clindamycin can also be used for the treatment of BV in a dose of 300 mg orally twice daily for 7 days, with a 93% efficacy at 1 week and 89% efficacy at 1 month (2). However, the side effects of clindamycin, including diarrhea and colitis, are significant and need to be considered if this drug is chosen.

TABLE 4. *Treatment options for bacterial vaginosis*

Oral Regimens
Metronidazole 500 mg PO b.i.d. for 7 d
Metronidazole 2 g PO in a single dose
Clindamycin 300 mg PO b.i.d. for 7 d
Topical regimens
Clindamycin cream 2%, one full applicator (5 g) intravaginally at bedtime for 7 d
Metronidazole gel 0.75%, one full applicator (5 g) intravaginally b.i.d. for 5 d

Modified from ref. 25, with permission.

Topical therapies may also be utilized for the treatment of BV. Topical therapies can be advantageous because there is less systemic absorption compared to oral therapy, which subsequently results in lower toxicity. Several topical therapies are available including clindamycin cream 2%. Clindamycin vaginal cream applied each evening for 7 days has similar efficacy to oral therapy but is more expensive (2). The efficacy of a 3-day course is being studied. Metronidazole gel 0.75%, twice daily for 5 days, can also be used in the treatment of BV and has been associated with higher intravaginal drug levels. A randomized study evaluating the efficacy of oral metronidazole, 500 mg twice daily for 7 days, metronidazole gel 0.75%, twice daily for 5 days, and clindamycin vaginal cream 2%, 5 g daily for 7 days, showed no significant difference in the cure rate when evaluated after 7 to 14 days of follow-up (17). However, this small study may have lacked the power to detect a significant difference between the above therapies.

After treatment, the recurrence rate of BV is high, and as many as 30% of treated patients have a recurrence within 3 months (4). It is unclear whether this is secondary to a reinfection or a relapse, and currently it is unclear how these patients should be managed. Patients should probably receive a longer course of therapy (i.e., 10 to 14 days); however, the clinician should keep in mind that long-term treatment with metronidazole can lead to a peripheral neuropathy. Several randomized, double-blind studies have shown that there is no benefit in treating partners to decrease the recurrence rate (18,19).

Currently, routine treatment of asymptomatic disease is not recommended; however, patients who are pregnant or about to have gynecologic surgery should be treated.

Trichomoniasis

Trichomoniasis, which is responsible for 10% to 25% of vaginal infections, affects 180 million women worldwide and 2 to 3 million women annually (20). It is seen in 30% to 40% of the male partners of infected women (4).

T. vaginalis, the infectious agent in trichomoniasis, is a motile protozoan with four flagella. This organism is transmitted sexually, and it has been reported to survive in hot tubs and pools (2). Many risk factors are associated with trichomoniasis, including a history of other STDs, lower socioeconomic status, increased number of sexual partners, tobacco use, and African-American race (2). *T. vaginalis* has also been reported to facilitate the transmission of the human immunodeficiency virus (21).

Clinical Presentation

The clinical presentation of trichomoniasis is variable. Many women with this infection are asymptomatic, while others have a more severe and acute presentation. Some studies suggest that as many as 25% to 50% of women who are culture-positive for *T. vaginalis* are asymptomatic (21). In contrast, patients may note a malodorous, yellow or green vaginal discharge, dyspareunia, external dysuria, internal dysuria (if there is coinfection of the urethra), and vaginal pruritus. Five percent to 10% will also present with abdominal pain. However, all these symptoms are also characteristic of other causes of vaginitis and therefore alone do not have enough sensitivity or specificity to make a diagnosis of trichomoniasis.

On pelvic examination, a copious, purulent, odorous, yellow or green discharge with a pH 5 to 6 can be seen. The vaginal wall may be inflamed, and in 2% of patients punctate hemorrhages may be noted on the cervix on visual inspection (versus 90% with colposcopy) (20). This latter sign is commonly referred to as a strawberry cervix.

Diagnosis

The wet mount remains the most cost-effective test to diagnose trichomoniasis. A wet mount should be done to look for motile trichomonads (Fig. 2); however, these may be seen in only 50% to 70% of culture-confirmed cases (22). The wet mount is also remarkable for an increased number of PMN leukocytes. While culture for *T. vaginalis* has a sensitivity of 95%, it is rarely used to diagnose trichomoniasis and is only indicated when there is a high vaginal pH and many PMN leukocytes on wet mount, but an absence of trichomonads (4). Pap smear has a sensitivity of approximately 60% in detecting *T. vaginalis*; however, there are many false-positives (22). Therefore, a positive result on Pap smear should be confirmed with a wet mount prior to treatment. Deoxyribonucleic acid (DNA) probes and monoclonal antibodies have high sensitivity and specificity, but they are used less frequently for diagnosis (23).

Treatment

The treatment of trichomoniasis is important because the infection can result in several complications, including premature rupture of membranes, posthysterectomy cellulitis, abnormal Pap smears, and neonatal respiratory tract infection (24). Further, trichomoniasis has been associated with pelvic inflammatory disease. It has been hypothesized that the motility of trichomonads facilitates the movement of other microorganisms from the vagina to the fallopian tubes (2).

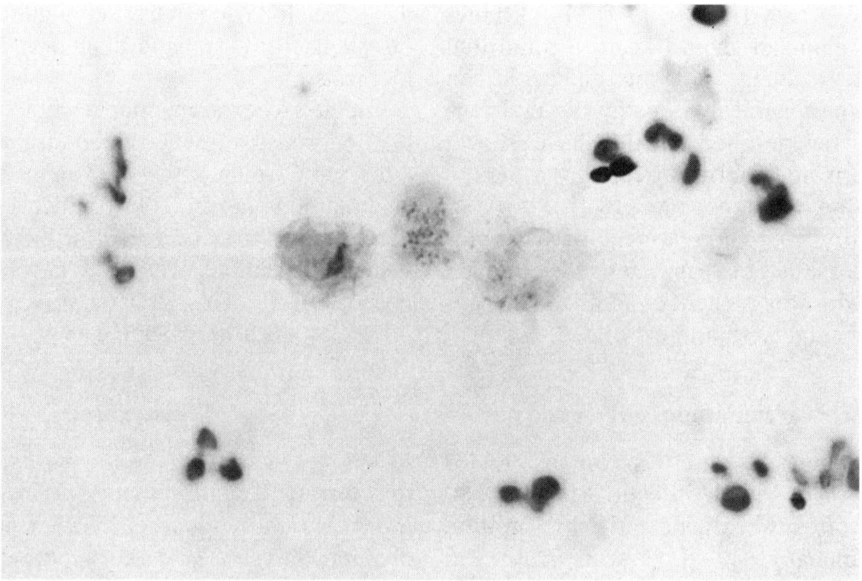

FIG. 2. Trichomonads. Small, pear-shaped organisms are seen with faint vesicular nuclei, cytoplasmic granules, and pseudoflagella. (Courtesy of Cindy McGrath, M.D., and Prabody Gupta, M.D., University of Pennsylvania Health System, Philadelphia, PA.)

The treatment of trichomoniasis consists of oral or topical metronidazole (Table 5). Oral metronidazole is better because it prevents an endogenous recurrence from the urethra and periurethral glands, where trichomonads may reside (4). The typical dose is 500 mg orally twice daily for 7 days, with an 85% to 90% cure rate. It may also be given as a single 2-g dose, with a cure rate of 82% to 88% (20). The cure rate increases to more than 90% when sexual partners are simultaneously treated. Advantages of the single-dose regimen are improved compliance, decreased candidal superinfection, and shorter period of alcohol abstinence to avoid a disulfiram-like reaction (4). However, the single oral dose is associated with a lower cure rate, and it is thus imperative to treat the partner if a single dose is chosen. Common side effects of metronidazole include a metallic taste, nausea (10%), transient neutropenia (7.5%), interactions with warfarin sodium (Coumadin), and peripheral neuropathy. Topical intravaginal metronidazole has been used to treat trichomoniasis, although it is typically less effective secondary to lower drug concentrations in the urethra and perivaginal glands (25).

TABLE 5. *Treatment options for trichomoniasis*

Typical infection
Metronidazole 500 mg PO b.i.d. for 7 d
Metronidazole 250 mg PO t.i.d. for 7 d
Metronidazole 2 g PO in a single dose
Resistant infection
Metronidazole 2–4 g PO b.i.d. for 10–14 d
Metronidazole 750 mg PO q.i.d. for 6–10 d
Combination oral metronidazole with vaginal metronidazole suppository (500 mg daily for 5 d)
Paromomycin sulfate (Humatin) 250 mg q.d. for 2 w

Modified from ref. 25, with permission.

In rare instances, trichomoniasis can be refractory to treatment. In this setting, it is important to assess the treatment compliance of both patient and partner. It is also important to determine whether the patient is using any medications that can decrease the efficacy of metronidazole, such as phenobarbital or phenytoin sodium (Dilantin). Cases of metronidazole-resistant trichomoniasis have been reported, and if this is suspected, it should be confirmed *in vitro* (26). Metronidazole-resistant trichomoniasis should be treated with higher doses of antibiotic: 2 to 4 g orally once daily for 10 to 14 days, or 650 mg four times daily for 6 to 10 days. Vaginal metronidazole may also be used in combination with oral therapy (21). When high doses of metronidazole are not effective, persistent infection may require treatment with paromomycin sulfate (Humatin), 250 mg daily for 2 weeks.

Vulvovaginal Candidiasis

The true incidence and prevalence of candidiasis are difficult to assess, given that many women self-diagnose the condition and self-treat with over-the-counter (OTC) medications. Candidiasis affects most adult women at least once in their lifetime, and by age 25 one-half of college women will have had at least one physician-diagnosed incident (4).

The majority (80% to 92%) of vulvovaginal yeast infections are caused by *Candida albicans*, although recently there has been an increased prevalence of infections caused by *Candida glabrata* and *Candida tropicalis* (27). These latter species, which were responsible for only 10% of yeast infections in the 1970s, were responsible for 20% of infections in the 1980s (28). Several theories have been proposed to explain this increased incidence of non–*C. albicans* infections. Some suggest that the increase is secondary to the increased use of OTC drugs and long-term suppressive azoles (4). Others suggest that short courses of antifungal drugs may select for strains that are not as sensitive to imidazoles; however, some studies refute this theory (29).

Vulvovaginal candidiasis is not considered an STD since many celibate women are diagnosed with it, and *Candida* species constitute a normal part of the vaginal flora (4). As many as 15% to 20% of women have asymptomatic colonization with yeast (2). It has been shown that there is no difference in strain type between those yeasts that cause symptoms and those that do not (30).

Frequency of infection increases when women begin regular sexual activity, which has led some to believe that *Candida* can be transmitted sexually. Yeast vaginitis may also be stress-induced and, in some women, may occur consistently before menstruation (2); the reason for this remains unclear.

While many candidal infections are sporadic and without an identifiable trigger, many occur in patients who have a recognizable risk factor. A thorough history can help identify these risk factors. Women with either diabetes mellitus or obesity are at particular risk. Antibiotics are an important risk factor, and certain antibiotics such as ampicillin, tetracycline, clindamycin, and the cephalosporins have been especially responsible because their antimicrobial spectrum is directed against the normal vaginal flora, thus permitting the overgrowth of yeast (2). High-estrogen states, whether from oral contraceptive use, pregnancy, or the premenstrual state, can increase the risk for candidal infection. Certain methods of contraception, such as IUDs and vaginal sponges, have been associated with yeast infections. Immunosuppressed patients, whether secondary to therapy with systemic steroids or from primary immunodeficiency, are also at increased risk.

Clinical Presentation

Vulvovaginal candidiasis commonly presents with symptoms of vulvar and perivaginal pruritus, vaginal soreness, and dyspareunia. Women may initially present with symptoms similar to cystitis, including frequency and dysuria. This external dysuria is caused by urine contact with an irritated vulva. A thick vaginal discharge is also a common symptom. The degree of symptomatology is not strictly related to the number of organisms; however, the majority of symptomatic women do have large numbers of yeast present (2).

Diagnosis

The diagnosis of vulvovaginal candidiasis relies on a complete history that focuses on the aforementioned risk factors. Pelvic examination reveals vulvar erythema, fissures, and scaling with inflamed vaginal rugations. The vaginal pH remains normal at 4 to 4.5, and the vaginal discharge is characteristically curdy white, adherent, and odorless. The amine test is negative. Saline wet-mount microscopy reveals fewer white blood cells than in other vaginal infections, and in 40% of patients pseudohyphae are present (31). A wet mount with 10% KOH, which is more sensitive than the saline wet mount for the identification of yeast, reveals pseudohyphae in 70% of cases (3) (Fig. 3). Finding pseudohyphae can be facilitated by preparation of a wet mount that has more vaginal discharge on the slide (2). However, despite the characteristic microscopy, the wet mount has an overall low sensitivity, so that it is not uncommon for a patient with a candidal infection to have negative microscopy (4).

Vaginal cultures have also been used in the detection of vulvovaginal candidiasis, although they are not routinely helpful. One circumstance in which vaginal cultures may be particularly useful is when a patient has classic symptoms of a yeast infection but a negative wet mount.

Treatment

Many treatment options are available for vulvovaginal candidiasis, and they can be divided into two categories of agents: OTC and prescription medications (Table 6). OTC medications are ideal for women with infrequent infections. The choice of preparation is important because different symptoms may respond to different preparations. Specifically, if the symptoms of vaginitis are greater than vulvitis, suppositories may be better than creams. The converse is true in that vulvar symptoms respond better to creams. Finally, if both vulvar and vaginal symptoms coexist, the combination of a cream and suppository may be useful (2). There are many different choices of agents, but the most commonly used treatments include miconazole (Monistat) or clotrimazole for 7 days. Three-day courses of miconazole may maximize compliance but may be associated with a higher recurrence rate (2). While the choice of products is vast, clinicians should be reassured that there is no difference in the efficacy of

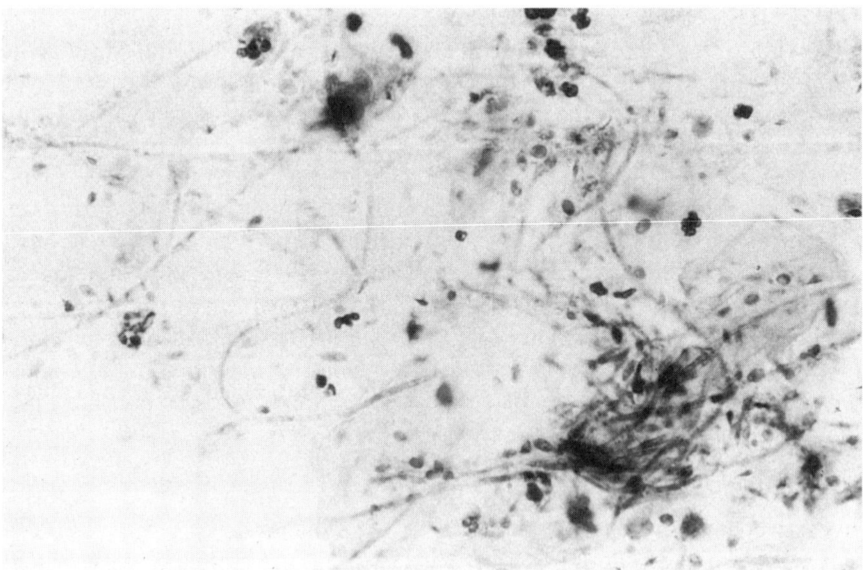

FIG. 3. Yeast vaginitis. Pseudohyphae and spores are seen characteristic of *Candida* species. (Courtesy of Cindy McGrath, M.D., and Prabody Gupta, M.D., University of Pennsylvania Health System, Philadelphia, PA.)

TABLE 6. *Recommended regimens for the treatment of vulvovaginal candidiasis*

Intravaginal agents[a]
Butoconazole (Femstat) 2% cream, 5 g intravaginally for 3 d
Clotrimazole (Gyne-Lotrimin Mycelex) 1% cream, 5 g intravaginally for 7–14 d
Clotrimazole 100 mg vaginal tablets for 7 d
Clotrimazole 100 mg vaginal tablet, one single tablet in a single application
Miconazole (Monistat) 2% cream, 5 g intravaginally for 7 d
Miconazole 200 mg vaginal suppository, one suppository for 7 d
Nystatin (Mycostatin) 100,000-unit vaginal tablet, one tablet for 14 d
Ticonazole (Vagistat) 6.5% ointment, 5 g intravaginally in a single application
Terconazole (Terazol) 0.4% cream, 5 g intravaginally for 7 d
Terconazole 0.8% cream, 5 g intravaginally for 3 d
Terconazole 80 mg vaginal suppository, one suppository for 3 d
Oral agent
Fluconazole (Diflucan) 150 mg tablet PO in a single dose

[a]With the exception of nystatin (Mycostatin), these agents are available over the counter.
Modified from ref. 4, with permission.

the different products and that most produce a cure rate of 80% (4). Most important, selection of a formulation should be based on patient preference. Boric acid vaginal suppositories, twice daily for 2 weeks, have been used, but only when other treatments are contraindicated (32). Gentian violet has also been used, but most patients find it unacceptable and severe allergic reactions have been associated with it (33).

Prescription medications are also used in the management of vulvovaginal candidiasis. These should be reserved for women who have multiple recurrences and are not responsive to OTC medications. They are also useful for women who have difficulty using the topical preparations or who are not compliant with the full course of topical therapy (2). Some studies comparing the efficacy of oral versus topical medications have found a higher cure rate with the former, although this may be secondary to the increased efficacy against *C. glabrata* (27). Currently, the only United States Food and Drug Administration (FDA)–approved oral medication for the treatment of vulvovaginal candidiasis is fluconazole (Diflucan) in a single 150-mg oral dose (34). This achieves therapeutic concentrations in vaginal secretions for as long as 72 hours (35). Reported side effects include headache, gastrointestinal discomfort (nausea, vomiting, and diarrhea), and rash. Although not FDA-approved, itraconazole (Sporanox) has also been used in a single 200-mg oral dose. It should be noted that in complicated infections, such as recurrent infections or those in diabetic or immunocompromised patients, a 10- to 14-day course of therapy may be needed with any of the above agents (34).

Recurrent Vulvovaginal Candidiasis

Recurrent vulvovaginal candidiasis, defined as more than four infections a year, occurs in fewer than 5% of healthy women but is more problematic in oncology patients who are immunosuppressed or receive multiple courses of antibiotics (4). The pathogenesis of recurrent infections is not certain, but several mechanisms have been proposed:

1. Recurrent infection may be secondary to the persistence of *C. albicans.* Longitudinal DNA typing has shown that most recurrent infections are secondary to vaginal relapses or endogenous reinfection with the identical strain (36).
2. The importance of the vaginal immune mechanism has been proposed (37). Forty percent to 70% of recurrent candidal vaginitis can be attributed to an acquired *Candida* antigen–specific cutaneous anergy characterized by a reduced T-lymphocyte reactivation to *Candida* antigen (2).
3. Recurrence may be secondary to a hypersensitivity reaction rather than an invasive infection (38). This has been supported by studies that have evaluated the vaginal washings of women with recurrent infection and have found IgE, suggesting an intermediate hypersensitivity response (38).
4. There have been reports suggesting an association between Lewis blood group anti-

gens and recurrent vulvovaginal candidiasis (39).

5. Infection with non—*C. albicans* species has been proposed as another cause of recurrent candidiasis (27).

It is important in the treatment of a patient with recurrent vulvovaginal candidiasis to look for and eliminate modifiable risk factors. This may include stopping the use of oral contraceptives or improving glycemic control in diabetic patients. Physicians should counsel patients to stop wearing nylon and tight-fitting undergarments. If infections routinely occur before menses, intravaginal medication several days prior to menstruation may be helpful. Ingestion of 8 ounces of yogurt with *Lactobacillus acidophilus* can also decrease candidal colonization and vaginitis (2).

Several therapeutic regimens are available for women with recurrent vulvovaginal candidiasis. Several studies have shown the effectiveness of antifungal maintenance suppressive therapy for 6 months after an initial induction regimen has resulted in negative cultures (2). Ketoconazole (Nizoral), 100 mg daily; itraconazole, 50 to 100 mg daily; fluconazole, 100 mg weekly; or clotrimazole, 500-mg suppository weekly, have all been used (2). Other agents that have been used are topical boric acid in a dose of 600 mg daily for 2 weeks or topical flucytosine (Ancobon) (2).

Atrophic Vaginitis

Atrophic vaginitis is a frequent cause of vaginitis and is typically seen with aging and in estrogen-deprived states such as menopause. The time between the onset of menopause and the development of atrophic vaginitis is variable (40). For some women, it occurs immediately after cessation of menses, while in others it can take years. It has also been shown that tobacco use may exacerbate atrophic changes (40).

As its name implies, atrophic vaginitis is characterized by atrophy of the vaginal skin and mucosal surfaces. With estrogen deprivation, the vaginal epithelium loses it rugae and becomes thin and pale in appearance. With estrogen deficiency, the vaginal epithelium can also become erythematous with petechial hemorrhage (40). The tissue becomes avascular, and increasing amounts of connective tissue result in a loss of elasticity (40). Further, there is a reduction in the amount of normal vaginal secretions. The decreased lubrication can cause dyspareunia and a subsequent avoidance of sexual intercourse, which can ultimately cause vaginal or introital contraction and rigidity (40). If estrogen deprivation is protracted, the genital tract can become permanently contracted with a narrow, contracted introitus and a friable, unrugated vagina (40). A urethral caruncle, characterized by dark-red tissue at the entrance of the urethra, may also be present

In patients with atrophic vaginitis, a vaginal smear displays a diminished number of superficial cells with an increased number of intermediate and parabasal cells (40) (Fig. 4). With estrogen deficiency, there is a decreased glycogen concentration in cells, leading to inhibition of lactobacilli. The decreased number of hydrogen peroxide–producing organisms increases the vaginal pH (40). The breakdown of the normal protective barrier also results in an overgrowth of organisms such as streptococci, staphylococci, coliforms, and diphtheroids.

Clinical Presentation

Atrophic vaginitis typically does not have a clinically significant presentation. In fact, most cases of mild to moderate atrophic vaginitis are clinically silent. When present, symptoms can be classified into vaginal symptoms and lower urinary tract symptoms, and the severity differs among women (40). Vaginal symptoms consist of vaginal dryness and itching, vulvar pruritus, burning leukorrhea, dyspareunia, and spotting. Burning is especially common after intercourse. Lower urinary tract symptoms include urgency, frequency, incontinence, and dysuria.

Diagnosis

During examination of a women in whom atrophic vaginitis is suspected, it is often

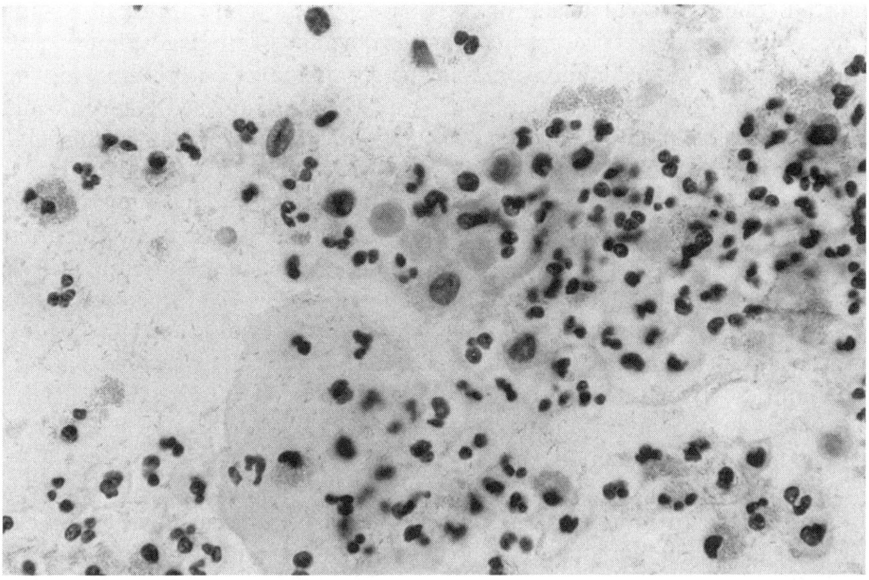

FIG. 4. Atrophic vaginitis. Marked acute inflammation and increased numbers of parabasal epithelial cells are evident. (Courtesy of Cindy McGrath, M.D., and Prabody Gupta, M.D., University of Pennsylvania Health System, Philadelphia, PA.)

helpful to use a small speculum to avoid damage to the atrophic tissues and decrease the patient's discomfort. The perivaginal skin should be examined for any signs of irritation caused by incontinence, and the vulva should be inspected for dystrophy. The labia minora, which are extremely estrogen-dependent, should be inspected for irritation and friability. It should be determined whether there is a complicating rectocele or cystocele. The vaginal mucosa should be inspected for evidence of thinning mucosa, diffuse redness, petechiae, or ecchymoses with decreased or absent vaginal folds (40).

In atrophic vaginitis, a serosanguineous or watery discharge may be present. During the pelvic examination, the pH should be measured using a pH-indicator strip inserted into the proximal one-third of the vaginal vault. The usual pH in atrophic vaginitis is 5 to 7, compared with a lower pH in premenopausal women. A wet mount should be performed to exclude an infectious etiology such as BV, trichomoniasis, or candidiasis. The wet mount typically reveals an increased number of PMN leukocytes with small rounded parabasal cells (2). These latter cells are immature squames that have not been exposed to sufficient estrogen. A mean maturation index is calculated by counting the number of parabasal, intermediate, and superficial cells per 100 cells.

Treatment

Once diagnosed, atrophic vaginitis is treated with estrogen replacement. This can be administered either locally or systemically. The most common method of administration is topical estrogen cream, although in controlled trials topical and oral estrogen were equally effective (40). Vaginal estrogen cream, compared to oral estrogen therapy, produces equivalent estrone and estradiol levels (40). Initially, systemic absorption of topical therapy may be suboptimal secondary to the atrophy and avascularity of the vaginal mucosa. With time, however, the vascularity of the mucosa improves, and systemic absorption increases. Normal epithelial function can be restored using one-fourth to one-half an applicator of estrogen cream twice weekly for 3 weeks (31). Other therapies include vaginal administration of estrogen in the form of rings, tablets, and gels. The estrogen patch and oral estrogen, as mentioned above, are additional options.

Radiation Effects on the Vulva and Vagina

Patients who have been treated with radiotherapy to the pelvis, vagina, or vulva frequently suffer a range of symptoms both acutely and chronically (41). Acutely, the skin of the vulva undergoes erythema, dry desquamation, moist desquamation, and ulceration. These changes are more commonly observed, however, when radiation was administered from lower energy sources. With modern radiotherapy equipment, it is more common for patients to acutely suffer erythema with pain or pruritus, followed chronically by radiation fibrosis. As it is throughout the body, the underlying mechanism is hypoxia in the affected tissues. Radiation damage to the vascular endothelial cells causes thrombosis and irreversibly decreases the caliber of affected arterioles. Ultimately, necrosis occurs, causing replacement of viable stromal cells and compliant collagen with inflammatory cells and fibrin (42). Clinically, the result is thinning and stiffening of the affected tissues, causing atrophy of the vulva and vagina that is often more severe than that seen in the setting of estrogen deficiency. Exacerbating the situation is the fact that in most women pelvic irradiation will have caused loss of ovarian function. The vulva may become tightened with loss of the architecture of the labia majora and minora. The vagina frequently becomes stenotic and shortened, causing dyspareunia and, in patients with pelvic malignancies, making it difficult for the practitioner to monitor pelvic anatomy by rectovaginal examination.

Diagnosis

The diagnosis of acute radiation effects on the vulva and vagina is often self-evident, based on the temporal relationship to radiation therapy. Chronically, however, there may be formation of polyps or cystic masses that must be distinguished from infection or malignancy. This distinction can usually be made by histopathology, which reveals arteriolar narrowing with thickening and fibrosis of the endothelial cells, a chronic inflammatory reaction, fibrin, and often bizarre-appearing stromal cells. The squamous epithelium is dramatically thinned, and there is loss of most underlying dermal structures.

Treatment

Acute radiation burns of the vulva or vagina are best treated with a topical application of silver sulfadiazine (Silvadene Cream) or a similar antiinflammatory preparation. Chronic changes are frequently treated with either systemic or topical estrogens in an attempt to increase the number and caliber of blood vessels (43). Because of the underlying irreversible changes to the vascular endothelium and other supporting structures, the response to this treatment is often undramatic, and many patients require long-term supportive care. Biofine ointment has been shown to promote healing of radiation-associated ulcerations. Patients receiving pelvic, vaginal, or vulvar radiation are generally given a regimen of estrogen applications and vaginal dilation in an attempt to prevent or palliate these effects. Ulceration and superinfection may occur, and these can usually be treated with sitz baths using warm saline or aluminum acetate solution (Domeboro). If ulceration, infection, or stenosis become intractable or extreme, surgical resection and reconstruction of the affected tissues by transposing well perfused, unirradiated tissues may be required (44,45).

Desquamative Inflammatory Vaginitis

Desquamative inflammatory vaginitis, also known as erosive lichen planus, is an idiopathic vaginitis, which has been described in either case reports or case series (33). It is a poorly defined disease that affects cutaneous and mucosal surfaces.

Clinical Presentation and Diagnosis

Common presenting symptoms of erosive lichen planus are severe dyspareunia, intractable pain, intense pruritus, and a profuse seropurulent vaginal discharge (33). In the absence of sexual activity, vaginal adhesions and stenosis can occur. The pelvic examination reveals a vaginal mucosa that is acutely inflamed and denuded of epithelium. Distinct patches of hyperemic, eroded vaginal mucosa may be especially noticeable in the areas of the vaginal fornices (33). A gray pseudomembrane on the vaginal surface and a seropurulent discharge are characteristic of inflammatory vaginitis (33). The inner labia minora and the vulvar vestibule can appear erythematous and eroded as well. Because oral lesions have been reported in as many as two-thirds of women with vulvovaginal disease, examination of the buccal mucosa is also important (33).

In women with erosive lichen planus, the vaginal pH is slightly increased (range, 5 to 7). A wet-mount examination of the vaginal discharge reveals a higher preponderance of basal and parabasal cells, indicating both exfoliation and cytolysis (33). Accompanying this is an absence of gram-positive bacilli and a marked increase in PMN leukocytes. Biopsy, if undertaken, reveals eroded mucosa with changes of chronic inflammation (33).

Treatment

Erosive lichen planus typically does not resolve spontaneously. Unfortunately, there is no effective treatment. The current recommendation for therapy is vaginal application of clindamycin cream 2% (4). Topical corticosteroids have been used with occasional success, and short courses of an oral corticosteroid are sometimes advocated (33).

Noninfectious Vaginitis/Vulvitis

Any chemical that contacts the vulvar or vaginal epithelium has the potential to be an irritant. The symptoms of noninfectious vaginitis are indistinguishable from infectious vaginitis, especially vulvovaginal candidiasis (4). These symptoms include pruritus, irritation, burning, soreness, and a variable discharge. The most important intervention in the management of noninfectious vaginitis is the elimination of offending agents and the avoidance of steroids, which can result in further burning. Women may obtain symptomatic relief from sitz baths and topical vegetable oils (4).

VULVITIS

Herpes Vulvovaginitis

Genital herpes is a widely prevalent disease, with at least 45 million cases diagnosed by serology in the United States (23). Genital herpes, a recurrent, incurable disease caused by the herpes simplex virus (HSV), is the most common cause of genital ulcers. HSV is a small DNA virus, and two serotypes, HSV-1 and HSV-2, are responsible for urogenital disease. Most cases of genital herpes are secondary to HSV-2, although HSV-1 accounts for 5% to 30% of first-episode cases (46). The infections of each serotype are clinically indistinguishable.

The transmission of HSV occurs from either oral or genital contact with an individual who is shedding the virus or from autoinoculation. Many individuals infected with HSV are asymptomatic; however, they can still be infectious during periods of asymptomatic viral shedding (47). After exposure, there is an incubation period of 3 to 7 days, followed by a period of viral shedding that can last 1 to 2 weeks.

An important feature of genital herpes is the high rate of recurrent disease. Recurrences are not secondary to reinfection, but rather to reactivation of latent virus that lies dormant in the sensory ganglia neurons (48). Recurrences typically occur at the sites of primary infection, although it still remains unknown what causes reactivation. Factors thought to contribute to reactivation include stress, concurrent infection, and immunosuppression (48). There are fewer recurrences with HSV-1 infection compared to HSV-2. More than 80% of individuals with primary HSV-2 infection have a recurrence, compared to 55% of those with primary HSV-1 infection (49).

Clinical Presentation

The clinical presentation of genital herpes varies, depending on whether it is a primary infection or a recurrence (Table 7). First-episode herpes infections are characterized by severe local symptoms caused by multiple painful vesicles that may be located on the vulva, vagina, cervix, urethra, and bladder. Inguinal lymphadenopathy and systemic features such as headache, myalgias, fever, malaise, gastrointestinal upset, and/or central nervous system involvement may also be present. Women with a primary herpetic infection may also present with a severe vulvovaginitis and urinary retention (46).

A burning or tingling sensation is often the initial symptom of genital herpes. Within 24 hours, one or more pruritic vesicles emerge, followed by vesicle rupture causing shallow ulceration. These ulcers, which are associated with increased pain, burning, itching, and dysuria, can become more symptomatic if bacterial superinfection occurs. The presence of herpetic lesions can also cause severe dyspareunia. Ulcers can coalesce to form larger ulcerations or bullae. Ruptured vesicles take approximately 12 days to heal and typically resolve without scarring, unless there is a coexistent bacterial superinfection. Labial adhesions, a potential long-term complication of genital herpes, can occur when contiguous ulcerated surfaces contact each other, ultimately forming a fibrotic scar.

Unlike primary infections that present with multiple vesicles and systemic symptoms, the clinical presentation of recurrences is typically less severe (33). In recurrent infection, lesions are smaller, the virus titer is lower, and there is less pain. The herpetic lesions tend to be more discrete with clusters of vesicles rather than diffuse involvement. Systemic symptoms are typically absent. Further, in contrast to primary infection, the duration of symptoms is shorter. Symptoms peak at 2 days, and virus is shed for approximately 5 days, with complete healing by 7 to 9 days (33).

Diagnosis

The diagnosis of HSV infection is usually made based on typical clinical manifestations and the presence of herpetic lesions on the vulva, vagina, cervix, or urethra. However, when there is a question about the diagnosis or a definitive diagnosis must be made, there are several mechanisms by which to identify HSV.

Specimens for definitive diagnosis can be obtained from either the vesicle or vesicle fluid. Vesicle fluid can be aspirated using a small syringe, or the roof of a vesicle can be removed and the base scraped with a Dacron swab. If pustules or ulcers are present, they

TABLE 7. *Characteristics of primary versus recurrent genital herpes*

Characteristics	Primary HSV	Recurrent HSV
Fever, headache, malaise, myalgias	Present (70%)	Usually absent
Local pain, burning, itching	Present (99%)	Present (88%)
Dysuria	Present (83%)	Uncommon (27%)
Tender inguinal lymphadenopathy	Present (81%)	Uncommon (31%)
Mean duration of local pain (d)	12	6
Mean duration of viral shedding (d)	12	4
Mean duration of lesions (d)	20	9
Shedding of virus from cervix (%)	88	12

HSV, herpes simplex virus.

Modified from Corey L. Genital herpes. In: Holmes KK, Mardh P-A, Sparing PF, Wiesner PJ, eds.: *Sexually transmitted diseases.* New York: McGraw-Hill, 1984:449–474; with permission.

should be cleaned with sterile saline prior to swabbing of the ulcer base (50).

Multinucleated giant cells with intranuclear inclusions can sometimes be found on Pap smear, but this is not recommended as a diagnostic tool (47). These cells can also be found in Tzanck preparations. The sensitivity of a Tzanck smear in identifying multinucleated giant cells is only 50% to 70% when the specimen is obtained from a vesicle; it is lower if the lesion has already crusted (50). The yield tends to be higher with a vulvar as compared to a cervical specimen (50). One difficulty with the Tzanck smear, however, is that this technique does not permit the differentiation of an HSV infection from varicella-zoster virus infection.

Viral tissue cultures have been used to document HSV infection. The best time to take these cultures is during the vesicular stage (47). Initial results are often available in 48 hours, although final results may not be available for 1 to 2 weeks (47). Test kits are available for detection of HSV monoclonal antibodies, as well as the enzyme-linked immunosorbent assay and Western blot assay to differentiate type 1 and type 2 viruses (47). Under routine circumstances, use of these tests is not necessary.

Treatment

Counseling is a very important part of managing any patient with genital herpes. It should begin at the first visit during the initial presentation and should include information on the natural history of the infection, including the possibility of recurrent episodes, the nature of asymptomatic shedding, sexual transmission, and means to reduce transmission (25). This counseling should be continued at follow-up visits. Patients need to learn that they should abstain from sexual activity both when lesions are present and when the prodromal symptoms are present. The patient should be instructed that condoms be used with all new or uninfected partners, even when the patient is asymptomatic (25).

Systemic antiviral drugs play an important role in the management of genital herpes. Antiviral drugs can help control symptoms and signs in primary episodes, as well as recurrent episodes, when used as daily suppressive therapy (Table 8). It should be remembered, however, that these drugs do not eradicate latent virus or affect the risk, frequency, or severity of recurrent events once the drug is discontinued (25). Randomized, controlled trials have shown that acyclovir (Zovirax), valacyclovir hydrochloride (Valtrex), and famciclovir (Famvir) provide clinical benefit in the treatment of genital herpes (25). Compared with acyclovir, both valacyclovir and famciclovir have increased oral bioavailability. Acyclovir also comes in a topical form, although this preparation is felt to be less efficacious, and currently its use is discouraged (25).

For the first clinical episode of genital herpes, there are four recommended regimens. These include acyclovir, 400 mg orally three times a day for 7 to 10 days; acyclovir, 200 mg orally five times a day for 7 to 10 days; famciclovir, 250 mg orally three times a day for 7 to 10 days; or valacyclovir, 1 g orally twice a day for 7 to 10 days. These regimens have been shown to shorten the duration of pain and viral shedding by 1 to 2 days (51).

TABLE 8. *Recommended treatment options for genital herpes infection*

First clinical episode of genital herpes[a]
Acyclovir (Zovirax) 400 mg PO t.i.d. for 7–10 d
Acyclovir 200 mg, PO 5 times daily for 7–10 d
Famciclovir (Famvir) 250 mg PO t.i.d. for 7–10 d
Valacyclovir HCl (Valtrex) 1 g PO b.i.d. for 7–10 d
Recurrent episodic infection
Acyclovir 400 mg PO t.i.d. for 5 d
Acyclovir 200 mg PO 5 times daily for 5 d
Acyclovir 800 mg PO b.i.d. for 5 d
Famciclovir 125 mg PO b.i.d. for 5 d
Valacyclovir 500 mg PO b.i.d. for 5 d
Daily suppressive therapy
Acyclovir 400 mg PO b.i.d.
Famciclovir 250 mg PO b.i.d.
Valacyclovir 500 mg PO once daily
Valacyclovir 1 g PO once daily
Severe disease
Acyclovir 5–10 mg/kg body weight IV q8h for 5–7 d or until clinical resolution is obtained

[a]Treatment may be extended if healing is incomplete after 10 days of therapy.

Modified from ref. 25, with permission.

Recurrent infections can be managed with episodic therapy. If treatment is begun during the viral prodrome or within 1 day after onset of lesions, many patients with recurrent disease benefit from episodic therapy (46). This necessitates that the patient be given a prescription for antiviral therapy so that there is no delay in starting therapy when initial symptoms occur. There are several recommended regimens that use either acyclovir, famciclovir, or valacyclovir (see Table 8).

Acyclovir prophylaxis is recommended for women with more than eight recurrences per year. Daily suppressive therapy has been shown to reduce the frequency of genital herpes recurrences by 75% in patients with frequent recurrences (defined as more than six recurrences per year) (25). Suppressive therapy regimens include acyclovir, 400 mg orally twice a day; famciclovir, 250 mg orally twice a day; valacyclovir, 500 mg orally once a day; or valacyclovir, 1 g orally once a day. For patients with more than 10 recurrences per year, a higher dose of valacyclovir has been shown to be more efficacious (25). Again, it is important to remember that suppressive therapy reduces but does not eliminate asymptomatic viral shedding (33). Safety has been documented for up to 7 years using acyclovir chemoprophylaxis (52). Since valacyclovir and famciclovir are newer drugs, their long-term safety has only been demonstrated for a shorter duration. To date, there has been no evidence to suggest the emergence of virus resistant to acyclovir in immunocompetent patients using chronic suppressive therapy (25).

Cyclic Vulvitis

Cyclic vulvitis is defined as variable vulvodynia. This syndrome is characterized by alternating periods of exacerbations and quiescence with a patient-specific pattern regarding her menstrual cycle. Cyclic vulvitis is associated with episodic vulvar erythema, pruritus, and discharge. There may be a relationship to candidiasis, and if so, long-term anticandidal therapy may play a role in treatment (38).

Vestibular Papillomatosis

Vestibular papillomatosis has been known by many names including pseudocondylomata, pruritic vulvar squamous papillomatosis, vestibular micropapillomas, benign squamous papillomatosis, and hirsutoid papillomas of the vulva. The prevalence is 1% among unselected outpatients attending a GU clinic (53). Most patients are asymptomatic, but others may present with pruritus, vulvodynia, superficial dyspareunia, and postcoital irritation (38). The physical examination is most remarkable for vestibular papillae that are numerous, smooth, pearly-white, soft excrescences causing a grainy appearance on affected surfaces. Typically, the papillae involve the inner aspects of the labia minora, vulvar vestibule, and fourchette. The lesions are usually bilateral and symmetric but also can be linear in appearance (38). While vestibular papillomatosis can usually be visualized without magnification, magnification and acetowhitening of the vulva with dilute acetic acid can facilitate lesion identification (53). The etiology of vestibular papillomatosis is unclear, and current controversy surrounds the etiologic significance of human papillomavirus (HPV) (38).

Zoon's Vulvitis

Zoon's vulvitis, also called vulvitis circumscripta plasmacellularis, was first described in 1954. This entity is much less common than its male counterpart, balanitis circumscripta plasmacellularis (38). Zoon's vulvitis represents a rare disorder, and the majority of the literature on this disease is from limited case reports. Women with Zoon's vulvitis range in age from 28 to 89 years (38). To date, the etiology remains unknown, although chronic irritation, poor personal hygiene, or persistent infection have been proposed as potential risk factors (38).

Clinical Presentation and Diagnosis

The presenting symptoms of Zoon's vulvitis vary among women. Common symptoms include burning, pruritus, soreness, and dyspareunia (38). However, other women are asymptomatic. Given the lack of symptom specificity, a clinical diagnosis is unreliable. Therefore, the diagnosis of Zoon's vulvitis should be based on the presence of typical lesions and suggestive biopsy findings. This is important because the differential diagnosis for Zoon's vulvitis is extensive, including lichen planus, genital Bowen's disease, extramammary Paget's disease, syphilis, a fixed drug eruption, and candidal vulvitis (38).

On pelvic examination, the characteristic lesions of Zoon's vulvitis can be identified. These lesions are shiny, glazed, erythematous patches with an orange hue, very similar to the lesions of Zoon's balanitis. They have been described as pinpoint purpuric "cayenne-pepper" spots, but they can also appear as shallow erosions (38). As mentioned previously, the lesions should be biopsied for diagnosis.

Microscopic evaluation of the biopsy specimen reveals several distinct epidermal changes. These include atrophy with loss of epidermal rete ridges, spongiosis, and elongated keratinocytes. A lichenoid infiltrate composed of plasma cells, lymphocytes, mast cells, neutrophils, and eosinophils can be seen in the mid- and upper dermis (38). The biopsy specimen may also reveal vascular proliferation with erythrocyte extravasation.

Treatment

Unfortunately, to date, no therapy has proven to be consistently effective in the treatment of Zoon's vulvitis. Topical corticosteroids have been used for treatment with a variable response. Interferon and topical cyclosporine (Sandimmune) have also been used with differing degrees of success.

Ulcerating/Blistering Diseases

Many different diseases can cause ulceration and blistering of the vagina and vulva. It is imperative to identify the etiology of the ulceration so that appropriate therapy can be instituted. The differential diagnosis for ulcerating disease includes granulomatous diseases, Crohn's disease, herpetic infections, syphilis, and traumatic lesions (54). The evaluation of ulcerative disease should include a rapid plasma reagin test and darkfield examination for syphilis, culture for HSV, *Chlamydia* culture, Giemsa stain of the ulcer base, oral evaluation, biopsy of the leading edge of the ulcer for malignancy, and photography (54).

Blistering diseases can also involve the vagina and more commonly the vulva. When blisters or bullae are present, the differential diagnosis includes pemphigus vulgaris, dermatitis herpetiformis, epidermolysis bullosa acquisita, cicatricial pemphigoid, and bullous pemphigoid (38). Evaluation and differentiation of the bullous disease relies heavily on biopsy and direct immunofluorescence. Immunofluorescence can also help autoantibodies directed against epithelium.

Lichen Planus

Another etiology of vulvitis is lichen planus, a papulosquamous disorder. Lichen planus typically involves the oral mucosa, but women may also have vulvovaginal involvement.

Clinical Presentation

Women with lichen planus describe burning, pain, pruritus, dyspareunia, and postcoital bleeding. Pelvic examination reveals vulvar lesions that are raised, whitish, reticulated papules and plaques (38). The vulva may also appear erythematous with erosions rimmed by white, lacy, epithelial lesions. The classic definition of lichen planus includes the five P's: purplish, pruritic, polygonal papules and plaques (55). In severe cases, the vulva may be extensively scarred and even mutilated (38). Occasionally, lichen planus may involve the vagina and cervix, causing a desquamative or erosive vaginitis. With vaginal involvement, intercourse can become difficult to impossible if adhesions and stenosis have formed (38).

The differential diagnosis of vulvar lichen planus should include pemphigus vulgaris, bullous and cicatricial pemphigoid, epidermolysis bullosa aquisita, Zoon's disease, and bullous lichen sclerosis (38). Vulvar lichen planus can be differentiated by the presence of colloid bodies on direct immunofluorescence. The white, reticulated periphery should be the site of biopsy because the eroded areas reveal only nonspecific changes.

Treatment

Unfortunately, there are very few effective treatment options for vulvar lichen planus. Agents that have been tried include topical and systemic corticosteroids, systemic retinoids, griseofulvin, dapsone and cyclosporine (38).

Contact Dermatitis

A very important and often overlooked cause of vulvitis is contact dermatitis. The vulvar skin is very susceptible to irritation by a variety of agents. Moisture, friction, urine, vaginal discharge, cosmetics, cleansing products, topical medications, spermicides, and noncotton underwear have all been implicated as causative agents in the development of vulvar contact dermatitis (38,54). Therefore, it is necessary to take a very detailed exposure history in the evaluation of a patient in whom contact dermatitis is suspected.

There are three types of contact dermatitis (38):

- Acute irritant dermatitis, in which the vulvar skin is exposed to a potent irritant. This is analogous to a chemical burn.
- Chronic or cumulative irritant dermatitis, which is secondary to repeated exposures to an otherwise weak irritant. An irritative dermatitis results because there is insufficient time to repair the vulvar epithelium between each exposure.
- Vulvar dermatitis, a sensory irritation in which the patient reports sensations of burning and stinging in the absence of skin changes.

Allergic contact dermatitis is a cell-mediated immunologic reaction that occurs days after an exposure to the offending agent (38). This makes identification of the causative agent difficult because the exposure is more remote. Ethylenediamine, neomycin, and clobetasol propionate (Temovate) have all been reported to cause allergic contact dermatitis (38,55).

The most important aspect of therapy is removal of the offending agent. Topical corticosteroids for 7 to 10 days may also provide relief. It should be remembered that potent topical steroids be restricted to short-term use to avoid complications associated with long-term use. Further, potent steroids themselves can cause a vulvar dermatitis characterized by burning and erythema (55).

Vulvar Vestibulitis

Vulvar vestibulitis is a condition known by many other names, including minor vestibular gland syndrome, focal vulvitis, vulvar vestibulitis syndrome, and periglandular vestibulitis.

The vulvar pain syndrome has been defined by the Seventh Congress of the International Society for the Study of Vulvar Disease as a chronic vulvar discomfort characterized by complaints of burning, stinging, irritation, and/or rawness (56). A subset of vulvodynia is the vulvar vestibulitis syndrome characterized by a constellation of symptoms, including severe pain on vestibular touch or attempted vaginal entry, tenderness to pressure localized to the vulvar vestibule, and erythema on physical examination (57).

The vestibule is located between the labia minora and is visualized when the labia are held apart. The area is defined superiorly by the clitoris and inferiorly by the posterior fourchette and fossa navicularis that extends inward to the hymen (58).

The incidence of the vulvar pain syndrome is unknown but has been estimated in some studies to be as high as 15% (59). Typically, 97% of patients are white and 62% are nulliparous. The syndrome has been identified in women from 11 to 75 years of age, but the mean age of onset is 32 years. Often, women have visited many physicians before the condition is diagnosed. Many have a history of sexual abuse, allergies, HPV infection, and recurrent candidal infections (58).

The etiology of the vulvar pain syndrome is still unknown. There have been many theories to explain it, although none has been proven. Possible etiologies include the presence of fixed candidal antigens, contact dermatitis, allergic response, sexual dysfunction, hormonal reaction, and infectious agents such as *Candida* or HPV (58). KY jelly, urine-borne oxalate crystals, and psychiatric diagnoses, particularly depression, have also been implicated (58).

Diagnosis

During examination of a patient with possible vulvar vestibulitis, it is important to map painful areas using a cotton swab. The patient will have exquisite point tenderness when a cotton swab is touched on the hymenal ring and posterior fourchette. Color changes in the vestibule should be quantified. Physical examination of patients with vulvar vestibulitis is characterized by minute spots (between 1 and 11) of erythema around the small vestibular glands. Occasionally, small ulcerations may be noted and are usually located in the lower half of the vestibule. Speculum examination with wet-mount microscopy and culture are very important to exclude an infectious etiology that would require appropriate management.

Histologic examination is characterized by a chronic inflammatory infiltrate of T lymphocytes and some small B lymphocytes. This cell infiltration is located in the mucosal lamina propria and periglandular and periductal connective tissue (60). In addition, there may be squamous metaplasia or nodular hyperplasia of the minor vestibular glands (60).

Treatment

Several treatment strategies are available for women given the diagnosis of vulvar vestibulitis. Unfortunately, many of these interventions have not been found to be consistently helpful. Sitz baths, topical steroids, lubrication, antiinflammatory agents, sex hormones, antibiotics, antimycotics, and retinoid compounds are not effective in the overwhelming majority of cases (58). Antidepressive medication has been helpful in some cases (61). Women with vulvar vestibulitis should undergo a complete psychiatric evaluation. A cornerstone of management is a strong physician–patient relationship, and frequent visits with the patient are useful in establishing a good patient–physician alliance.

It is crucial to have the patient stop using all topical vulvar medications and review vulvar hygiene, such as wearing cotton underwear and avoiding constricting garments. Topical lidocaine hydrochloride 2% jelly (Xylocaine 2% Jelly) has been reported to provide some relief to patients (58). Oral calcium citrate plus a low-oxalate diet (to inhibit formation of calcium oxalate crystals) may be of benefit (62). Surgery, including perineoplasty and excision by carbon dioxide laser surgery, has been utilized in some cases for symptomatic relief (63). Short-term results have been more encouraging than long-term follow-up data (58). It is important to recognize that in 50% of cases there is spontaneous resolution; therefore, in managing a patient with vulvar vestibulitis, it is very important to consider conservative therapy. Surgical therapy should only be considered as a last resort.

Other treatments that have been used include topical or intralesional corticosteroids and interferon. Again, it is of utmost importance that any woman diagnosed with vulvar vestibulitis receive strong psychologic support.

CERVICITIS AND URETHRITIS

Gonorrhea

More than 1.3 million cases of gonorrhea are reported each year in the United States (64). *N. gonorrhoeae* is the causative agent, and transmission is via sexual contact with an infected individual. The risk factors for gonorrhea include low socioeconomic status, living in an inner city, multiple sexual partners, failure to use barrier contraceptive methods, and age younger than 30 years (47). The risk of male-to-female transmission during a single sexual encounter is 80% to 90% (46). *N. gonorrhoeae* infects both transitional and columnar epithelial surfaces; therefore, infection of the cervical and urethral epithelium results in cervicitis, urethritis, and/or a periurethral infection. After infection, there is a subsequent incubation period of 3 to 7 days.

Clinical Presentation

Unlike men, the majority of women with gonorrhea are asymptomatic. One-third of women have a purulent vaginal discharge, intermenstrual bleeding, or lower abdominal discomfort. Gonorrhea may also present as a urethritis or cystitis with dysuria, urgency, frequency, pyuria, and rarely hematuria. This presentation describes the acute urethral syndrome when it occurs in the absence of bacteriuria. In 0.5% to 3% of patients, gonorrhea disseminates, causing fever, arthralgias, arthritis, and skin lesions (50). Local complications of gonorrhea include pelvic inflammatory disease, which can occur in up to 10% to 20% of infected women, and abscesses of the Bartholin glands (46). On pelvic examination, the cervix appears erythematous, edematous, and friable, with a mucopurulent discharge coming from the cervical os.

Diagnosis

After the pelvic examination, the saline wet mount is performed to identify PMN leukocytes. The vaginal discharge in gonorrhea is characterized by more than 30 white blood cells per high-power field. A Gram stain, if performed, reveals gram-negative kidney bean–shaped diplococci extracellularly and intracellularly within neutrophils. The Gram stain, however, is not recommended for the diagnosis of gonococcal cervicitis because the normal flora of the female genital tract can appear similar to *N. gonorrhoeae* (50).

Traditionally, bacterial culture has been the standard for the diagnosis of gonorrhea. The endocervix, rectum, and pharynx can all be cultured using a rayon- or Dacron-tipped swab. There are important considerations for the culturing of gonorrhea. First, one must use swabs treated with charcoal, which inhibits any antibacterial substances that may be present on the swab fibers, thereby enhancing the recovery of organisms (50). Second, *N. gonorrhoeae* is a fastidious and fragile organism and requires an enriched medium for growth. Therefore, a culture must be performed using a modified Thayer-Martin medium. This is a selective medium that inhibits the growth of other, more rapidly growing bacteria. A single endocervical swab will identify about 90% of cases of gonorrhea (46).

Enzyme immunoassays (EIA) using urethral and endocervical specimens have also been used to diagnose gonorrhea. However, for endocervical specimens, the sensitivity is less than that of culture, and there is a high rate of false-positive test results (50).

Most recently, at many institutions, DNA probes have become the most frequently used tool for the diagnosis of gonorrhea. This commercial acridinium ester–labeled DNA probe is able to detect *N. gonorrhoeae* in endocervical and urethral specimens (50). Several studies have shown that the reliability of the DNA probe is comparable to culture, with the advantage that the probe provides more rapid results (65,66). A second advantage is that *C. trachomatis* can be detected using the same probe. Drawbacks to the probe include its cost and the inability to perform susceptibility testing should *N. gonorrhoeae* be detected (50).

Treatment

Since coinfection with *C. trachomatis* is common in women diagnosed with gonorrhea, a patient treated for gonorrhea should simultaneously be treated for chlamydia (discussed in the next section).

Several treatment options are available for gonorrhea (Table 9), including the cephalosporins—cefixime (Suprax) or ceftriaxone sodium (Rocephin)—and the quinolones—ciprofloxacin (Cipro) or ofloxacin (Floxin). Although cefixime and ceftriaxone have similar antimicrobial spectrums, cefixime has a lower and less sustained bactericidal level, compared to intramuscular ceftriaxone (25). In uncomplicated infections, cefixime has a 97.1% cure rate compared to a 99.1% cure rate with ceftriaxone. The quinolones have been shown to be safe and inexpensive, with a cure rate between 98% and 99% in uncomplicated infections. However, cases of gonorrhea resistant to fluoroquinolones have been reported throughout the United States (25). Therefore, it is most important to consider local susceptibility patterns in the selection of antimicrobial therapy.

Several alternative regimens can be used for the treatment of gonorrhea, including spectinomycin hydrochloride (Trobicin), 2 g intramuscularly in a single dose, other cephalosporins that can be given in a single intramuscular injection, and other single-dose quinolones (see Table 9).

TABLE 9. *Recommended treatment options for uncomplicated gonococcal infections of the cervix and urethra*

Recommended regimens
Cefixime (Suprax) 400 mg PO in a single dose
Ceftriaxone sodium (Rocephin) 125 mg IM in a single dose
Ciprofloxacin (Cipro) 500 mg PO in a single dose
Ofloxacin (Floxin) 400 mg PO in a single dose plus
Azithromycin (Zithromax) 1 g PO in a single dose
Doxycycline 100 mg PO b.i.d. for 7 d
Alternative regimens
Spectinomycin HCl (Trobicin) 2 g IM in a single dose
Single-dose cephalosporins
Ceftizoxime sodium (Cefizox) 500 mg IM
Cefotaxime sodium (Claforan) 500 mg IM
Cefotetan disodium (Cefotan) 1 g IM
Cefoxitin sodium (Mefoxin) 2 g IM with probenecid (Benemid) 1 g PO
Single-dose quinolones
Enoxacin (Penetrex) 400 mg PO
Lomefloxacin HCl (Maxaquin) 400 mg PO
Norfloxacin (Noroxin) 800 mg PO

Modified from ref. 25, with permission.

An essential component in the management of gonorrhea is referral of the patient's sexual contacts for evaluation and possible treatment. All partners diagnosed with gonorrhea should be treated for both gonorrhea and chlamydiosis. Patients diagnosed with gonorrhea also need to be instructed to avoid sexual intercourse until antimicrobial therapy is completed for all partners.

Chlamydia

C. trachomatis is an obligate intracellular organism that is the causative agent in chlamydial infection. It is one of the most common causes of STDs in the United States (67). *C. trachomatis* infects the columnar epithelium of the endocervical canal, causing cervicitis. *Chlamydiae* can also infect transitional epithelium of the urinary tract, resulting in urethritis. The mechanism of infection is sexual contact with an infected individual. Several risk factors for infection have been identified, including low socioeconomic status, age less than 24 years, and sexual intercourse with a new partner within the prior 2 months (68).

Clinical Presentation

The majority of women with chlamydial infection are asymptomatic. Both asymptomatic and symptomatic infections can persist for months, during which complications and sexual transmission can occur. These complications of infection include chronic pelvic pain, infertility, and ectopic pregnancy. Symptoms, when present, include vaginal discharge and intermenstrual bleeding. In addition to cervicitis, chlamydia can cause urethritis with frequency, urgency, dysuria, and pyuria. Finally, women may present with endometritis or pelvic inflammatory disease.

On pelvic examination, a mucopurulent discharge from the cervical os may be present, and a urethral discharge may be seen as well. The cervix may appear edematous and erythematous.

Diagnosis

The following guidelines are recommended for obtaining endocervical specimens for examination for chlamydia (69):

1. Specimens should be obtained after specimens for the Pap smear and gonorrhea are obtained.
2. Prior to specimen collection, any secretions or discharge should be removed from the endocervical os.
3. An appropriate swab should be inserted 1 to 2 cm into the endocervical canal past the squamocolumnar junction and rotated against the wall of the endocervical canal several times for 10 to 30 seconds. A wooden shaft should not be used because it is toxic to *C. trachomatis*; therefore, a plastic or wire shaft with tips made of cotton, rayon, Dacron, or calcium alginate should be used (50). Nonculture tests often have appropriate swabs supplied by the manufacturer.
4. The swab should be withdrawn without touching the surface of the vaginal wall and placed on the appropriate medium. Specimens used for culture must contain an adequate number of infected cells; purulent discharge alone is not an appropriate specimen for the detection of *Chlamydiae*.

In chlamydia, the wet-mount specimen usually reveals more than 30 white blood cells per high-power field. A Gram stain is typically not needed for diagnosis but, if done, reveals gram-negative intracellular diplococci.

Cell culture has been the standard diagnostic tool against which other tests have been compared. The sensitivity of a single culture is 70% to 90% (69). The sensitivity decreases when the specimen is handled improperly. However, the specificity of the *Chlamydia* culture is 100%, which means that regardless of the prevalence of disease in the population, when the test is positive, the clinician can be certain that the disease is present (70). Unfortunately, the *Chlamydia* culture is difficult to process, and results may not be available for at least 7 days.

Many nonculture tests are available for the diagnosis of chlamydia, including EIAs such as Chlamydiazyme (Abbott Laboratories, Abbott Park, Illinois), direct fluorescent antibody tests, and nucleic acid hybridization tests. The advantages of these tests are that they are easier to transport and have a shorter processing time. The greatest disadvantage of nonculture tests is the decreased specificity compared with culture (50). The sensitivity of nonculture tests typically ranges between 70% and 90% (70). Office-based rapid-test kits based on EIA technology are also used to diagnose chlamydia. The advantage of these tests is that they take only 10 to 30 minutes to perform, and are less expensive than the commercial tests. The current office-based tests have a sensitivity of 81% to 94% and a specificity of 97% to 99% (70).

Treatment

Treatment for chlamydial infection should also include treatment for gonorrhea, which has been described above. As with gonorrhea, sexual partners of infected patients also need to be treated, and patients should be instructed to abstain from sexual intercourse until both partners have completed the course of antibiotics.

The current recommended treatment regimens for chlamydia include either azithromycin (Zithromax) 1 g orally in a singe dose, or doxycycline 100 mg twice daily for 7 days. Both these regimens are equally efficacious, as long as the patient complies with the 7-day course of doxycycline (25). Alternative regimens include erythromycin and ofloxacin (Table 10). Patients often have a difficult time

TABLE 10. *Recommended regimens for treatment of chlamydial cervicitis and urethritis*

Recommended regimens
Azithromycin (Zithromax) 1 g PO in a single dose
Doxycycline 100 mg PO b.i.d. for 7 d
Alternative regimens
Erythromycin base 500 mg PO q.i.d. for 7 d
Erythromycin ethylsuccinate 800 mg PO q.i.d. for 7 d
Ofloxacin (Floxin) 300 mg PO b.i.d. for 7 d

Modified from ref. 25, with permission.

completing the course of erythromycin because of gastrointestinal side effects. Ofloxacin is equally efficacious to doxycycline and azithromycin but can be more expensive.

Urinary Tract Infections

Urinary tract infections (UTIs) are a very common problem for women of all ages. There are approximately 7 million episodes of cystitis per year in the United States with approximately 250,000 episodes of pyelonephritis per year (71). Approximately 25% to 35% of women aged 20 to 40 years have had at least one uncomplicated UTI diagnosed (1). Furthermore, these numbers most likely underestimate the true prevalence largely because of underreporting. UTIs encompass infections of the bladder (cystitis), collecting system, and kidney. Bacteria are responsible for most infections; however, viruses and fungi have also been implicated.

TABLE 11. *Classification of complicated urinary tract infections*

Obstruction
Nephrolithiasis
Tumors
Urethral strictures
Congenital anomalies
Bladder diverticuli
Renal cysts
Pelvic calyceal junction obstruction
Calculi
Foreign bodies
Indwelling catheter
Urethral stent
Nephrostomy tubes
Impaired host responses
Transplant recipients
Neutropenia
Immunodeficiency syndromes
Congenital
Acquired
Metabolic disorders
Diabetes mellitus
Renal failure
Functional abnormalities
Neurogenic bladder
Vesicoureteral reflux
Other
Urinary instrumentation
Urinary diversions

Modified from ref. 79, with permission.

Classification

Traditionally, UTIs have been classified as uncomplicated or complicated. Uncomplicated infections typically occur in women who have no underlying condition that would increase their likelihood of having a UTI, and no condition that would increase their chance of failing therapy. The most common example of a patient with an uncomplicated UTI is the premenopausal, sexually active, and nonpregnant woman who has not used antibiotics recently and has not had GU instrumentation (1).

Many factors suggest the possibility of a complicated UTI (Table 11), including older age, hospital-acquired infections, infections occurring during pregnancy, the presence of an indwelling catheter, or recent GU instrumentation. Any history of a functional or anatomic urinary tract abnormality or a history of childhood UTIs indicates a complicated UTI. Finally, a history of recent antibiotic use, the presence of symptoms more than 7 days prior to presentation, diabetes, or immunosuppression is also more suggestive of a complicated UTI. Using this definition, most oncology patients would be diagnosed with a complicated UTI.

Unfortunately, the terms *complicated* and *uncomplicated* have not been scientifically validated (72). While women with recurrent cystitis after sexual intercourse or cystitis associated with pregnancy and diabetes mellitus are traditionally thought of as having a complicated UTI, many studies suggest that antibiotic courses of 3 days to 2 weeks cure the majority of these patients (72). It may be that the term *complicated* UTI should be reserved for patients who fail therapy secondary to either relapse or persistent infection (72).

Pathogenesis

Several mechanisms have been implicated in the pathogenesis of UTIs. The most common mechanism is an ascending infection by organisms located around the periurethral tissue. The urinary system can also become infected through a hematogenous or lymphatic route, although these mechanisms are felt to be less responsible (73). Critical in the pathogenesis of UTIs are bacterial virulence factors, such as the fimbrial adhesions responsible for bacterial adherence.

Host defense mechanisms are also important in diminishing the survival of bacteria in the urinary tract. Several characteristics of the urine, such as urea salts, low pH, and high osmolarity, inhibit bacterial activity (73). In contrast, glucose in the urine can facilitate the multiplication of *Escherichia coli* (71). Adequate urine flow and bladder emptying are other important host factors. Efficient bladder emptying is essential to eliminate transient bacteriuria (73).

Several risk factors increase the likelihood of infection of the urinary tract. In addition to anatomy- and patient-related factors characteristic of complicated UTIs, several other important risk factors have been implicated. In a prospective study of sexually active young women, the risk for UTI was strongly and independently associated with recent sexual intercourse, recent use of a diaphragm with spermicide, and a history of recurrent UTI (74).

Many different bacteria can cause cystitis (Table 12). *E. coli* is the cause of 70% to 95% of UTIs, especially in the setting of a first infection (75). Other common organisms include *Staphylococcus saprophyticus*, *Proteus mirabilis, Klebsiella* species, and *Enterococcus* species (76).

TABLE 12. *Microorganisms isolated in patients with complicated urinary tract infection*

Gram-negative
Escherichia coli
Klebsiella spp.
Citrobacter spp.
Enterobacter spp.
Proteus mirabilis
Providencia spp.
Pseudomonas aeruginosa
Gram-positive
Enterococcus spp.
Group B streptococci
Coagulase negative staphylococci
Staphylococcus aureus

Clinical Presentation

Many women with cystitis present with acute dysuria. The presence of dysuria is not specific because dysuria can also seen with urethritis (secondary to *C. trachomatis, N. gonorrhoeae*, or HSV) and vaginitis (75). While there is considerable overlap in the presenting symptoms of urethritis, vaginitis, and cystitis, a detailed history of clinical symptoms, physical examination, and urinalysis may be useful in differentiating among these entities (1) (Table 13). Whereas women with cystitis typically present with frequency, urgency, suprapubic pain, and hematuria, women with vaginitis are more likely to report pruritus, vaginal odor, and dyspareunia with fewer symptoms of frequency and urgency. Women with urethritis are more likely to report a new sexual partner, a sexual partner with symptoms, subacute onset over several weeks, and accompanying symptoms such as a vaginal discharge.

Diagnosis

The first step in the diagnosis of a UTI is to determine whether there is pyuria on microscopy or whether dipstick testing of a midstream urine collection is positive for leukocyte esterase. The presence of leukocyte esterase has a sensitivity of 75% to 96% and a specificity of 94% to 98% for detecting pyuria. The test has a positive predictive value of only 50%, but it has a negative predictive value of 92% (77). Therefore, even with a negative leukocyte esterase test, a UTI cannot be completely ruled out, and microscopy with culture should be performed if the patient is symptomatic (75). Microscopic evaluation of the urine specimen is valuable for identifying white blood cells and red blood cells; however, microscopy for bacteriuria is insensitive because pathogens are often present in low quantities.

TABLE 13. *Differentiation of infectious conditions responsible for dysuria in women*

Condition	Symptoms	Signs	Pyuria	Hematuria
Cystitis	Abrupt onset Severe symptoms Dysuria Frequency Urgency Suprapubic pain Low-back pain	Suprapubic tenderness	Usually	Sometimes
Urethritis	Gradual onset Mild symptoms Vaginal discharge Vaginal bleeding Low-abdominal pain	Cervicitis or herpetic lesions on examination	Usually	Rarely
Vaginitis	Vaginal discharge Vaginal odor Pruritus Dyspareunia External dysuria No frequency No urgency	Vulvovaginitis on examination	Rarely	Rarely

Modified from ref. 1, with permission.

In the setting of an uncomplicated UTI, the general consensus is that a pretreatment urine culture does not need to be obtained and that empiric therapy can be initiated (1,75). It is felt that this management strategy is efficacious, safe, and cost-effective. A decision analysis showed, for example, that routine pretreatment urine culture in patients with an uncomplicated, acute cystitis increased the cost of care by 39% but only decreased duration of symptoms by 10% (78). However, in patients with a complicated UTI, and especially in those with structural abnormalities of the urinary tract or immunosuppression, a pretreatment culture should be obtained (75).

The definition of what constitutes bacteriuria remains controversial. Traditionally, a uropathogen count greater than 10^5/mL in a midstream collection has been diagnostic of cystitis; however, a recent evaluation has shown this to be insensitive in the presence of symptoms. Approximately one-third to one-half patients with acute cystitis have a uropathogen count less than 10^5/mL (1). For the diagnosis of acute cystitis, a uropathogen count of 10^2/mL or greater has better sensitivity (95%) at the expense of lower specificity (85%) (1). The Infectious Disease Society of North America consensus definition of cystitis is the presence of 10^3 colony-forming units/mL or greater (1). This has a sensitivity of 80% and a specificity of 90%.

Treatment

The management of cystitis depends on both the causative organism and whether the infection is considered complicated or uncomplicated. The most marked difference between the management of uncomplicated and complicated UTIs is the duration of therapy. Uncomplicated infections typically require 3 to 5 days of antimicrobial therapy, while complicated infections usually necessitate a longer course of 7 to 14 days (79). Generally, however, the antimicrobial agents used for treatment do not differ between complicated and uncomplicated infections. An algorithm for the management of acute cystitis is presented in Table 14.

The clinician should consider several factors when selecting antimicrobial therapy:

1. Knowing the patterns of drug sensitivity in the area where the clinician practices is important for recognizing the prevalence of resistant organisms.

TABLE 14. *Management of acute cystitis*

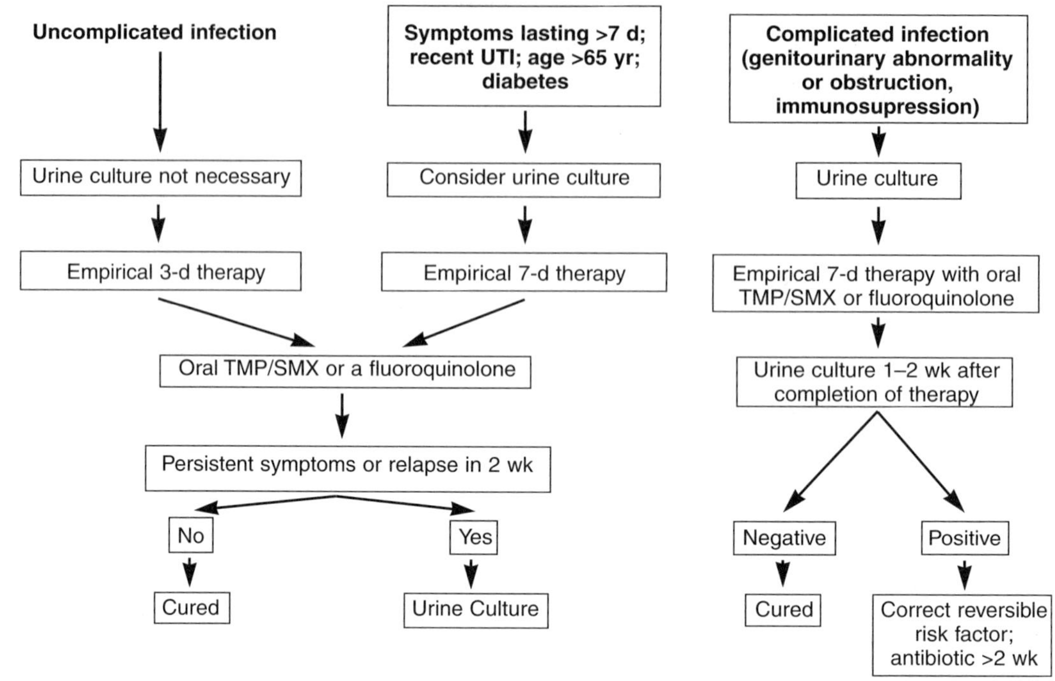

TMP/SMX, trimethoprim/sulfamethoxazole; UTI, urinary tract infection.
Modified from ref. 76, with permission.

2. The pharmacokinetics of different antibiotics are important to consider so that medications with less frequent dosing intervals are chosen.
3. An antibiotic that provides adequate drug urinary levels for an appropriate duration of time should be chosen.
4. Side effects, cost, and potential drug interactions should be considered.
5. If empiric therapy is started, the antibiotic selection should be reevaluated once the results of the urine culture and sensitivity profile become available.

Many antibiotics can be used to treat cystitis (Table 15). In general, as long as the organism is sensitive to the antibiotic chosen, it is not clear that any specific antibiotic or antibiotic class has superior efficacy (79). The most commonly selected antibiotics tend to be trimethoprim/sulfamethoxazole (TMP/SMX) and the fluoroquinolones, which are effective in eradicating gram-negative organisms. In acute, uncomplicated cystitis in a young woman, a 3-day course of TMP/SMX has been shown to be more effective and less expensive than 3-day courses of amoxicillin, nitrofurantoin, and cefadroxil (80).

The organisms isolated from individuals with complicated UTIs tend to be more varied and demonstrate a higher prevalence of resistance to antimicrobial therapy (79). Increased resistance reflects the fact that women with complicated UTIs tend to have a history of either recurrent infections requiring antibiotics or a history of hospitalizations with the potential for the nosocomial acquisition of resistant organisms.

Additional therapeutic interventions may be needed in the management of cystitis. In women with severe dysuria, phenazopyridine hydrochloride (Pyridium) can be added for 1 to 2 days to decrease dysuria. Women should be warned that this drug will turn the color of their urine orange. It is controversial whether increased hydration plays a role in the man-

TABLE 15. *Antimicrobial agents for the treatment of urinary tract infection*

Oral
Amoxicillin 500 mg t.i.d.
Amoxicillin potassium clavulate (Augmentin) (500 mg amoxicillin) t.i.d.
Nitrofurantoin 50–100 mg q.i.d.
Cephalexin 500 mg q.i.d.
Cefaclor (Ceclor) 500 mg q.i.d.
Cefadroxil 1 g q.d. or b.i.d.
Cefixime (Suprax) 400 mg q.d.
Cefuroxime axetil (Ceftin) 125–250 mg b.i.d.
Cefpodoxime proxetil (Vantin) 100–400 mg q12h
Trimethoprim/Sulfamethorazole 160/800 mg b.i.d.
Norfloxacin (Noroxin) 400 mg b.i.d.
Ciprofloxacin (Cipro) 250–500 mg b.i.d.
Ofloxacin (Floxin) 200–400 mg b.i.d.
Enoxacin (Penetrex) 200 mg b.i.d.
Lomefloxacin HCl (Maxaquin) 400 mg q.d.
Fleroxacin 400 mg q.d.
Fluconazole (Diflucan) 200 mg q.d.
Parenteral
Gentamicin 1–1.5 mg/kg q8h or 4–5 mg/kg q24h
Tobramycin sulfate (Nebcin) 1–1.5 mg/kg q8h or 4–5 mg/kg q24 h
Amikacin sulfate (Amikin) 5 mg/kg q8h or 15 mg/kg/d
Aztreonam (Azactam) 1–2 g q6h
Cefazolin sodium 1–2 g t.i.d.
Cefotaxime sodium (Claforan) 1–2 g q8h
Ceftriaxone sodium (Rocephln) 1–2 g q.d.
Cefepime HCl (Maxipime) 2 g b.i.d.
Ceftazadime 0.5–2 g t.i.d.
Piperacillin sodium (Pipracil) 3 g q4h
Piperacillin/tazobactam sodium (Zosyn) 4 g–500 mg q8h
Imipenem/cilastatin sodium (Primaxin) (500 mg imipenem) q6h
Meropenem (Merrem) 500 mg q8h
Amphotericin B (Fungizone) 0.3–0.5 mg/kg/d

Modified from ref. 79, with permission.

agement of UTIs. Some believe that it increases uropathogen removal, while others feel that it decreases the urinary concentration of the antimicrobial agent.

Recurrent Urinary Tract Infections

Many women experience recurrent UTIs. Several mechanisms are responsible for the development of recurrent UTIs. In some instances, recurrence is secondary to a persistent focus of infection; however, exogenous reinfection is typically responsible for 90% of cases.

Risk factors for recurrence include use of diaphragms and spermicides (the latter may facilitate the colonization of the vagina with *E. coli*) and nonsecretion of blood group antigens (81,82). Postmenopausal women are also at increased risk for UTI (83). This may be secondary to incomplete voiding (from bladder or uterine prolapse) or to increased vaginal colonization with *E. coli.* In the postmenopausal state, estrogen deficiency is associated with a relative loss of lactobacilli, thereby increasing vaginal pH (84).

Recurrent UTIs can be a difficult problem to manage. All recurrent infections must be confirmed with culture at least once. Certain individuals may require continuous prophylactic antibiotics to prevent recurrent infection. Typically, prophylactic antibiotics are given at a low dose for a longer duration (usually longer than 6 months). A potential problem with the use of prophylactic antibiotics is the emergence of resistant microorganisms with subsequent infections. If infections recur after sexual intercourse, postcoital prophylaxis can be used (85,86). Another treatment strategy is for the patient to initiate therapy with symptom onset (87). An algorithm for

TABLE 16. *Management of recurrent cystitis*

Recurrent cystitis

- *Relapse—* Seek occult source of infection or urologic abnormality
  - Treat longer (2–6 wk)
- *Reinfection—* If woman uses a diaphragm and spermicide, consider changing contraceptive method
  - Urologic evaluation not routinely indicated
    - ≥3 UTI/yr
      - No relation to coitus → Daily or thrice weekly prophylaxis
        - Recommended regimens:
          - Trimethoprim 100 mg
          - TMP/SMX 40/200 mg
          - Nitrofurantoin 50–100 mg
          - Norfloxacin (Noroxin) 200 mg
          - Cephalexin 250 mg
      - Temporally related to coitus → Postcoital prophylaxis
        - Recommended regimens:
          - TMP/SMZ 40/200 mg
          - Cephalexin 250 mg
          - Nitrofurantoin 50–100 mg
    - <2 UTI/yr → Patient-initiated therapy for symptomatic episodes
      - Single dose or 3-d regimen

TMP/SMX, trimethoprim/sulfamethoxazole; UTI, urinary tract infection.
Modified from ref. 75, with permission.

managing recurrent cystitis that incorporates the above strategies has been proposed (75) (Table 16). In postmenopausal women with recurrent cystitis, topical estrogen therapy may be an effective preventive measure (84).

URINARY PROBLEMS IN THE CANCER PATIENT

Women with cancer frequently develop hematuria and/or UTIs due to both direct and indirect effects of cancer and cancer treatments. The major syndromes encountered in these women are an increased susceptibility to UTIs due to both physical and immunologic effects of treatment, hemorrhagic cystitis caused by chemotherapeutic urothelial toxins, and urinary problems caused by both acute and chronic effects of radiation therapy.

Various factors conspire to dramatically increase the incidence of UTIs among cancer patients. It is not infrequent for women who have borne children to have a slightly diminished capacity to void due to alterations in both the physical support and innervation of the bladder. In such cases, patients often compensate for this diminished contractile function by bearing down to increase intraabdominal pressure, and sometimes even by applying direct suprapubic pressure to assist with voiding. The presence of a pelvic or intraabdominal mass or of an abdominal incision interferes with this compensation and results in significant and sometimes undiagnosed urinary retention. Occasionally, women with pelvic malignancies initially present with urinary frequency or retention caused by impingement of a mass on both the bladder itself and its innervation. The need for frequent or prolonged catheterizations either to drain the bladder or to monitor urine output also increases the rate of bladder contamination and infection.

Effects of Radiation Therapy on the Bladder

Patients receiving pelvic radiotherapy may develop cystitis as they reach a dose of 3000 cGy to the bladder. This condition causes inflammation and swelling of the bladder mucosa and often spasm of the muscular bladder wall. These findings are accompanied by suprapubic tenderness, dysuria, urinary frequency, and incontinence (88). With modern radiotherapy, this full-blown syndrome is uncommon, and it is imperative that the practitioner encountering such a patient ensure that she does not have an infection. Since this is a complicated UTI, optimal treatment involves urine culture before or at the initiation of antibiotic therapy.

As patients reach doses to the bladder greater than 6000 cGy, they are at some risk, both acutely and chronically, for hemorrhagic cystitis, chronic cystitis, fibrosis with decreased bladder capacity, and fistula formation.

Hemorrhagic cystitis is usually the result of bleeding from bladder telangiectasias, which form as a result of the poor perfusion that ensues as a result of radiation-induced obliterative endarteritis. In most patients, this syndrome may be managed conservatively, but some will have significant bleeding with anemia. Cystoscopy with diathermic coagulation of the affected vessels is an effective treatment in this case, although some patients will have extensive, diffuse hemorrhage not amenable to diathermy. Such patients are best treated with bladder irrigations containing a contact procoagulant, such as a very dilute formalin solution.

Chronic cystitis due to irradiation is a troublesome clinical scenario. If a patient has adequate bladder function, treatment is symptomatic. Mild urothelial anesthetics, such as phenazopyridine may be given, or the patient may be treated with nonsteroidal antiinflammatory drugs, amitriptyline hydrochloride, or mild narcotics to make the symptoms more manageable. The practitioner must again remain alert for the possibility of a concomitant infection, which will exacerbate the patient's symptoms. Patients with intractable symptoms may benefit from bladder irrigation with dilute formalin.

Although it is rarely seen with modern radiotherapy techniques, fibrosis of the bladder with diminished bladder capacity and urinary incontinence occasionally develops in patients treated with radical pelvic radiotherapy. Once recognized, this syndrome can usually be managed through a regimen of bladder training, in which the patient is taught to void on a regular basis and may be able to gradually increase the interval between voiding. If this regime becomes unmanageable or intolerable, however, surgical augmentation of the bladder may be performed using a segment of colon, ileum, or stomach sewn to the dome of the bladder to increase the compliance and capacity of the bladder (89).

Any patient with a current or past history of pelvic irradiation and urinary incontinence or recurrent UTIs must be carefully evaluated for the development of a ureteral, vesical, or urethral fistula. This workup usually includes physical examination, either computed tomography of the pelvis or intravenous pyelogram combined with voiding cystourethrogram, and directed cystourethroscopy by a trained urologist or other pelvic surgeon.

Effects of Chemotherapy on the Bladder

Many chemotherapeutic agents or their metabolites are irritants to the urothelium (90). The clinician needs to be aware of the most toxic agents to the urothelium: cyclophosphamide and ifosfamide. Ifosfamide is an alkylating agent that is effective in the first-line treatment of advanced-stage cervical carcinoma and uterine sarcomas and is used as second-line treatment for ovarian cancer. Ifosfamide is metabolically activated to yield cytotoxic metabolites, as well as acrolein, a highly potent bladder irritant. It is important therefore to keep the patient well hydrated during and after the infusion of ifosfamide and to concurrently administer the urothelial protectant mesna (Mesnex). Cyclophosphamide has similar toxicity in the bladder to ifosfamide, but the effect is much less at equivalent doses and vigorous hydration is generally adequate prophylaxis.

Significant and occasionally dose-limiting hematuria will develop in some patients, however. Treatment is usually with aggressive hydration and supportive care. Occasionally, patients may require cystoscopic electrocautery of the bleeding portion of bladder mucosa. If no discrete bleeding vessels are found, bladder irrigation with a dilute formalin solution may be more effective.

REFERENCES

1. Hooton TM, Stamm WE. Diagnosis and treatment of uncomplicated urinary tract infection. *Infect Dis Clin North Am* 1997;11:551–581.
2. Carr PL, Felsenstein D, Friedman RH. Evaluation and management of vaginitis. *J Gen Intern Med* 1998;13: 335–346.
3. Schaaf VM, Perez-Stable EJ, Borchardt K. The limited value of symptoms and signs in the diagnosis of vaginal infections. *Arch Intern Med* 1990;150:1929–1933.
4. Sobel JD. Vaginitis. *N Engl J Med* 1997;337:1896–1903.
5. Eschenbach DA, Hillier S, Critchlow C, et al. Diagnosis and clinical manifestations of bacterial vaginosis. *Am J Obstet Gynecol* 1988;158:819–828.
6. Hill GB. The microbiology of bacterial vaginosis. *Am J Obstet Gynecol* 1993;169:450–454.
7. Moi H. Prevalence of bacterial vaginosis and its association with genital infections, inflammation, and contraceptive methods in women attending sexually transmitted disease and primary health clinics. *Int J STD AIDS* 1990;1:86–94.
8. Gardner JJ. Comparison of the vaginal flora in sexually abused and non-abused girls. *J Pediatr* 1992;120:872–877.
9. Bump RC, Buesching WJ. Bacterial vaginosis in virginal and sexually active adolescent females: evidence against sexual transmission. *Am J Obstet Gynecol* 1988; 158:935–939.
10. Nilsson U, Hellberg D, Shoubnikova M, Nilsson S, Mardi PA. Sexual behavior risk factors associated with bacterial vaginosis and *Chlamydia trachomatis* infection. *Sex Transm Dis* 1997;24:241–246.
11. Amsel R, Tolten PA, Spiegel CA, et al. Non-specific vaginitis: diagnostic criteria and microbial and epidemiological associations. *Am J Med* 1983;74:14–22.
12. Hillier SL, Nugent RP, Eschenbach DA, et al. Association between bacterial vaginosis and preterm delivery of a low birth weight infant. *N Engl J Med* 1995;333: 1737–1742.
13. Spiegel CA, Amsel R, Holmes KK. Diagnosis of bacterial vaginosis by direct gram stain of vaginal fluid. *J Clin Microbiol* 1983;18:170–177.
14. Nugent RP, Krohn MA, Hillier SL. Reliability of diagnosing bacterial vaginosis is improved by a standardized method of gram stain interpretation. *J Clin Microbiol* 1991;29:297–301.
15. Schwebke JR, Hillier SL, Sobel JD, et al. Validity of the vaginal gram stain for the diagnosis of bacterial vaginosis. *Obstet Gynecol* 1996;88:573–576.
16. Hay PE. Therapy of bacterial vaginosis. *J Antimicrob Chemother* 1998;41:6–9.
17. Ferris DG, Litaker MS, Woodward L, et al. Treatment of bacterial vaginosis: a comparison of oral metronidazole, metronidazole vaginal gel, and clindamycin vaginal cream. *J Fam Pract* 1995;41:443–449.
18. Moi H, Erkkola R, Jerve F, et al. Should male consorts of women with bacterial vaginosis be treated? *Genitourin Med* 1989;65:263–268.
19. Vejtorp M, Bollerup AC, Vejtorp L, et al. Bacterial vaginosis: a double-blind randomized trial of the effect of treatment of the sexual partner. *Br J Obstet Gynaecol* 1988;95:920–926.
20. Heine P, McGregor JA. *Trichomonas vaginalis: a reemerging pathogen.* Clin Obstet Gynecol 1993;36: 137–144.
21. Petrin D, Delgaty K, Blatt R, Garber G. Clinical and microbiological aspects of *Trichomonas vaginalis. Clin Microbiol Rev* 1998;11:300–317.
22. Krieger JN, Tam MR, Stevens CE, et al. Diagnosis of trichomoniasis: comparison of conventional wet mount examination with cytologic studies, cultures and monoclonal antibody staining of direct specimens. *JAMA* 1988;259:1223–1227.
23. Demeo LR, Draper DL, McGregor JA, et al. Evaluation of deoxyribonucleic acid probe for the detection of *Trichomonas vaginalis* in vaginal secretions. *Am J Obstet Gynecol* 1996;174:1339–1342.
24. Cotch MF, Pastorek JG, Nugent RP, et al. *Trichomonas vaginalis* associated with low birth weight and preterm delivery. *Sex Transm Dis* 1997;24:353–360.
25. Centers for Disease Control and Prevention. 1998 Guidelines for the treatment of sexually transmitted diseases. *MMWR* 1998;47(RR-1).
26. Narcisi EM, Secor WE. *In vitro* effect of tinidazole and furaxolidone on metronidazole-resistant *Trichomonas vaginalis. Antimicrob Agents Chemother* 1996;40:1121–1125.
27. Horwitz BJ, Giaquinta D, Ito S. Evolving pathogens in vulvovaginal candidiasis: implications for patient care. *J Clin Pharmacol* 1992;32:248–255.
28. Kent HL. Epidemiology of vaginitis. *Am J Obstet Gynecol* 1991;165:1168–1176.
29. O'Connor MI, Sobel JD. Epidemiology of recurrent vulvovaginal candidiasis: identification and strain differentiation of *Candida albicans. J Infect Dis* 1986;154: 358–363.
30. Sobel JD. Epidemiology and pathogenesis of recurrent vulvovaginal candidiasis. *Am J Obstet Gynecol* 1985; 152:924–935.
31. Sobel JD. Vaginitis in adult women. *Obstet Gynecol Clin North Am* 1990;17:851–879.
32. Jovanovich R, Congema E, Nguyen HT. Antifungal agents vs. boric acid for treating chronic mycotic vulvovaginitis. *J Reprod Med* 1991;36:593–597.
33. Brown D Jr, Kaufman RH. Vulvovaginitis. In: Robert H. Glass, ed. *Office Gynecology,* 4th ed. Baltimore: Williams & Wilkins, 1993:25–54.
34. Sobel JD, Brooker D, Stein GE, et al. Single oral dose fluconazole compared with conventional clotrimazole topical therapy of *Candida* vaginitis. *Am J Obstet Gynecol* 1995;172:1263–1268.
35. Houang ET, Chappatte O, Byrne D, et al. Fluconazole levels in plasma and vaginal secretions of patients after a 150-milligram single oral dose and rate of eradication of infection in vaginal candidiasis. *Antimicrob Agents Chemother* 1990;34:909–910.
36. Vazquez JA, Sobel JD, Demitriou R, et al. Karyotyping of *Candida albicans* isolates obtained longitudinally in women with recurrent vulvovaginal candidiasis. *J Infect Dis* 1994;170:1566–1569.
37. Fidel PJ Jr, Sobel JD. Immunopathogenesis of recurrent vulvovaginal candidiasis. *Clin Microbiol Rev* 1996;9: 335–348.
38. Kamarashev JA, Vassileva SG. Dermatologic diseases of the vulva. *Clin Dermatol* 1997;15:53–65.

39. Hilton E, Chandrasekaran V, Rindos P, et al. Association of recurrent candidal vaginitis and inheritance of Lewis blood group antigens. *J Infect Dis* 1995;172: 1616–1619.
40. Pandit L, Ouslander JG. Postmenopausal vaginal atrophy and atrophic vaginitis. *Am J Med Sci* 1997;314:228–231.
41. Perez CA, Hall EJ, Purdy JA, Williamson J. Biologic and physical aspects of radiation oncology. In: Hoskins WJ, Perez CA, Young RC, eds. *Principles and practice of gynecologic oncology,* 2nd ed. Philadelphia: Lippincott–Raven Publishers, 1997:305–380.
42. Zaino RJ, Robboy SJ, Bently R, Kurman RJ. Diseases of the vagina. In: Kurman RJ, ed. *Blaustein's pathology of the female genital tract.* New York: Springer-Verlag, 1994:131–184.
43. Pitkin RM, Van Voorhis LW. Post-irradiation vaginitis: an evaluation of prophylaxis with topical estrogen. *Radiology* 1971;99:417–420.
44. Crawley WA, Grumbine FC, Dorsey JH. Flap reconstruction of the stenotic vagina. *J Am Coll Surg* 1994; 178:47–51.
45. Morrow CO, Curtin JP. *Gynecologic cancer surgery.* New York: Churchill Livingstone, 1996.
46. Landers DV, Sweet RL. Sexually transmitted infections. In: Robert H. Glass, ed. *Office Gynecology,* 4th ed. Baltimore: Williams & Wilkins, 1993:1–23.
47. Youngkin EQ. Sexually transmitted diseases: current and emerging concerns. *J Obstet Gynecol Neonatal Nurs* 1995;24:743–758.
48. Prober CG. Herpetic vaginitis in 1993. *Clin Obstet Gynecol* 1993;36:177–187.
49. Corey L, Spear PG. Infections with herpes simplex viruses. *N Engl J Med* 1986;314:749–757.
50. Woods GL. Update on laboratory diagnosis of sexually transmitted diseases. *Clin Lab Med* 1995;15:665–684.
51. Bryson YJ, Dillon MM, Lovett M, et al. Treatment of first episode of genital herpes simplex virus infections with oral acyclovir. *N Engl J Med* 1983;308:916–921.
52. Rooney JF, Straus SE, Mannix ML, et al. Oral acyclovir to suppress frequently recurrent herpes labiales: a double-blind, placebo-controlled trial. *Ann Intern Med* 1993;118:268–272.
53. Welch JM, Nayagam M, Parry G, et al. What is vestibular papillomatosis? A study of its prevalence, aetiology and natural history. *Br J Obstet Gynaecol* 1993;100: 939–942.
54. Foster DC. Vulvitis and vaginitis. *Curr Opin Obstet Gynecol* 1993;5:726–732.
55. McKay M. Vulvitis and vulvovaginitis: cutaneous considerations. *Am J Obstet Gynecol* 1991;165:1176–1182.
56. Burning vulvar syndrome: report of the International Society for the Study of Vulvar Disease. *J Reprod Med* 1984;29:457.
57. Friedrich EG Jr. Vulvar vestibulitis syndrome. *J Reprod Med* 1987;32:110–114.
58. Braggish MS, Miklos JR. Vulvar pain syndrome: a review. *Obstet Gynecol Surv* 1995;50:618–627.
59. Goetsch MF. Vulvar vestibulitis: prevalence and historic features in a general gynecologic practice population. *Am J Obstet Gynecol* 1991;164:1609–1616.
60. Pyka RE, Wilkinson EJ, Friedrich EG Jr, et al. The histopathology of vulvar vestibulitis syndrome. *Int J Gynecol Pathol* 1988;7:249–257.
61. McKay M. Dysesthetic essential vulvodynia: treatment with amitriptyline. *J Reprod Med* 1993;38:9–11.
62. Solomon CC, Melmed MH, Heitler SM. Calcium citrate for vulvar vestibulitis. *J Reprod Med* 1991;36:879–882.
63. Davis GD. The management of vulvar vestibulitis syndrome with the CO laser. *J Gynecol Surg* 1989;5:87–91.
64. Centers for Disease Control and Prevention. 1993 Sexually transmitted diseases treatment guidelines. *MMWR* 1993;42(RR-14).
65. Panke ES, Yang LI, Leist PA, et al. Comparison of Genprobe DNA test and culture for the detection of *Neisseria gonorrhoeae* in endocervical specimens *J Clin Microbiol* 1991;29:883–888.
66. Vlaspolder F, Mutsaers JAEM, Blog F, et al. Value of a DNA probe assay (Gen-probe) compared with that of a culture for diagnosis of gonococcal infection. *J Clin Microbiol* 1993;31:107–110.
67. Majeroni BA. Chlamydia cervicitis: complications and new treatment options. *Am Fam Phys* 1994;49: 1825–1832.
68. Majeroni BA, Schank JN, Horwitz M, Valenti J. Use of wet mount to predict *Chlamydia trachomatis* and *Neisseria gonorrhoeae* cervicitis in primary care. *Fam Med* 1996;28:580–583.
69. Centers for Disease Control and Prevention. Recommendations for the prevention and management of *Chlamydia trachomatis* infections 1993. *MMWR* 1993; 42(RR-12):1–39.
70. Skolnik NS. Screening for *Chlamydia trachomatis* infection. *Am Fam Phys* 1995;51:821–826.
71. Patton JP, Nash DB, Abrutyn E. Urinary tract infection: economic considerations. *Med Clin North Am* 1991;75: 495–513.
72. Ronald AR, Harding GKM. Complicated urinary tract infections. *Infect Dis Clin North Am* 1997;11:583–592.
73. Sobel JD. Pathogenesis of urinary tract infection: role of host defenses. *Infect Dis Clin North Am* 1997;11: 531–549.
74. Hooton TM, Scholes D, Hughes JP, et al. A prospective study of risk factors for symptomatic urinary tract infection in young women. *N Engl J Med* 1996;335: 468–474.
75. Stamm WE, Hooton TM. Management of urinary tract infection in adults. *N Engl J Med* 1993;329:1328–1334.
76. Hooton TM. A simplified approach to urinary tract infection. *Hosp Pract* 1995;30:23–30.
77. Pappas PG. Laboratory in the diagnosis and management of urinary tract infections. *Med Clin North Am* 1991;75:313–325.
78. Carlson KJ, Mulley AG. Management of acute dysuria: a decision analysis model of alternative strategies. *Ann Intern Med* 1985;102:244–249.
79. Nicolle LE. A practical guide to the management of complicated urinary tract infection. *Drugs* 1997;53: 583–592.
80. Hooton TM, Winter C, Tiu F, Stamm WE. Randomized comparative trial and cost analysis of 3-day antimicrobial regimens for treatment of acute cystitis in women. *JAMA* 1995;273:41–45.
81. Hooton TM, Hillier S, Johnson C, Roberts PL, Stamm WE. *Escherichia coli* bacteriuria and contraceptive method. *JAMA* 1991;265:64–69.
82. Sheinfeld J, Schaeffer AJ, Cordon-Cardo C, Rogatkoa A, Fair WR. Association of the Lewis blood group phenotype with recurrent urinary tract infections in women. *N Engl J Med* 1989;320:773–777.
83. Nicolle LE, Ronald AR. Recurrent urinary tract infec-

tion in adult women: diagnosis and treatment. *Infect Dis Clin North Am* 1987;1:793–806.
84. Raz R, Stamm WE. A controlled trial of intravaginal estriol in postmenopausal women with recurrent urinary tract infections. *N Engl J Med* 1993;329:753–756.
85. Stapleton A, Latham RH, Johnson C, Stamm WE. Postcoital antimicrobial prophylaxis for recurrent urinary tract infection: a randomized, double-blind, placebo-controlled trial. *JAMA* 1990;264:703–706.
86. Pfau A, Sacks T, Englestein D. Recurrent urinary tract infections in premenopausal women: prophylaxis based on an understanding of the pathogenesis. *J Urol* 1983; 129:1153–1157.
87. Wong ES, McKevitt M, Running K, Counts GW, Turck M, Stamm WE. Management of recurrent urinary tract infections with patient-administered single-dose therapy. *Ann Intern Med* 1985;102:302–307.
88. Zimmern PE. Bladder dysfunction after radiation and radical pelvic surgery. In: Raz S, ed. *Female urology,* 2nd ed. Philadelphia: WB Saunders, 1996:214–218.
89. Wheeless CR Jr. *Atlas of pelvic surgery,* 3rd ed. Baltimore: Williams & Wilkins, 1997.
90. Walther MM. Cystitis. In: Devita VT, Hellman S, Rosenberg SA, eds. *Cancer: principles and practice of oncology,* 4th ed. Philadelphia: JB Lippincott Co, 1993:2358–2361.

7

Breast Cancer: Gynecologic, Reproductive, and Hormonal Issues

Deborah K. Armstrong and *Edward L. Trimble

*Department of Oncology, Johns Hopkins Hospital and Johns Hopkins University School of Medicine, Baltimore, Maryland 21287; *Division of Cancer Treatment and Diagnosis, National Cancer Institute, Bethesda, Maryland 20892; and Departments of Gynecology, Obstetrics, and Oncology, Johns Hopkins University School of Medicine, Baltimore, Maryland 21287*

The breast is a reproductive organ. Not surprisingly, reproductive issues and hormonal factors influence the incidence of breast cancer and its subsequent course. In addition, treatment of breast cancer may have profound effects on reproductive, hormonal, and sexual function. Clinicians caring for women with breast cancer, including surgeons, radiation and medical oncologists, internists, obstetrician-gynecologists, nurse-midwives, and nurse-oncologists, should have an understanding of how reproductive issues interact with breast cancer.

PREGNANCY AND REPRODUCTIVE FACTORS IN BREAST CANCER

The incidence of breast cancer rises as a woman passes from decade to decade. About age 50 years, or around the time of menopause, the rate of this increase slows (1) (Fig. 1). The risk of breast cancer also appears to be linked to the length of time a woman experiences the normal adult endocrine function of the ovary. Women who have a longer period between onset of ovulation with menarche and cessation of ovulation with menopause are at increased risk for breast cancer, compared to women who experience later menarche and earlier menopause (1) (Fig. 2).

Over the last century, the median age of menarche has progressively decreased, largely due to improved nutritional factors and childhood disease prevention (2). More recently, the median age at first birth has increased due to social, economic, professional, and educational factors, as well as the availability of effective, reliable birth control. In the 16-year period from 1970 to 1986, the National Center for Health Statistics reported that the number of first births to women ages 30 to 34 years increased by 140% and by 124% to women ages 35 to 39 years (3). While early menarche alone has long been a recognized risk factor for breast cancer, it has also been postulated that the time between menarche and first birth may be a significant factor in the development of breast cancer (4). Thus, as women defer childbearing into their 30s and 40s, when breast cancer incidence begins to rise, the dual factors of increased risk of breast cancer and pregnancy at an age when breast cancer more commonly develops will overlap. These changing demographic patterns suggest that pregnancy-associated breast cancer will become more common.

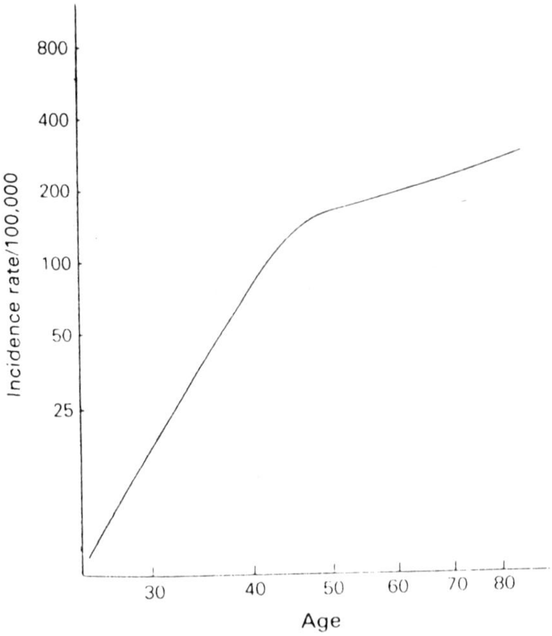

FIG. 1. Age–incidence curve of breast cancer (from data for U.S. white females 1969–1971, ref. 1).

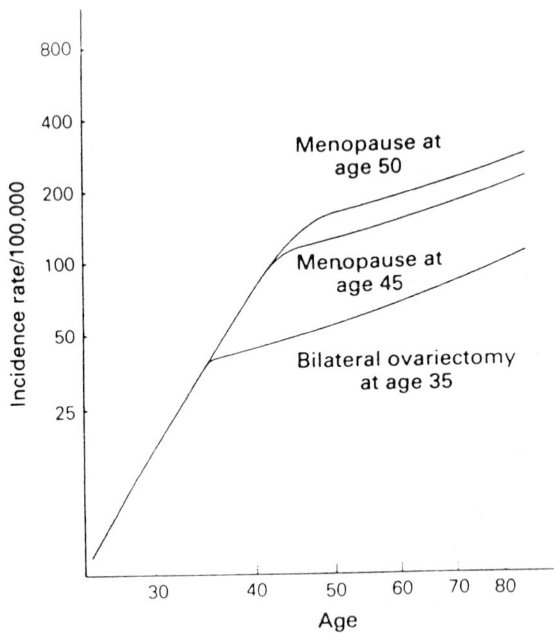

FIG. 2. Age–incidence curves of breast cancer for (working from top curve down) women with natural menopause at age 50 years, at age 45 years, and with a bilateral ovariectomy at age 35 years, respectively (with no hormone replacement therapy given to any group) (from ref.1).

Effect of Pregnancy and Hormonal Factors on Breast Cancer Risk

Young age at first pregnancy appears to convey protection against the development of breast cancer. This protection is evident when first full-term pregnancies occur before age 30 years and is strongest when a first full-term pregnancy occurs before age 20 years. First full-term pregnancy later in life appears to convey little protection and may actually be associated with an increased breast cancer risk (5,6). The beneficial effect of early first full-term pregnancy is felt to be due to the induction of differentiation of normal mammary cells. It has also been observed that the first full-term pregnancy is associated with an initial, short-term increase in breast cancer risk. This effect is most pronounced in women who are older at the time of the first delivery. This effect is felt to be due to the stimulatory effects on the breast epithelium of the markedly increased levels of bioavailable estradiol during pregnancy (7). In the long-term, however, this effect appears to be nullified by the protective effects of pregnancy-associated terminal differentiation of breast cells. In addition, each full-term birth after the first continues to reduce the risk of breast cancer, although this effect is weaker than younger age at first pregnancy.

From large studies conducted in the United States, it is unclear whether breast-feeding conveys protection against the development of breast cancer (6,8). These studies are complicated by the low cumulative number of months of nursing and the rarity of prolonged nursing. However, studies from China, where longer duration of nursing is more common, show that breast cancer risk was reduced by approximately 30% for each 5 years of nursing (9).

It has previously been hypothesized that an interrupted pregnancy might increase the risk of breast cancer due to proliferative stimulation of breast cells by hormonal changes in the first trimester but without breast cell differentiation. In a recent population-based study from Denmark, Melbye et al. (10) found no overall effect of elective abortion on the risk of breast cancer.

Oral contraceptives, when used for a long time early in life, appear to slightly increase the risk of breast cancer (8,11–13). This risk is outweighed by the decreased risk of pregnancy-associated morbidity, as well as protection from ovarian and endometrial cancer associated with the use of oral contraceptives (14). There does not appear to be an increased risk of breast cancer associated with injectable or implanted contraceptives, such as intramuscular medroxyprogesterone acetate (Depo-Provera) or levonorgestrel implants (Norplant System) (15).

Late age of natural menopause is also associated with an increased rate of breast cancer. Furthermore, women who undergo surgical removal of the ovaries before menopause have a decreased risk of breast cancer that is more profound the earlier the age of oophorectomy (16–18). This effect is felt possibly to be due to the abrupt decline in endogenous hormones associated with surgical oophorectomy in premenopausal women (18).

Estrogen replacement therapy (ERT) is associated with an increase in the risk for breast cancer (19). The use of combined estrogen and progesterone replacement does not decrease this risk. The breast cancer risk associated with menopausal ERT increases with time and, possibly, with estrogen dose. It is important to point out, however, that all-cause mortality for women using menopausal ERT is dramatically decreased. This is largely due to the beneficial effects on cardiovascular morbidity and mortality that are felt to far outweigh the carcinogenic potential of menopausal estrogen. Other positive health benefits associated with ERT include protection from osteoporosis and Alzheimer's disease, as well as control of menopausal symptoms. ERT may also cause the breasts to appear more dense on mammography, thus decreasing the sensitivity and specificity of mammography.

The information presented above points to the common etiologic factor of exposure of the breast to estrogen. More prolonged exposure or higher levels of exposure result in increased risk of breast cancer due to stimulation of these hormones on the breast epithelium, which may be exacerbated by progesterone.

Evaluation of the Breast during Pregnancy

The first prenatal visit should include a thorough breast examination, conducted both while the patient is seated and while she is lying supine. Any suspicious masses should be immediately referred to a surgeon and/or radiologist with expertise in the diagnosis of breast cancer. Masses associated with nipple retraction, fixation to skin, skin thickening, skin dimpling, or axillary lymphadenopathy are particularly worrisome. Women should be advised to report any new masses at once to their obstetrician, nurse-midwife, or family practitioner. Most breast masses diagnosed in pregnancy will turn out to be benign. The differential diagnosis includes cysts, fibroadenomas, lipomas, galactoceles, localized infarcts, and inflammation. Lactating adenomas, galactoceles, infarcts, and mastitis are generally unique to pregnancy and lactation (20).

During pregnancy, the weight of the breasts almost doubles, while blood flow increases 180%. The mammary epithelium proliferates and differentiates into mature milk-producing cells under the influence of cortisol, insulin, prolactin, estrogen, and progesterone (20). These changes make physical examination of the breast much less reliable for both the patient and the clinician.

Bloody nipple discharges are common during pregnancy and lactation. They should be evaluated with cytologic study of the discharge. If the discharge is associated with a mass, then the mass should be evaluated as described below. If the cytology is unremarkable and there are no associated masses, then a woman with a bloody nipple discharge may be observed for 1 to 2 months after delivery. If the discharge persists, then it should be evaluated with mammography postpartum.

With proper abdominal shielding, mammography can be performed with minimal fetal radiation exposure. However, increased breast density during pregnancy limits the clinical utility of mammography. Max and Klamer (21) examined mammograms of eight pregnant women with biopsy-proven carcinomas and found that the malignancies were detectable in only two cases. Thus, although not absolutely contraindicated, mammography appears to be relatively less sensitive in the gravid breast. Furthermore, a negative mammogram in a pregnant patient with a breast mass should not be considered reassuring, nor should it delay further evaluation of the mass. Ultrasound may be useful in determining whether a mass is cystic or solid and in guiding biopsy. Although breast magnetic resonance (MR) imaging appears to be safe, the role of MR imaging in evaluating breast masses has not been established in the general population.

As in nonpregnant patients, fine-needle aspiration (FNA) will help distinguish a cystic mass from a solid mass. FNA cytology in pregnancy may yield a false-positive result, however, due to cellular atypia as a result of hormonal influences (22). Novotny et al. (22) reported a series of 25 pregnant women with breast masses who underwent FNA. They diagnosed nine lactating adenomas, seven fibroadenomas with lactational change, five galactoceles, two infiltrating duct carcinomas, one juvenile fibroadenoma with lactational change, and one case with atypical reactive duct cells with lactational change.

A solid breast mass diagnosed in pregnancy should be promptly evaluated via an open biopsy. Because of increased vascularity, biopsy of the pregnant or lactating breast requires meticulous hemostasis. Local anesthesia, while safe, may be challenging in the enlarged breast. Stopping lactation before a biopsy will decrease the risk of infection and milk fistula. Binding the breasts, applying ice packs to the breasts, and ceasing to breastfeed will generally stop lactation. Bromocriptine mesylate (Parlodel) can also be used to lower prolactin levels. If a woman chooses to continue lactation, then she should pump and discard her breast milk for the 24 hours after surgery. This will protect the infant from potential exposure to perioperative antibiotics or anesthetic agents.

Several retrospective series have documented frequent delays in diagnosis of pregnancy-associated breast cancer. Petrek et al. (23), for example, found that more than one-half of patients diagnosed with breast cancer postpartum had breast masses that had been palpated during pregnancy. Those masses diagnosed postpartum were larger (mean diameter, 3.5 cm) than those diagnosed during pregnancy (mean diameter, 2 cm). These delays are thought due to the difficulty in appreciating breast lumps in enlarged breasts, the clinicians' and the patients' lack of suspicion for breast cancer, and a presumptive diagnosis of mastitis during lactation.

Treatment of Breast Cancer during Pregnancy

A diagnosis of breast cancer during pregnancy is obviously devastating to a patient and her family and will present difficult medical, ethical, and emotional issues for her and her health care providers. When approaching a pregnant breast-cancer patient, it is important for clinicians to consider her, the pregnancy, the fetus, and the disease process. All treatment options and alternatives must be carefully laid out. The risks of any procedure or therapy, including the risks of delaying or deferring these treatments, must be discussed. This approach requires a multidisciplinary team that may include an obstetrician, a breast surgeon, a medical oncologist, a radiation oncologist, and a pediatrician. In some cases, a medical ethics committee may become involved.

Pregnancy-associated breast cancer is defined as breast cancer diagnosed during pregnancy or within 1 year postpartum. As discussed previously, the postponement of childbearing not only increases the risk for breast cancer but results in a larger number of women who are becoming pregnant in their 30s and 40s when breast cancer is more common. Thus, the incidence of pregnancy-associated breast cancer will undoubtedly continue to rise. Currently, about 15% of breast cancer occurs in women of childbearing age (24). When pregnancy and breast cancer occur together, they do so almost always in women between ages 25 and 40 years. If the average woman has two pregnancies, she would be pregnant for 18 of the 180 months between ages 25 and 40 years, or 10% of the total time at risk for breast cancer in this period. As a number of authors have pointed about, the incidence of pregnancy among young women with breast cancer is in fact about 10%; thus, it does not appear that breast cancer in premenopausal women is more common during pregnancy (24). The overall incidence of pregnancy-related breast cancer is low, however, and has been estimated to occur in 1 in 3000 to 1 in 10,000 pregnancies (25).

Once breast cancer is diagnosed, the clinician must decide what further imaging studies to recommend for staging. The most common sites of metastatic breast cancer are the liver, lung, bone, brain, and adrenal glands. In the absence of neurologic signs or symptoms, imaging of the central nervous system is not recommended. A chest radiograph can be obtained using pelvic and abdominal shielding. Hepatic ultrasound can be considered if liver imaging is desired. In nonpregnant patients with apparent early-stage breast cancer, a bone scan is rarely revealing. Measurement of serum alkaline phosphatase may be misleading, as it is frequently elevated in pregnancy. Conventional radiographs of symptomatic bony sites at a distance from the abdomen and pelvis can also be considered. For pregnant patients with symptoms of bone pain or with more advanced disease, a bone scan may be obtained in the third trimester or postpartum. Low-back pain is frequent in the second and third trimesters of pregnancy, however, and should not automatically trigger a bone scan. If symptoms or abnormal laboratory studies indicate further evaluation for possible metastatic disease, MR imaging may be helpful. MR imaging can be particularly helpful in evaluating the spine, other bony sites, and the brain, if indicated, and in confirming suspicious lesions detected by ultrasound or conventional radiographs. Recent reports suggest that fetal exposure to MR imaging have not been associated with any adverse events.

The first issue to be discussed with a patient is termination of the pregnancy. This is clearly a complex decision, but even patients with a strong moral or religious objection to elective termination of pregnancy should be aware that this is a medical option. Although reports on elective termination of pregnancy are small and anecdotal, there is no evidence that termination has any beneficial influence on disease outcome. It will, however, simplify breast cancer treatment decisions. Many patients will elect to terminate pregnancy to minimize the largely unknown factors associated with cancer diagnosis and treatment in pregnancy. Decisions regarding termination should be individualized, based primarily on the wishes of the patient.

Patients with apparent localized disease should undergo surgery. There is now an extensive body of literature documenting the safety of anesthesia during pregnancy. Up to 2% of pregnant women undergo anesthesia for nonobstetric surgery (25). As discussed above, meticulous hemostasis is necessary in the enlarged breast. From 24 gestational weeks onward, obstetric monitoring for uterine contractions and fetal heart rate should be performed at time of surgery and for several hours afterward.

If breast cancer is diagnosed in the first or second trimester of pregnancy, then continuing the pregnancy precludes breast-conserving surgery with radiation. It is clear that the dosage of radiation used during breast radiation therapy results in unacceptable exposure to the fetus. Standard radiation to the breast and axilla will deliver 5000 cGy, from which a fetus in the first trimester will receive 10 to 15 cGy. In the third trimester, the fetus could receive as much as 200 cGy. Even with shielding, the internal scatter from maternal bones will deliver a significant amount of radiation to the developing fetus (27). Microcephaly, growth retardation, congenital malformations, and spontaneous abortion have been observed with fetal exposures higher than 5 cGy (28).

In addition to concerns about fetal radiation exposure, it may not be prudent to extrapolate to pregnant patients data regarding lumpectomy and radiation in nonpregnant patients. The gravid breast has markedly increased vascularity, as well as changes in lymphatic and ductal architecture, that may predispose to spread of disease within the breast. There are in fact no data regarding the efficacy of breast-conserving therapy in pregnant women. For these reasons, modified radical mastectomy is generally recommended for pregnant breast cancer patients, and breast-conserving therapy is not routinely employed during pregnancy.

Radiation therapy may also be recommended after mastectomy for patients with multiple positive lymph nodes or other risk factors for increased local recurrence, such as pectoral muscle involvement, positive surgical margins, or locally advanced (stage III) tumors. The dosage of radiation used postmastectomy is similar to that used after breast-conserving therapy, and the same precautions apply. For these patients, radiation therapy is deferred until after pregnancy or until late in pregnancy when the risk to the fetus is lessened.

Patients with locally advanced disease at the time of diagnosis should be treated with neoadjuvant chemotherapy (see below) followed by surgery. Patients should receive appropriate and coordinated counseling from their obstetrician, surgeon, oncologist, and neonatologist on these issues (25).

Adjuvant systemic therapy is recommended for many patients with stage I and most patients with stage II breast cancer. For most premenopausal patients, chemotherapy is recommended because tumors in these patients are less commonly hormone receptor–positive. There is very little information about steroid hormone receptors during pregnancy, and one may question the accuracy of the few available data. Elevated estrogen and progesterone levels in pregnancy may result in down-regulation of steroid hormone receptors. In addition, some assays require that receptors be unbound from ligand; thus, the elevated hormone levels encountered during pregnancy may result in false-negative receptor assays (25). The efficacy of hormonally directed therapy in pregnancy-associated breast cancer is brought into question by one series of 32 patients with pregnancy-associated breast cancer, none of whom responded to oophorectomy (29). Tamoxifen citrate (Nolvadex), the most commonly used hormonal agent for the treatment of breast cancer was originally developed as an abortifacient. The safety of tamoxifen in pregnancy has not been established. For these reasons, hormonal therapy is not generally recommended for pregnant breast cancer patients. Women diagnosed with breast cancer during pregnancy should receive adjuvant chemotherapy for the same indications as nonpregnant women with breast cancer (30).

Chemotherapy during pregnancy presents clear concerns regarding the safety to the fetus. Chemotherapy administered to the mother will enter the fetal circulation via the placenta (31). While there are few firm data regarding chemotherapy during pregnancy, several points have become clear. The first is that, when possible, chemotherapy should be avoided during the first trimester of pregnancy. While the risk of delaying chemotherapy until the second trimester is unknown, it is clear that the teratogenic effects of chemotherapeutic agents are most potent during early fetal development. The rapidly dividing cells of early fetal development are more sensitive to cytotoxic agents. In the first 2 weeks after conception, the blastocyst is relatively resistant because circulation is not yet established. *In utero* drug exposure shortly after circulation develops may result in spontaneous abortion. Organogenesis extends from the fifth to the tenth gestational weeks. During this time, 10% to 20% of fetuses exposed to chemotherapeutic agents will have major congenital malformations, compared with 3% of fetuses in the general population (32). During the second and third trimesters, exposure to chemotherapeutic agents does not cause significant malformations but can impair fetal growth and development (31). Retrospective studies suggest that infants exposed to chemotherapy in the second and third trimesters do face an increased risk for low birthweight.

While any chemotherapeutic agent may be teratogenic, folic acid antagonists, such as methotrexate, which is used for the treatment of ectopic pregnancies and gestational trophoblastic disease, have been more frequently associated with fetal abnormalities during the first trimester than any other agents. The folic acid antagonists should be avoided altogether during pregnancy (31). While some combination chemotherapy regimens for the treatment of breast cancer use methotrexate, such as cyclophosphamide, methotrexate, and 5-fluorouracil (CMF), equal or improved efficacy can be obtained using a non–methotrexate-containing regimen such as doxorubicin (Adriamycin) and cyclophosphamide (AC).

Supportive care during chemotherapy will need to be tailored to pregnant patients. Use of blood transfusions or erythropoietin may be necessary to maintain maternal hematocrit at about 25% to 30%. Antibiotics typically used during aplasia or for the treatment of neutropenic fevers may need to be modified in pregnant patients.

There is no reason why a wanted pregnancy cannot be continued until term. Effective coordination among the oncologist, the obstetrician, and the neonatologist will facilitate the appropriate treatment of a woman's cancer and the timely delivery of a healthy infant. It is reasonable to alter the normal schedule of chemotherapy administration to facilitate safe delivery of the infant. Sufficient time should have elapsed since chemotherapy administration to ensure drug clearance from the fetal circulation because neonatal organs may be incapable of metabolizing or excreting any remaining drug that might have otherwise been cleared by the placenta and maternally metabolized. In addition, the risk for maternal peripartum bleeding or infection should be minimized by timing chemotherapy so that hematologic recovery has taken place by the time of delivery. These arrangements may require delivery by induction of labor at or near term or by elective cesarean section to maximize safety and minimize treatment delays.

Long-term data on children exposed to chemotherapeutic agents *in utero* are not available (33). As noted above, children exposed to chemotherapy in the second and third trimesters of pregnancy appear to have minimal risk of teratogenesis, although there does appear to be an increased risk of low birthweight. Zemlickis et al. (34) found a statistically significant lower mean birthweight, lower mean gestational age, and higher rate of preterm birth among babies born to mothers with breast cancer compared to matched control mothers who had been exposed to nonteratogenic drugs or chemicals.

Concern has been raised about the possible transmission of tumor to the fetus. While there have been reports of fetal metastases from melanoma and sarcoma, there have been no reports of fetal metastases from breast cancer. However, the placenta has been reported as a site of metastatic breast cancer and should be carefully examined both grossly and microscopically, as the presence of placental metastasis from breast cancer may have a significant impact on future therapy and maternal prognosis.

Few prospective or retrospective data on the long-term consequences of exposure to chemotherapy *in utero* are available. Of particular concern are potential late effects on growth, intellectual function, pubertal development, and reproductive function. It is important that these children should have careful medical follow-up with close attention to physical and intellectual development. Dr. John Mulvihill at the University of Pittsburgh (phone: 412-624-9951; fax: 412-624-3020; e-mail: jjm@helix.hgen.pitt.edu) maintains a registry of children who experienced *in utero* chemotherapeutic drug exposure.

Impact of Pregnancy on Breast Cancer Outcome

In retrospective studies, women diagnosed with breast cancer during pregnancy or in the postpartum period have the same survival as age-matched nonpregnant peers after adjustment for stage at diagnosis. Petrek et al. (23) reported 10-year survival of 77% for pregnant patients with negative lymph nodes, compared to 75% for nonpregnant women with negative lymph nodes. Zemlickis et al. (34) reported identical survival for 102 pregnant women with breast cancer and 269 controls matched for age, stage, and other prognostic factors (Fig. 3). As mentioned above, however, women diagnosed with breast cancer during pregnancy are more likely to present with larger tumors, higher stage, and more frequent metastatic disease than those who are not pregnant (34). Women with pregnancy-related breast cancer are more likely to have lymph node involvement than those who are not pregnant. In addition, younger women with breast cancer have a worse prognosis stage for stage than older women. Younger women, both pregnant and nonpregnant, are also more likely to have estrogen receptor (ER)–negative tumors than older women. Thus, a young woman's stage and tumor characteristics at diagnosis of breast cancer determine her risks for recurrence and survival, while the coincidental pregnancy has little effect on prognosis.

Pregnancy after Breast Cancer

Given the increasing number of women who are deferring childbearing and the frequency of breast cancer in premenopausal women, it should not be surprising that many women may wish to become pregnant after completing therapy for breast cancer. Pregnancy after breast cancer can be an emotion-laden topic for patients and health care providers, as the women face the prospect of bearing and raising children with a potentially limited life expectancy. The specter of a breast cancer recurrence during pregnancy or in a patient with a young child may prompt both patients and physicians to avoid pregnancy after breast cancer. However, for many women, bearing children may be a hallmark of return to normalcy, and they will seek advice from

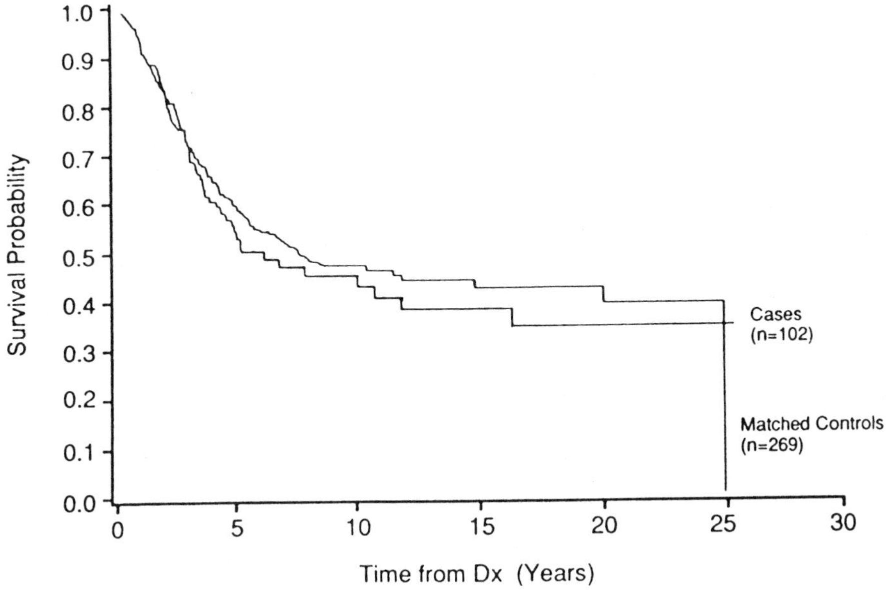

FIG. 3. Kaplan-Meier cause-specific survival curve for breast cancer comparing women who were pregnant and had breast cancer (n=102) against matched nonpregnant controls (n=269) (p=0.6).

health care providers about the potential risks pregnancy may pose for disease recurrence and their chances for successful conception and delivery.

For many years, women were counseled to avoid pregnancy after a diagnosis of breast cancer because of a possible adverse disease outcome due to the hormonal changes of pregnancy. The profound changes in estrogen and progesterone were hypothesized to permit the growth of occult, otherwise quiescent breast cancer cells. The main determinant of hormone sensitivity is the presence or absence of hormone receptors detected in breast cancers at the time of diagnosis. Although premenopausal patients are less likely than postmenopausal patients to have detectable hormone receptors on their tumors, a substantial number of young women diagnosed in the reproductive years will have tumors that are positive for ER or progesterone receptor (PR). Their disease course has the potential to be affected by hormonal factors, including pregnancy.

Clinical data regarding the risks of pregnancy after breast cancer are hampered by small numbers. Many premenopausal women will cease menstruation as a result of the ovarian effects of chemotherapy (see below). Furthermore, it has been estimated that only 7% of women who are fertile postmastectomy will have children (24). With few clinical data available, however, it appears that subsequent pregnancy does not affect the risk of breast cancer recurrence. In a study from the Danish Breast Cancer Cooperative Group, Kroman et al. (35) reported on 5725 women with breast cancer who were 45 years of age or younger at time of diagnosis. Information on subsequent pregnancies was obtained from national birth and abortion registries. Women were followed for a total of 35,067 patient-years. After adjustment for age, stage, and reproductive history before diagnosis, women who had a full-term pregnancy after breast cancer treatment had a nonsignificantly reduced risk of death, compared to women who had no subsequent pregnancy. However in this study, only 173 (3%) of the 5725 women became pregnant. Other reports in the literature have primarily been single-institution, retrospective studies. Sutton et al. (36) reported 33 pregnancies among 25 breast cancer survivors. The median interval between the completion of chemotherapy and pregnancy was 12 months. Of the 25 women who became pregnant, recurrence of breast cancer developed in seven women and three died. Compared to their peers who did not experience pregnancy, disease-free and overall survival was not adversely affected by pregnancy. Von Schoultz et al. (37) reported good survival among 50 women with breast cancer who subsequently became pregnant. Malamos et al. (38) reported 21 women who became pregnant after treatment for breast cancer diagnosed when they were younger than age 35. The majority (17 of 21) had adjuvant chemotherapy after lumpectomy or mastectomy. Seven chose to terminate the pregnancies, while 14 delivered 16 healthy children. At a median age of 51 months, all children had normal growth. Three patients experienced cancer recurrences, and one patient had a primary ovarian cancer 5 years after mastectomy. Recurrence rates and survival did not differ from women of the same age who did not become pregnant. Clark and Chua (39) reported a 71% 5-year survival rate among 136 patients with stage I to III disease who subsequently became pregnant. Danforth (40) summarized eight prior studies and identified a 71.5% 5-year survival rate among 465 women with breast cancer who subsequently became pregnant. None of these studies demonstrated an effect of hormone-receptor status on relapse.

Many clinicians have held the belief that the rate of recurrence of breast cancer is highest in the first 2 years after treatment. Thus, health care providers have sometimes recommended that women wait 2 or more years following the diagnosis of breast cancer before attempting pregnancy. While rapid recurrence may be the rule for patients with aggressive tumors, locally advanced disease, or multiple positive lymph nodes, the annual risk of recurrence of node-negative breast cancer is generally linear over the first 10 to 12 years after treatment (41). Such recommendations have led to the general impression among both lay and medical communities that pregnancy would itself increase the risk of recurrence. It would seem more appropriate to inform a woman who had been treated for breast cancer of her risk of recurrence based on her stage at diagnosis and other prognostic factors and of the fact that there is currently no evidence that pregnancy affects this risk. Furthermore, for many women, such delays may compromise fertility.

HORMONAL EFFECTS OF CHEMOTHERAPEUTIC AGENTS

Chemotherapeutic agents are known to affect ovarian function, although the magnitude of this effect and its implications for therapeutic outcome, long-term toxicities, and quality-of-life issues are not always clearly appreciated. This is of particular importance for premenopausal women undergoing adjuvant chemotherapy for breast cancer, a group that has grown dramatically in numbers over the last two decades. In the face of a life-threatening disease such as breast cancer, the significance of the hormonal effects of treatment may be underestimated. However, as these women approach life after chemotherapy, addressing issues such as reproductive capacity, menopause, and sexual function, the effect of their treatment on hormonal function takes on a more profound importance.

Mechanism of Ovarian Toxicity of Chemotherapeutic Agents

Oogenesis occurs exclusively *in utero.* The ovarian toxicity of chemotherapeutic agents is primarily against replicating follicular cells rather than nonreplicating germ cells. In ovulating, premenopausal women, follicular cells are damaged by exposure to cytotoxic drugs. This results in decreased estrogen and progesterone secretion and a resultant increase in follicle-stimulating hormone (FSH) and luteinizing hormone (LH). The increased gonadotropin levels in turn lead to accelerated follicular recruitment. Further exposure at this time results in a cycle of increased follicular cell damage and ultimately progressive deterioration of ovarian function. Since follicular cell reserve is a function of age, older patients will be more likely to experience permanent primary ovarian failure with exposure of chemotherapeutic agents.

Alkylating agents are a mainstay of most chemotherapeutic regimens in use for treatment of breast cancer. These drugs appear to bear the primary responsibility for ovarian ablation. Cyclophosphamide is the agent most commonly linked to destruction of ovarian follicles. (42,43). Cyclophosphamide alone causes premature ovarian failure. Koyama et al. (42) demonstrated that 15 of 18 premenopausal breast cancer patients who received 8.4 to 39.9 g of cyclophosphamide developed permanent amenorrhea. Damewood and Grochow (44) also reported premature ovarian failure in more than one-half of patients treated with cyclophosphamide at doses of 40 to 120 mg per day. It appears that both total cumulative dose and the duration of therapy, as well as patient age, are key factors in the development of permanent ovarian failure (42,45).

Most adjuvant chemotherapy regimens involve the use of a combination of chemotherapy drugs, the two most common being CMF and AC. Few data are available on the gonadal toxicity of doxorubicin alone. However, in the treatment of Hodgkin's disease, doxorubicin-containing combination chemotherapy regimens have not been associated with ovarian failure (46). Methotrexate and 5-fluorouracil also do not appear to induce permanent ovarian failure either alone or in combinations without alkylating agents (42,47). The largest body of data regarding combination chemotherapy–associated amenorrhea in breast cancer is with the CMF regimen.

To date, no effective method of ovarian protection against chemotherapeutic agents has been identified, although both oral contraceptives and gonadotropin-releasing hormome (Gn-RH) analogs have been used in such an effort. It is possible that the combined use of oral contraceptives and Gn-RH analogs may provide more complete ovarian suppression, although this has not been rigorously tested. In the treatment of breast cancer, however, use of estrogen and progesterone, as in oral contraceptives, would be contraindicated. Harvest of ovarian tissue before chemotherapy with subsequent reimplantation after chemotherapy has been proposed for young women strongly desiring to retain fertility. Such a technique, however, has not been validated in a large, multicenter evaluation.

Menopause Induced by Chemotherapeutic Agents

As noted above, adjuvant chemotherapy commonly results in amenorrhea. Although ovulation and menstruation may resume in some women, standard adjuvant chemotherapy may result in permanent ovarian failure in many women. Such ovarian ablation is more common with increasing age at the time of adjuvant chemotherapy. For CMF, amenorrhea occurs in 94% of women older than age 45 years, in 84% of women aged 35 to 44 years, and in 53% of women younger than 35 years (48). In 86% of women younger than 40 years and in 96% of women age 40 or older, this amenorrhea is permanent. Very young women, those younger 30 years, may have no menstrual abnormalities (43). An inverse relation has also been noted between age and duration of treatment required to induce ovarian suppression, with older women experiencing amenorrhea after a shorter duration of therapy (49). Since breast cancer incidence increases with age, it must be kept in mind that even within the category of premenopausal patients, the largest numbers of patients will be found in the older age ranges. Thus, it is estimated that, overall, 60% to 80% of premenopausal breast cancer patients will experience permanent ovarian failure with adjuvant chemotherapy. As discussed below, ovarian ablation caused by adjuvant chemotherapy often has a negative impact on sexual functioning (50).

Potential Therapeutic Effects of Chemotherapy-induced Menopause

It was recognized as early as the 1960s that adjuvant chemotherapy for treatment of breast cancer was more effective in delaying the onset of treatment failures in premenopausal than in postmenopausal patients (51). Since that time similar findings have been replicated in a large number of clinical trials. It was also observed that many premenopausal patients will cease menstruating and undergo menopause as a result of adjuvant chemotherapy. These observations led to the hypothesis that the effects of chemotherapy on ovarian function might be responsible for some of the therapeutic effects of chemotherapy.

It seems likely that the beneficial effects of adjuvant chemotherapy cannot be attributed to the induction of early menopause alone. If the benefits of chemotherapy in premenopausal patients were due solely to induction of ovarian failure, patients with hormone receptor–negative tumors would not be expected to benefit. It is clear, however, that these patients do benefit from adjuvant chemotherapy. The Milan group tested CMF in premenopausal patients with ER-negative tumors and found significantly improved disease-free and overall survival (46). Furthermore, even when chemotherapy-induced ovarian failure is associated with a survival advantage, this advantage is not confined to patients with receptor-positive tumors. In a trial from the Eastern Cooperative Oncology Group, development of amenorrhea was associated with an improvement in survival (52). This improvement was more significant for ER-negative than for ER-positive patients.

If all the beneficial effects of adjuvant chemotherapy in premenopausal patients are due to ovarian suppression, then older women, who are more likely to have ovarian function affected by chemotherapy, should have greater benefit. Fisher et al. (51) compared women age 39 years or younger with women 40 to 49 years of age who were entered in a trial comparing adjuvant chemotherapy to placebo. Amenorrhea occurred in only 22% of women in the younger age group compared with 73% in the older age group. However, women in the younger age group showed a greater improvement in 4-year disease-free survival—32% (placebo) versus 69% (chemotherapy)—than did those in the older age group—48% (placebo) versus 61% (chemotherapy). Thus, while the beneficial effects of chemotherapy were more profound in the younger patients, the ovarian effects of chemotherapy were more profound in the older premenopausal patients. Evidence that adjuvant chemotherapy does not work by ovarian ablation alone comes from data from some studies indicating that surgical oophorectomy does not improve outcome (53,54). Finally, although the effects are less pronounced than in premenopausal patients, it is clear that postmenopausal patients derive benefit from adjuvant chemotherapy, indicating that therapeutic response in this group is not mediated via hormonal effects (49).

When premenopausal patients are counseled regarding adjuvant chemotherapy, it is imperative that they understand both the short-term and long-term hormonal effects of this therapy. Table 1 provides a summary of the salient points to be made in such a discussion. First, the risk of chemotherapy-induced ovarian failure is related to patient age, with older patients being at highest risk. Second, the risk may be related to the specific drugs used, their dosage, and the duration of therapy. Third, even patients who continue to menstruate or have return of normal menses may have compromised fertility. Fourth, the

TABLE 1. *Issues of note in the counseling of patients regarding the risk of chemotherapy and ovarian failure*

Risk of ovarian failure increases with patient age.
Risk of ovarian failure depends on the chemotherapeutic agents used, the drug dosage, and the duration of therapy.
Women who maintain normal menses or who have return of normal menses may still have impaired fertility and early onset of menopause.
The effects of premature ovarian failure include increased risks for osteoporosis, heart disease, sexual dysfunction, and Alzheimer's disease.
Ovarian failure has potential beneficial effects on the risk of breast cancer recurrence.

effects of premature ovarian failure must be discussed. Finally, there may be beneficial effects of ovarian ablation on survival.

HORMONAL THERAPY OF BREAST CANCER

Adjuvant hormonal therapy has been shown to decrease the risk of relapse, primarily in older postmenopausal patients and those with ER-positive tumors. Hormonal therapy is also used in the treatment of overt metastatic breast cancer. In the setting of metastatic disease, breast cancer is not curable with current therapies. Thus, palliation of symptoms becomes the focus of treatment for many patients. Given the lower toxicity profile of hormonal therapy in comparison with chemotherapy, this is the initial approach in women who are predicted to respond to such treatment.

Indications for Hormonal Therapy

One of the most important characteristics determining whether or not hormonal therapy is appropriate for treatment of a patient with breast cancer is the hormone-receptor status of the tumor. Although there is some controversy as to the exact subcellular location of unbound ER protein, it is clear that the nucleus is the primary site of action of activated ER. When lipid-soluble estrogen diffuses passively into the cell, it binds to ER. This estrogen–ER complex then binds to hormone-response elements on deoxyribonucleic acid that control transcription of specific target genes. One such estrogen-regulated gene is the progesterone-receptor (PgR) gene. A cell with a functional, activated ER would be expected to express PgR. For this reason, breast tumor tissue that expresses ER but not PgR may have mutated or nonfunctional ER and thus be less hormone-responsive. Conversely, the rare tumor specimen that expresses PgR but not ER may have a false-negative ER if PgR synthesis is indeed estrogen-dependent. Table 2 summarizes the distribution of ER and PgR in primary breast tumors and the response to endocrine therapy based on ER and PgR in women with advanced, measurable disease. It should be noted that, besides PgR, there are a number of ER target genes, such as the transforming growth factors α and β and insulin-like growth factors, that may be mediators of estrogen action and may, in the future, provide prognostic information or function as therapeutic targets.

TABLE 2. *Distribution of ER and PgR in breast cancer and response to endocrine therapy by receptor status*

Receptor status	Patients (%)	Response rate (%)
ER+, PgR+	35–45	65–75
ER+, PgR–	25–35	30–35
ER–, PgR+	<5	35–45
ER–, PgR–	25–30	10

ER, estrogen receptor; PgR, progesterone receptor.

Ovarian Ablation as Hormonal Therapy of Breast Cancer

It has been over 100 years since Beatson performed the first surgical oophorectomy to treat inoperable breast cancer. The goal of castration is to prevent hormone production by the functioning ovary. Thus, the benefits of this therapy are limited to post- or perimenopausal women who retain ovarian function. Until recently, surgery or radiotherapy were the only means of ovarian ablation. Recently, luteinizing hormone–releasing hormone (LH-RH) analogs have shown promise as a means of achieving a medical oophorectomy. These drugs are thought to function, at least in part, by persistent and prolonged stimulation of the pituitary LH-RH receptor, ultimately leading to inhibition of receptor function. Treatment is therefore associated with an early, transient surge in LH and FSH levels followed by prolonged gonadotropin inhibition. The fall in serum estradiol levels seen with this treatment is ascribable to this indirect pituitary effect, as well as a possible direct inhibitory effect on ovarian estradiol release.

Ovarian ablation appears to be associated with a survival benefit in breast cancer patients. In some individual trials, as well as a large metaanalysis, ovarian ablation appears to convey both recurrence-free and overall survival advantage among premenopausal women. This advantage persisted even in the presence of adjuvant chemotherapy (41,52, 55–58). As expected, older, postmenopausal patients had no significant benefit from this therapeutic approach. Although oophorectomy is both effective and well tolerated as treatment for premenopausal patients, these patients will also respond to antiestrogen therapy such as tamoxifen. Several randomized studies comparing oophorectomy to tamoxifen have failed to show a clear benefit of one therapy over the other with regard to response rate, duration of response, or survival.

Pharmacologic Agents for Hormonal Therapy of Breast Cancer

For postmenopausal breast cancer patients, the most commonly employed endocrine therapy is tamoxifen. Tamoxifen, a synthetic antiestrogen, has been shown to decrease the incidence of new primary breast cancer in women at high risk for breast cancer, to reduce the risk of recurrence and death when given as adjuvant therapy after primary surgery for localized breast cancer, and to effect a 30% to 50% response rate in women with metastatic disease (59,60). Tamoxifen exerts its antitumor activity by binding to ER protein and competitively inhibiting estrogen action. In estrogen-dependent tumors, this blockade of estrogen action results in growth arrest (cytostatic effect) and possibly tumor cell death (cytotoxic effect). Although it is clear that tamoxifen blocks estrogen binding in human breast tumors, it has additional non–receptor-mediated mechanisms of action that may include modulation of growth factor secretion and altered immune function. These latter mechanisms may explain the activity of tamoxifen in patients whose tumors lack ER expression.

In addition to being a competitive estrogen inhibitor, tamoxifen may act in some tissues as a partial estrogen agonist. Tamoxifen, for example, increases lumbar spine and hip mineral density among postmenopausal women. Among premenopausal women, however, tamoxifen has been reported to decrease bone mineral density in these areas (61,62). Tamoxifen also appears to convey some protection against coronary heart disease. Costantino et al. (63) reported that tamoxifen appears to reduce the hazard rate of death from definite fatal heart disease to 0.66, compared to placebo. Although this difference was not statistically significant, it is consistent with other reports of slightly decreased coronary heart disease among women taking tamoxifen.

The estrogenic activity of tamoxifen may explain the increase in endometrial cancer associated with tamoxifen use in some series. Women taking tamoxifen appear to have an increased incidence of endometrial polyps, endometrial hyperplasia, and endometrial cancer. The risk for endometrial cancer appears to be 1 per 1000 women per year (64). Thus, a woman who takes tamoxifen for 5 years would have a 0.5% chance for the development of endometrial cancer. Women in whom endometrial cancer develops while taking tamoxifen appear to have the same spectrum of histologies noted among women not taking tamoxifen (65).

There is no indication for routine endometrial sampling in women taking tamoxifen (66). In addition, as tamoxifen has a proliferative effect on endometrial stroma, transvaginal ultrasound will not accurately determine the endometrial thickness. The finding of an endometrial stripe of 5 mm or less is reassuring but does not guarantee a normal uterine cavity. Women in whom abnormal bleeding or spotting develops while taking tamoxifen should be evaluated with hysteroscopy or saline-infusion sonography. Use of a progesterone-releasing intrauterine device (IUD) (Progestasert) to counteract endometrial stimulation by tamoxifen is currently under investigation.

About one-half of premenopausal women taking tamoxifen will continue to ovulate. Of those women in whom amenorrhea develops while taking tamoxifen, almost 90% will resume normal ovulation after stopping tamoxifen. Premenopausal women taking tamoxifen should be encouraged to use effective contraception. Tamoxifen is generally a very well tolerated drug with mild vasomotor symptoms of estrogen withdrawal, such as hot flashes and night sweats, particularly in the pre- or perimenopausal patient. Other, more serious toxicities include endometrial and liver cancer, thrombophlebitis, keratopathy, and optic neuritis.

Tamoxifen is the first in a family of drugs now referred to as selective estrogen-receptor modulators (SERMs). In clinical trials of tamoxifen versus placebo, it was noted that the incidence of contralateral, second primary breast cancers was reduced in women taking tamoxifen. This led to the concept that tamoxifen might play a role in breast cancer prevention. To test this hypothesis, the National Surgical Adjuvant Breast and Bowel Project (NSABP) initiated the Breast Cancer Prevention Trial (BCPT) in 1992 (67). In this trial, women with an elevated risk of breast cancer were randomly assigned to receive placebo or tamoxifen, 20 mg per day. Tamoxifen reduced the risk of invasive breast cancer by 49% and the risk of noninvasive breast cancer by 50%. The decreased risk occurred in women in all age groups and in those with any category of predicted 5-year risk. The reduction in breast cancer was limited to ER-positive tumors; no difference was noted in the occurrence of ER-negative tumors. Tamoxifen administration did not alter the incidence of ischemic heart disease; however, a reduction in fractures was observed. Endometrial cancer incidence was increased in the tamoxifen group. In addition, the rates of thromboembolic vascular events, such as stroke, pulmonary embolism, and deep vein thrombosis, were elevated in the tamoxifen group. Two other trials of tamoxifen as a preventive agent for breast cancer have been reported. These trials are smaller than the BCPT and had significantly different eligibility criteria. The Italian trial was limited to women who had had a hysterectomy and no identifiable risk factors for breast cancer (68). The British trial limited eligibility to women with a strong family history of breast cancer (62). In both of these European trials, women were allowed to take estrogen along with tamoxifen. Neither trial documented a decrease in breast cancer with tamoxifen. Table 3 summarizes the data from these three trials.

Raloxifene (Evista), a second member of the SERM family, is approved for the treatment of osteoporosis. While it has not been tested as an antitumor agent in breast cancer, in a randomized trial of raloxifene versus placebo, 7704 postmenopausal women with osteoporosis were randomized to raloxifene or placebo. Patients receiving raloxifene were found to have a significantly decreased incidence of breast cancer: 11 in women taking raloxifene and 21 in women taking placebo. In addition, women taking raloxifene had a reduced incidence of endometrial cancer, suggesting that the drug might avert one of the major toxicities of tamoxifen (69). With the observation that tamoxifen is effective in preventing breast cancer in patients at high risk for the disease (67), the NSABP has undertaken a prevention trial, the

TABLE 3. *Tamoxifen breast cancer prevention trials*

Trial	Reference	Patients	Woman-years follow-up	Breast cancers per 1000 woman-years: Placebo	Breast cancers per 1000 woman-years: Tamoxifen
Breast Cancer Prevention Trial	Fisher et al. (1998)	13,388	46,858	6.6	3.6
Royal Marsden Hospital Study	Powles et al. (1998)	2472	12,355	5.0	4.7
Italian Tamoxifen Prevention Study	Veronesi et al. (1998)	5408	20,731	2.3	2.1

Study of Tamoxifen and Raloxifene (STAR). As noted above, however, raloxifene has not been tested for antitumor activity in breast cancer either in the adjuvant setting or for metastatic disease. Table 4 lists the estrogenic and antiestrogenic properties of these two drugs along with the properties of the ideal SERM. It is hoped that the newer-generation SERMs may be able to more closely approach the characteristics of the ideal SERM, with antiestrogenic activity in the breast and endometrium coupled with the maintenance of estrogenic activity in bone, vagina, liver, and the central nervous system.

Of the hormonal agents, only tamoxifen has undergone extensive testing in the adjuvant setting. For metastatic breast cancer, other hormonal agents have been used. Patients in whom treatment with hormonal therapy initially fails are unlikely to respond to a second endocrine manipulation. Patients who initially respond to hormonal therapy but then progress may benefit from an alternate hormonal treatment. After tamoxifen, the most frequently utilized hormonal therapies are the progestational agent megestrol acetate (Megace) and the aromatase inhibitors.

The antitumor mechanism of action of the progestins is unknown. Progestins have a variety of effects on secretion of other hormones, including gonadotropins, cortisol, estradiol, and dehydroepiandrosterone, and on expression of ER. Progestins have also been shown to have androgenic properties. Any of these secondary hormonal effects of progestins may account for observed antitumor responses. Alternatively, there may be direct cytotoxic effects on tumor cells. The common side effects of progestational agents include increased appetite, weight gain, and fluid retention.

In postmenopausal women, the principal source of estrogen is from the conversion of adrenally generated androgen to estrogen in peripheral tissues. Aromatase (estrogen synthetase) is a cytochrome P-450 enzyme that catalyzes multiple hydroxylation steps in the conversion of androgen to estrogen. Inhibition of aromatase activity results in suppression of circulating estradiol levels. In patients with estrogen-dependent tumors, this estrogen deprivation may result in a beneficial antitumor effect. Animal studies have documented an increase in ovarian weight and elevated circulating androgens after treatment with aromatase inhibitors (70). These drugs are thus contraindicated in premenopausal patients or women in whom menopausal status is unknown.

In addition to tamoxifen, megestrol acetate, and the aromatase inhibitors, several other hormonal agents have been utilized for treatment of breast cancer. The available hormonal therapies for breast cancer are listed in Table 5. Because quality-of-life issues are a clear priority in patients with metastatic breast cancer, toxicity of therapy should be of primary concern. Tamoxifen is the best tolerated of these agents, followed in order of toxicity by the aromatase inhibitors, the progestins, estrogens, and androgens. There is little experience at this time with antiprogestins as hormonal therapy of breast cancer, but they appear to have considerable toxicity.

In women with bony metastases, hormonal therapies may induce a "flare" in the disease

TABLE 4. *Selective estrogen receptor modulators (SERMs)*

Organ	Tamoxifen	Raloxifene	Ideal SERM
Breast	AE	AE	AE
Endometrium	E	AE	AE
Vagina	AE	AE	E
Central nervous system (hot flashes)	AE	AE	E
Liver (cholesterol)	E	E	E
Bone	E	E	E

AE, antiestrogenic activity; E, estrogenic activity.

TABLE 5. *Hormonal agents used for treatment of breast cancer*

Category	Drug
Estrogen	Diethylstilbestrol Ethinyl estradiol (Estinyl)
Antiestrogen	Tamoxifen citrate (Nolvadex)
Progestin	Megestrol acetate (Megace) Medroxyprogesterone acetate
Antiprogestin	Mifepristone/RU 486
Androgen	Fluoxymesterone (Halotestin)
Antiandrogen	Flutamide (Eulexin)
Aromatase inhibitor	Anastrozole Letrozole
Gonadotropin-releasing hormone analogs	Goserelin acetate (Zoladex) Leuprolide acetate (Luprox)

that is manifested as an acute onset of musculoskeletal pain, frequently associated with hypercalcemia, occurring in the first month of therapy. It is widely held that this reaction is a positive prognostic sign indicating a hormone-sensitive tumor, although there are no data to clearly support this view. It is apparent, however, that therapy can safely be continued and symptoms will usually resolve as long as adequate supportive care is provided.

GYNECOLOGIC ISSUES IN BREAST CANCER PATIENTS

Contraception

Breast cancer has been considered a contraindication to hormonal contraception. The exogenous administration of estrogen and progesterone have been thought to put women with breast cancer at increased risk of recurrence. Women treated for breast cancer therefore have a restricted list of options for control of fertility. It is unclear whether a progestin alone, such as medroxyprogesterone acetate, would be safe in women with breast cancer. Medroxyprogesterone acetate is the active agent in Depo-Provera, which is injected every 3 months, as well as in the Norplant System, composed of Silastic capsules that release the progestin over 5 years. Barrier contraceptives, such as diaphragm or condoms, are less effective than oral or injectable contraceptives, although efficacy can be improved with the concomitant use of a spermicidal jelly. In monogamous, parous women, an IUD would be a reasonable option. The Progestasert IUD, which slowly releases medroxyprogesterone acetate in the endometrial cavity, may also be considered. The device does not elevate systemic progestin levels. The Progestasert IUD may also reverse endometrial hyperplasia associated with prolonged tamoxifen administration. Permanent contraceptive options would include vasectomy for a partner, tubal ligation, or bilateral oophorectomy.

Gynecologic Follow-up of Breast Cancer Patients

Examination

Breast cancer patients should undergo gynecologic examinations yearly. Abnormal uterine bleeding should be evaluated promptly with office endometrial biopsy and transvaginal ultrasound. Menopausal breast cancer patients should be questioned routinely about menopausal symptoms, including hot flashes, insomnia, vaginal dryness, dyspareunia, and urinary incontinence.

Papanicolaou Smear

Women with breast cancer should continue with regular Papanicolaou (Pap) smear screening as otherwise indicated. Those with known risk factors for cervical cancer, such as documented history of cervical dysplasia, infection with human papillomavirus, multiple sexual partners, high-risk sexual partners, and chronic immunosuppression, should be screened yearly. Those women without such risk factors who have had three normal yearly Pap smears can be screened every 2 to 3 years. Women who never had cervical dysplasia or cervical cancer and have had hysterectomies do not need Pap smears of the vaginal cuff, although they should continue to have regular gynecologic examinations. It is unclear at what age Pap smears may be safely omitted in older women.

Mammography

Mammography after a diagnosis of breast cancer is used for the detection of local relapse in women who have undergone breast-conserving therapy, and for the detection of new primary tumors. The radiographic changes in the breast after lumpectomy and radiation are profound, and distinguishing between malignant and benign changes may be difficult. However, 30% to 50% of local recurrences in women who have undergone breast-conserving therapy are detected solely by mammography (71); thus, vigilant screening must continue throughout life. Mammography is a key element in the follow-up of these patients, along with breast self-examination and provider physical examination. Overall, the incidence of local recurrence after breast-conserving therapy is 10% to 20%, and the cumulative risk continues to rise for at least 20 years (72,73). When detected early, local recurrences can be salvaged with mastectomy. Thus, close follow-up is mandatory, as an undiscovered local recurrence may lead to disease dissemination.

The overall incidence of new primary breast cancers is approximately 1% per year. Women who have strong family history of breast cancer or a genetic predisposition to breast cancer may have a higher rate of new primary breast cancer. In women who have undergone breast-conserving therapy, a new diagnosis outside the originally involved quadrant or tumor occurring in the same quadrant many years later is felt to represent a new primary cancer.

Management of Gynecologic Issues in Breast Cancer Patients

Abnormal Uterine Bleeding

The most common causes of abnormal uterine bleeding are hormonal and structural. Evaluation of abnormal uterine bleeding therefore should begin with a complete menstrual history followed by endometrial biopsy and transvaginal ultrasound. Endometrial biopsy should give evidence of the hormonal milieu of the uterus. Transvaginal ultrasound will be able to identify uterine leiomyomata, as well as a thickened endometrial stripe. Women taking tamoxifen, however, often have a thickened endometrial stripe due to tamoxifen stimulation of the subendometrial stroma. In these women, saline-infusion sonography or hysteroscopy may be necessary to fully evaluate the endometrium.

If structural abnormalities are found, then surgical interventions may be required to control abnormal bleeding. Such interventions might include removal of endometrial or endocervical polyps via hysteroscopy, myomectomy, endometrial ablation, or hysterectomy.

As mentioned above, most clinicians are uncomfortable giving breast cancer patients prolonged courses of estrogens and progestins, as with oral contraceptives or hormonal contraception. A short course of progestins, such as medroxyprogesterone acetate, 10 mg per day for 10 days, may be useful to curtail endometrial bleeding associated with anovulation. The Progestasert IUD is currently under evaluation for the control of abnormal uterine bleeding in women with breast cancer.

Premenstrual Syndrome

Premenstrual symptoms can include altered emotional state, behavioral changes, somatic symptoms, altered appetite, and motor effects. To confirm the diagnosis, there must be cyclicity of the patient's symptoms, with worse symptomatology during the premenstrual rather than the preovulatory weeks. In addition, moderate to severe mood changes must be present. The symptoms must be relieved after menstrual flow, and there should be a symptom-free period after menstruation. Premenstrual symptoms should recur every menstrual cycle for at least 9 to 12 months, although the severity and constellation of symptoms may vary from month to month.

Premenstrual symptoms should be evaluated prospectively before the diagnosis of premenstrual syndrome is confirmed. In addition, the physician should elicit a thorough psychiatric history, as well as personal and social history. Family and work stresses can exacerbate or present as premenstrual symptoms. Patients should keep a menstrual calendar recording symptoms for at least three cycles. Review of the calendar by the health care provider will help differentiate premenstrual syndrome from various psychiatric disorders, such as chronic depression and anxiety disorder.

To date, no one single treatment has emerged for the management of premenstrual symptoms. Education and reassurance for women and their families are critical. Empiric treatments that have helped some patients include low-dose oral contraceptives, such as norgestimate/ethinyl estradiol (Ortho-Cyclen, Ortho Tri-Cyclen), prostaglandin-synthetase inhibitors, and selective serotonin-reuptake inhibitors.

Sexual Function in Breast Cancer Patients

Ovarian ablation from chemotherapy appears to be responsible for the majority of sexual dysfunction among breast cancer patients. Decreased desire for sex, vaginal dryness, and dyspareunia all appear linked to loss of ovarian function. While surgical issues, such as lumpectomy versus mastectomy, appear to be less important, the overall emotional impact of the diagnosis of breast cancer and the perceived and actual changes in the body associated with treatment are poorly studied (74).

Pozo et al. (75) reported on a small prospective study that followed 63 women who underwent primary surgery for breast cancer. Twenty-four underwent mastectomy following the strong recommendations of their physicians, 24 choose mastectomy for other reasons, and 15 choose lumpectomy. Mood disturbance, perceived quality of life, life satisfaction, marital satisfaction, perceptions of social support, and self-rated adjustment were assessed by interview before surgery, 10 days after surgery, then at 3 months, 6 months, and 12 months. Surgical groups differed in only one respect: Women who underwent lumpectomy reported a higher-quality sex life at 6 and 12 months than women who underwent mastectomy.

Young-McCaughan (50) reported on a cross-sectional survey of 67 women with stages I, II, or III breast cancer treated with chemotherapy and/or endocrine therapy or no adjuvant therapy. After control for endocrine therapy, the women treated with chemotherapy were 3.6 times more likely than women not treated with chemotherapy to report hot flashes (p=0.02), 6.5 times more likely to report mood swings (p=0.001), 5.7 times more likely to report vaginal dryness (p=0.001), 3.0 times more likely to report decreased libido ($p = 0.04$), 5.5 times more likely to report dyspareunia ($p = 0.003$), and 7.1 times more likely to report difficulty achieving orgasm ($p = 0.004$). There was a significant negative effect of chemotherapy on body image ($p = 0.01$), affects ($p = 0.001$), psychologic symptoms ($p = 0.001$), and overall sexual functioning ($p = 0.02$). After control for chemotherapy, there was no significant impact of endocrine therapy on sexual functioning. Endocrine therapy did not appear to affect sexual functioning in this small survey.

Schag et al. (76) reported that a specific quality-of-life instrument, the Cancer Rehabilitation Evaluation System, can distinguish, among women with stage I and II breast cancer, those who are at risk for psychosocial morbidity and those who are not at risk for such morbidity. When this instrument was used in a sample of 227 newly diagnosed, early-stage breast cancer patients, both groups reported substantial sexual problems related to interest in and performance of sexual activity. Patients considered at risk, however, had more difficulty in their sexual relationship than those considered not at risk. Among the at-risk patients, for example, fully one-third of all patients indicated that they perceived their partners as not seeing them as sexually attractive at 1 year after cancer diagnosis. One-half of those in both groups, however, continued to have sexual dysfunction 1 year after diagnosis. This study suggests that sexual rehabilitation needs to form a critical part in the ongoing care of breast cancer patients.

MENOPAUSAL ISSUES IN BREAST CANCER PATIENTS

Adjuvant chemotherapy in premenopausal breast cancer patients is clearly associated with ovarian failure. Furthermore, the increased life expectancy of both pre- and postmenopausal patients as a result of adjuvant therapies suggests that the number of menopausal years will be increased in survivors of breast cancer. For some of these women, the medical consequences of the low-estrogen state of menopause may have a greater impact on quality of life and life span than their diagnosis of breast cancer.

Management of Menopause in Breast Cancer Patients

Hormone-replacement Therapy

During menopause, women may experience unwanted and sometimes debilitating symptoms. Women with a history of breast cancer are no exception. In fact, women who experience menopausal symptoms due to the ovarian effects of chemotherapy may have more severe symptoms. As with surgical menopause, the decline in ovarian hormone synthesis from medical menopause may be more abrupt than with spontaneous menopause. In addition to the troublesome early symptoms of menopause, the long-term consequences of estrogen deficiency, including osteoporosis and resultant fractures, elevated total cholesterol, elevated low-density lipoprotein cholesterol, decreased high-density lipoprotein cholesterol, and increased coronary artery disease, may prove fatal. It has been known for several decades that hormone replacement therapy (HRT) can ameliorate the symptoms of menopause. Over the last decade, it has become clear that the all-cause mortality for menopausal women is decreased by the use of HRT.

In an analysis from the Nurses' Health Study, Grodstein et al. (77) examined the relationship between the use of postmenopausal hormones and mortality. They found that current hormone users had a lower risk of death (relative risk, 0.63) than subjects who had never taken hormones. This benefit decreased with long-term use because of an increase in mortality from breast cancer among long-term hormone users. In spite of the overall benefits of HRT, most clinicians have felt uncomfortable prescribing it to breast cancer survivors. The standard of care in the United States is to discourage the use of HRT in patients with a history of breast cancer (48).

What are the specific risks of HRT in women with a history of breast cancer? First, HRT may increase breast density in some women (78). This may make mammographic detection of recurrent disease or a new primary breast cancer difficult. Second, long-term ERT appears to increase the risk of primary breast cancer in an unselected population (77). Third, the use of ERT has been postulated to increase the risk of a recurrence of breast cancer. The hypothesis is that dormant tumor cells might be given a growth advantage by exposure to circulating estrogen. If this hypothesis were true, one would expect that women diagnosed with breast cancer while taking estrogen would have a worse prognosis. In fact, the prognosis of women who took ERT before diagnosis is better than that of women with no history of exogenous estrogen use (48).

What clinical data examining the use of estrogen in patients with breast cancer are available? There have been some retrospective reports and phase II studies in which HRT was prescribed, primarily for women with ER-negative and PR-negative tumors who were free of disease after primary therapy for more than 5 years. Unfortunately, these studies are characterized by retrospective analysis, anecdotal reporting, or a limited number of patients (79). However, these studies have failed to show adverse effects of ERT or an estrogen–progestin replacement therapy after treatment of breast carcinoma. In fact, some studies have demonstrated a positive effect in recurrence-free survival (80). One Danish study randomized women with breast cancer who had been treated with simple mastectomy and radiation therapy to placebo, tamoxifen, or diethylstilbestrol (DES) (81). There was no significant difference between the relapse rates for the tamoxifen (24%) and the DES (18%) groups, while those on placebo had a recurrence rate of 37%.

In the absence of definitive prospective studies, however, we cannot conclude that HRT is safe for breast cancer survivors (82–84). The clinician and breast cancer survivor must together define the deficits and risks associated with menopause and put together a comprehensive strategy to manage them. Table 6 lists some of these potential factors for consideration.

Nonhormonal Treatment of Menopausal Symptoms

Many symptoms of menopause may be treated with nonhormonal approaches. Maintaining a cool environment at home and at work, wearing layered clothing that can be removed as necessary to remain cool, and regular exercise will reduce the incidence of hot flashes. In addition, an increase in the intake of dietary soy protein may also decrease the incidence of hot flashes. Vasomotor symptoms such as hot flashes will spontaneously abate within 2 years in most women. Pharmacologic approaches, such as megestrol acetate, clonidine hydrochloride (Catapres), and the combination of ergotamine tartrate, belladonna, and phenobarbital (Bellergal-S), have been used with some success, but these agents have side effects that frequently limit their use. These agents may be helpful in transiently easing vasomotor symptoms for some women. Vaginal dryness and dyspareunia may be treated with vaginal lubricants, such as the over-the-counter preparations Replens and Astroglide. Use of a vaginal estrogen cream or an estradiol vaginal ring (Estring) may ameliorate symptoms of genitourinary atrophy. After estrogen-induced cornification of the vagina occurs, there appears to be little systemic exposure from vaginal estrogen.

TABLE 6. *Potential risks and benefits of hormone replacement therapy in women with a history of breast cancer*

Risks
Increased breast cancer recurrence
New primary breast cancer
Less reliable mammography
Benefits
Control of menopausal symptoms
Vasomotor symptoms (hot flashes)
Sleep disruption
Cystitis, urinary frequency, and urinary incontinence
Vaginal dryness and dyspareunia
Decreased risk of heart disease
Improved cholesterol profile
Decreased risk of osteoporosis and fracture
Decreased risk of Alzheimer's disease

Osteoporosis

There have been significant recent gains in the treatment and prevention of osteoporosis. Although systemic estrogen or an estrogen–progesterone combination is the most effective means of preventing menopausal bone loss, the use of bisphosphonates, such as alendronate sodium (Fosamax), is an effective alternative. Raloxifene has also been found to protect bone mineral density, but not to the extent of estrogen or alendronate. Adequate calcium intake and exercise are important adjuncts to these therapies but do not prevent osteoporosis when used alone in most women (85). The National Institutes of Health Consensus Development Panel on Optimal Calcium Intake (86) has recommended that postmenopausal women not taking estrogen should take at least 1500 mg of calcium daily, while postmenopausal women taking estrogen should take 1000 mg of calcium daily.

Hyperlipidemia and Cardiovascular Disease

Cardiovascular disease is the major health threat to older women in this country, including survivors of breast cancer. Among women in whom ERT is contraindicated, prevention and treatment of hyperlipidemia and cardiovascular disease should follow the recommendations for the general population. Lifestyle modifications, including cessation of smoking, regular exercise, weight control, and a diet low in saturated fats, will all contribute to decreasing cardiovascular risk. Careful attention to screening for hypertension and hyperlipidemia, as well as prompt medical treatment of these disorders, remains imperative.

REFERENCES

1. Pike MC, Ross RK, Lobo RA, et al. LH-RH agonists and the prevention of breast and ovarian cancer. *Br J Cancer* 1989;60:142–148.
2. Frisch R, McArthur J. Menstrual cycles: fatness as a determinant of minimum weight for height necessary for their maintenance or onset. *Science* 1974;185:949–954.
3. Ventura SJ. First births to older mothers, 1970-1986. *Am J Public Health* 1989;79:1675–1680.
4. Henderson BE, Ross RK, Judd HL, et al. Do regular ovulatory cycles increase breast cancer risk? *Cancer* 1985;56:1206–1212.
5. Kampert JB, Whittemore AS, Paffenbarger RS. Combined effect of childbearing, menstrual events and body size on age-specific breast cancer risk. *Am J Epidemiol* 1988;128:962–979.
6. Layde PM, Webster LA, Baughman AL, et al. The independent associations of parity, age at first full-term pregnancy, and duration of breast-feeding with the risk of breast cancer. *J Clin Epidemiol* 1989;42:963–973.
7. Lambe M, Hsieh C, Trichopoulos D, et al. Transient increase in the risk of breast cancer after giving birth. *N Engl J Med* 1994;331:5–9.
8. Colditz GA. Epidemiology of breast cancer. *Cancer* 1993;71(suppl):1480–1489.
9. Yuan MJ, Yu MC, Ross RK, et al. Risk factors for breast cancer in Chinese women in Shanghai. *Cancer Res* 1988;48:1949–1953.
10. Melbye M, Wohlfahrt J, Olsen JH, et al. Induced abortion and the risk of breast cancer. *N Engl J Med* 1997; 336:81–85.
11. Oral-contraceptive use and the risk of breast cancer. The Cancer and Steroid Hormone Study (CASH) of the Centers for Disease Control and the National Institute of Child Health and Human Development. *N Engl J Med* 1986;315:405–411.
12. Olsson H, Moller TR, Ranstam J. Early oral contraceptive use and breast cancer among premenopausal women: final report from a study in southern Sweden. *J Natl Cancer Inst* 1989;81:1000–1004.
13. Wingo PA, Lee NC, Ory HW, et al. Age-specific differences in the relationship between oral contraceptive use and breast cancer. *Cancer* 1993;71:1506–1517.
14. Schlesselman JJ. Net effect of oral contraceptive use on the risk of cancer in women in the United States. *Obstet Gynecol* 1995;85:793–801.
15. Kaunitz AM. Depot medroxyprogesterone acetate contraception and the risk of breast and gynecologic cancer. *J Reprod Med* 1996;41(5 suppl):419–427.
16. Hirayama T, Wynder E. A study of the epidemiology of cancer of the breast. II. The influence of hysterectomy. *Cancer* 1962;28–38.
17. Trichopoulos D, MacMahon B, Cole P. Menopause and breast cancer risk. *J Natl Cancer Inst* 1971;48:605–613.
18. Brinton LA, Schairer C, Hoover RN, et al. Menstrual factors and risk of breast cancer. *Cancer Invest* 1988;6: 245–254.
19. Colditz GA, Hankinson SE, Hunter DJ, et al. The use of estrogens and progestins and the risk of breast cancer in premenopausal women. *N Engl J Med* 1995;332: 1589–1593.
20. Sorosky JI, Scott-Conner CE. Breast disease complicating pregnancy. *Obstet Gynecol Clin North Am* 1998;25: 353–363.
21. Max, MH, Klamer TW. Pregnancy and breast cancer. *South Med J* 1983;76:1088–1090.
22. Novotny DB, Maygarden SJ, Shermer RW, et al. Fine-needle aspiration of benign and malignant breast masses associated with pregnancy. *Act Cytol* 1991;35: 676–686.
23. Petrek JA, Dukoff R, Rogatko A. Prognosis of pregnancy-associated breast cancer. *Cancer* 1991;67: 869–872.
24. Saunders CM, Baum M. Breast cancer in pregnancy: a review. *J R Soc Med* 1993;86:162–166.
25. Petrek JA. Breast cancer during pregnancy. *Cancer* 1994;74:518–527.
26. Petrek JA. Pregnancy safety after breast cancer. *Cancer* 1994;74:528–531.
27. Mayr NA, Wen BC, Saw CB. Radiation therapy during pregnancy. *Obstet Gynecol Clin North Am* 1998;25: 301–321.
28. Brent, RL. The effect of embryonic and fetal exposure to x-ray, microwaves, and ultrasound: counseling the pregnant and nonpregnant patient about these risks. *Semin Oncol* 1989;16:347–368.
29. Merkel DE. Pregnancy and breast cancer. *Semin Surg Oncol* 1996;12:370–375.
30. Hortobagyi GN. Treatment of breast cancer. *N Engl J Med* 1998;339:974–984.
31. Doll DC, Ringenberg QS, Yarbro JW. Antineoplastic agents and pregnancy. *Semin Oncol* 1989;5:337–346.
32. Buekers TE, Lallas TA. Chemotherapy in pregnancy. *Obstet Gynecol Clin North Am* 1998;25:323–329.
33. Garber JE. Long-term follow-up of children exposed in utero to antineoplastic agents. *Semin Oncol* 1989;16: 437–444.
34. Zemlickis D, Lishner M, Degendorfer P, et al. Maternal and fetal outcome after breast cancer in pregnancy. *Am J Obstet Gynecol* 1992;166:781–787.
35. Kroman N, Wohlfahrt J, Andersen KW, Mouridsen HT, Westergaard T, Melbye M. Time since childbirth and prognosis in primary breast cancer: population based study. *BMJ* 1997;315:851–855.
36. Sutton R, Buzdar AU, Hortobagyi G. Pregnancy and

offspring after adjuvant chemotherapy in breast cancer patients. *Cancer* 1990;60:847–850.
37. Von Schoultz E, Johansson H, Wilking N, et al. Influence of prior and subsequent pregnancy on breast cancer prognosis. *J Clin Oncol* 1995;13:430–434.
38. Malamos NA, Stathopoulos GP, Keramopolous A, Papadiamantis J, Vassilaros S. Pregnancy and offspring after the appearance of breast cancer. *Oncology* 1996;53:471–475.
39. Clark RM, Chua T. Breast cancer and pregnancy: the ultimate challenge. *J R Coll Radiol* 1989;1:11–18.
40. Danforth D. How subsequent pregnancy affects outcome in women with a prior breast cancer. *Oncology* 1991;5:23–35.
41. Early Breast Cancer Trialists Collaborative Group. Systemic treatment of early breast cancer by hormonal, cytotoxic, or immune therapy. *Lancet* 1991;339:1–15,71–85.
42. Koyama H, Wata T, Nishizawa H, et al. Cyclophosphamide-induced ovarian failure and its therapeutic significance in patients with breast cancer. *Cancer* 1977;39:1403–1409.
43. Hortobagyi GN, Buzdar AU, Marcus CE, et al. Immediate and long-term toxicity of adjuvant chemotherapy regimens containing doxorubicin in trials at M.D. Anderson Hospital and Tumor Institute. *NCI Monogr* 1986;1:105–109.
44. Damewood MD, Grochow LB. Prospects for fertility after chemotherapy or radiation for neoplastic disease. *Fertil Steril* 1986;45:443–459.
45. Reyno LM, Levine MN, Skingley P, et al. Chemotherapy-induced amenorrhea in a randomized trial of adjuvant chemotherapy duration in breast cancer. *Eur J Cancer* 1992;29A:21–23.
46. Bonadonna G, Valagussa P. Current status of adjuvant chemotherapy for breast cancer. *Semin Oncol* 1987;14:8–22.
47. Shamberger RC, Rosenberg SA, Seipp CA, et al. Effects of high-dose methotrexate and vincristine on ovarian and testicular functions in patients undergoing postoperative adjuvant treatment for osteosarcoma. *Cancer Treat Rep* 1981;65:739–743.
48. Cobleigh MA, Berris RF, Bush T, et al. Estrogen replacement therapy in breast cancer survivors: a time for change. *JAMA* 1994;272:540–545.
49. Dnistrian AM, Schwartz MK, Fraccia AA, et al. Endocrine consequences of CMF adjuvant therapy in premenopausal and postmenopausal breast cancer patients. *Cancer* 1983;51:803–807.
50. Young-McCaughan S. Sexual functioning in women with breast cancer after treatment with adjuvant therapy. *Cancer Nurs* 1996;19:308–319.
51. Fisher B, Sherman B, Rockette H, et al. L-Phenylalanine mustard (L-PAM) in the management of premenopausal patients with primary breast cancer. *Cancer* 1979;44:847–857.
52. Tormey DC, Gray R, Kennedy G, et al. Adjuvant chemohormonal therapy with cyclophosphamide, methotrexate, 5-fluorouracil, and prednisone (CMFP) or CMFP plus tamoxifen compared with CMF for premenopausal breast cancer patients. *Cancer* 1990;65:200–206.
53. Tengrup I, Nitby LT, Landberg T. Prophylactic oophorectomy in the treatment of carcinoma of the breast. *Surg Gynecol Obstet* 1986;162:209–214.
54. Ravolin RG. Results of a clinical trial concerning the work of prophylactic oophorectomy for breast carcinoma. *Surg Gynecol Obstet* 1970;131:1055–1064.
55. Ludwig CU, Hartmann D, Landmann R, et al. Unaltered immunocompetence in patients with non-disseminated breast cancer at the time of diagnosis. *Cancer* 1985;55:1673–1678.
56. Richards MA, O'Reilly SM, Howell A, et al. Adjuvant cyclophosphamide, methotrexate, and fluorouracil in patents with axillary node-positive breast cancer: an update of the Guy's/Manchester trial. *Clin Oncol* 1990;8:2032–2039.
57. Bianco AR, Del Mastro L, Gallo C, et al. Prognostic role of amenorrhea induced by adjuvant chemotherapy in premenopausal patients with early breast cancer. *Br J Cancer* 1991;63:799–803.
58. Early Breast Cancer Trialists Collaborative Group. Ovarian ablation in early breast cancer: overview of the randomised trials. *Lancet* 1996;348:1189–1196.
59. Osborne CK. Tamoxifen in the treatment of breast cancer. *N Engl J Med* 1998;339:1609–1618.
60. Early Breast Cancer Trialists Collaborative Group. Tamoxifen for early breast cancer: an overview of the randomised trials. *Lancet* 1998;351:1451–1467.
61. Love RR, Barden HS, Mazess RB, Epstein S, Chappell RJ. Effect of tamoxifen on lumbar spine bone mineral density in postmenopausal women after 5 years. *Arch Intern Med* 1994;154:2585–2588.
62. Powles T, Eeles R, Ashley S, et al. Interim analysis of the incidence of breast cancer in the Royal Marsden Hospital tamoxifen randomised chemoprevention trial. *Lancet* 1998;352:98–101.
63. Costantino JP, Kuller LH, Ives DG, et al. Coronary heart mortality and adjuvant tamoxifen therapy. *J Natl Cancer Inst* 1997;89:776–782.
64. Fisher B, Costantino JP, Redmond CK, et al. Endometrial cancer in tamoxifen-treated breast cancer patients: findings from the National Surgical Adjuvant Breast and Bowel Project (NSABP) B-14. *J Natl Cancer Inst* 1994;86:527–537.
65. Barakat RR, Wong G, Curtin JP, Vlamis V, Hoskins WJ. Tamoxifen use in breast cancer patients who subsequently develop corpus cancer is not associated with a higher incidence of adverse histologic features. *Gynecol Oncol* 1994;55:164–168.
66. Neven P, Vergote I. Should tamoxifen users be screened for endometrial lesions? (editorial) *Lancet* 1988;351:155–157.
67. Fisher B, Costantino JP, Wickerham DL, et al. Tamoxifen for prevention of breast cancer: report of the National Surgical Adjuvant Breast and Bowel Project P-1 Study. *J Natl Cancer Inst* 1998;90:1371–1388.
68. Veronesi U, Maisonneuve P, Costa A, et al. Prevention of breast cancer with tamoxifen: preliminary findings from the Italian randomised trial among hysterectomised women. Italian Tamoxifen Prevention Study. *Lancet* 1998;352:93–97.
69. Cummings SR, Norton L, Eckert S, et al. Raloxifene reduces the risk of breast cancer and may decrease risk of endometrial cancer in postmenopausal women: two-year findings from the Multiple Outcomes of Raloxifene Evaluation (MORE) Trial. Proc ASCO 1998;2a.
70. Sinha S, Kaseta J, Santner SJ, et al. Effect of CGS 20267 on ovarian aromatase and gonadotropin levels in the rat. *Breast Cancer Res Treat* 1998;48:45–51.
71. Orel SG, Fowble BL, Solin LJ, et al. Breast cancer re-

currence after lumpectomy and radiation therapy for early-stage disease: prognostic significance of detection method. *Radiology* 1993;188:189–193.
72. Fowble B, Solin L, Schulta D, et al. Ten-year results of conservative surgery and irradiation for stage I and II breast cancer. *Int J Radiat Oncol Biol Phys* 1991;21: 269–275.
73. Fouquet A, Campana F, Zafrani B, et al. Prognostic factors of breast recurrence in the conservative management of early breast cancer: a 25-year follow-up. *Int J Radiat Oncol Biol Phys* 1989;17:719–724.
74. Schover LR. Sexuality and body image in younger women with breast cancer. *NCI Monogr* 1994;16: 177–182.
75. Pozo C, Carver CS, Noriega V, et al. Effects of mastectomy versus lumpectomy on emotional adjustment to breast cancer: a prospective study of the first year post-surgery. *J Clin Oncol* 1992;10:1292–1298.
76. Schag CA, Ganz PA, Polinsky ML, et al. Characteristics of women at risk for psychosocial distress in the year after breast cancer. *J Clin Oncol* 1993;11:783–793.
77. Grodstein F, Stampfer MD, Colditz GA, et al. Postmenopausal hormone therapy and mortality. *N Engl J Med* 1997;336:1769–1775.
78. Berkowitz JE, Gatewood OM, Goldblum LE, et al. Hormonal replacement therapy: mammographic manifestations. *Radiology* 1990;174:199–201.
79. Vassilopoulou-Sellin R, Theriault R, Klein MJ. Estrogen replacement therapy in women with prior diagnosis and treatment for breast cancer. *Gynecol Oncol* 1997;65:89–93.
80. Braendle W. Hormone replacement therapy in women with breast cancer. *Anticancer Res* 1998;18: 2253–2255.
81. Palshof T, Mouridsen HT, Daehnfeldt JL. Adjuvant endocrine therapy of bresast cancer—a controlled clinical trial of oestrogen and anti-oestrogen: preliminary results of the Copenhagen breast cancer trials. *Recent Results Cancer Res* 1980;71:185–189.
82. Marchant DJ. Estrogen-replacement therapy after breast cancer. Risks versus benefits. *Cancer* 1993;71(6 Suppl): 2169–2176.
83. DiSaia PJ. Hormone-replacement therapy in patients with breast cancer. A reappraisal. *Cancer* 1993;71(4 Suppl):1490–1500.
84. Bluming AZ. Hormone replacement therapy: benefits and risks for the general postmenopausal female population and for women with a history of previously treated breast cancer. *Semin Oncol* 1993;20:662–674.
85. Andrews WC. What's new in preventing and treating osteoporosis? *Postgrad Med* 1998;104:89–92,95–97.
86. NIH Consensus Development Panel on Optimal Calcium Intake. Optimal calcium intake. *JAMA* 1994;272: 1942–1948.

8

Cervical Cancer in Pregnancy

Robert E. Bristow and F.J. Montz

Department of Gynecology and Obstetrics, Johns Hopkins Hospital and Johns Hopkins University School of Medicine, Baltimore, Maryland 21287

Cancer is the second most common cause of death among women aged 15 to 34 years and is the leading cause of death among women 35 to 54 years (1). It is estimated that one in 1000 to 1500 live births is complicated by a maternal malignancy. Cervical cancer is the most common malignancy in pregnancy, with a reported incidence ranging from one in 1200 to one in 2200 pregnancies (1.6 to 10.6 cases per 10,000 pregnancies), depending on the inclusive postpartum interval (2,3). Conversely, one of every 34 patients with invasive cervical cancer is pregnant at the time of diagnosis (2). For practical purposes, cases of cervical carcinoma diagnosed within 6 months of an antecedent pregnancy should be considered to have been coexistent with pregnancy. This definition is somewhat arbitrary, however; and clinical lesions diagnosed within 12 or even 18 months of delivery may have been present during pregnancy.

While the mean age at diagnosis for invasive cervical carcinoma is 52.2 years, the distribution of cases is bimodal, with peaks at 35 to 39 years and 60 to 64 years (4). This bimodal age distribution is indicative of the significant proportion of women diagnosed with cervical carcinoma in the reproductive-age group, with 30% of all cases occurring in women age 35 years or younger (5). Also significant is that as many as 39% of younger patients have reported being pregnant during the year preceding cervical cancer diagnosis (5). As women continue to delay childbearing, the frequency of cervical carcinoma during pregnancy will likely increase. It is therefore important for clinicians caring for women in the reproductive-age group to be familiar with the complex issues surrounding the diagnosis and management of a pregnant woman with cervical cancer.

EPIDEMIOLOGY AND RISK FACTORS

Worldwide, carcinoma of the cervix is the second most common solid malignant neoplasm in women, with more than 471,000 cases diagnosed annually (6). Only breast carcinoma has a higher incidence and mortality. In the United States, cervical carcinoma is the sixth most common solid malignant neoplasm in women. The American Cancer Society estimates that in 1997 there were 14,500 new cases of cervical carcinoma, with 4800 deaths attributable to the disease (1).

While women pregnant at the time of cervical cancer diagnosis tend to be somewhat younger (33.8 years) than their nonpregnant counterparts (48 years), epidemiologic risk factors for cervical carcinoma in pregnancy are similar to those in the nonpregnant state (2). As can be seen from Table 1, lower levels of education or income and nonwhite race are associated with a two- to threefold increase in cervical cancer risk. The risk for cervical cancer is also intimately associated with a

TABLE 1. *Risk factors for cervical cancer*

Factors influencing risk	Estimated RR
Older age	2
Residence in Asia, Africa, and certain parts of Latin America	2–6
Lower levels of education or income	2–3
African-American, Hispanic, American Indian ancestry	2
Multiparity	2–4
Early age at first sexual intercourse	2–4
Multiple sexual partners	2–5
Presence of detectable human papillomavirus	4–40
Previous sexually transmitted disease	2–10
Long-term smoking	2–4
Long-term oral contraceptive use	1.5–2
No prior regular cervical cytologic screening	2–6
Diet low in carotene, vitamin C	2–3

RR, relative risk.
From ref. 7, with permission.

woman's prior reproductive history. A multiparous woman is two to four times more likely to develop cervical cancer than a woman who has never been pregnant, while early age at first intercourse and a history of multiple sexual partners increase the relative risk two- to fivefold. Although the precise mechanisms are not known, long-term smoking appears to be associated with an increased risk for cervical cancer.

During the past decade, epidemiologic evidence has accumulated, implicating infection with human papillomavirus (HPV) as the most likely causative agent of squamous carcinoma of the cervix and related precursor lesions. As perhaps the most significant risk factor for cervical cancer, HPV infection increases the relative risk by four- to tenfold (see Table 1). Recent studies have indicated a proportionately higher frequency of cervical HPV infection in pregnant women (28% to 31%) compared with the measured or expected frequency in nonpregnant controls (12.5% to 18.6%) (8,9). Not all investigators have confirmed this finding, however (10). Rando et al. (11) reported an increased frequency of HPV deoxyribonucleic acid (DNA) detectability by Southern blot hybridization in exfoliated cervical cells during pregnancy, an increase in the percentage of HPV DNA–positive patients from the first trimester (20.9%) to the third trimester of pregnancy (46%), and a dramatic decrease in detection of HPV DNA in the postpartum state (17.5%). The down-regulation of cell-mediated immunity during pregnancy and pregnancy-related active metaplasia of cervical epithelium are likely contributing factors to these observations (12, 13). The cervix is most susceptible to HPV infection during periods of active metaplasia. It is also possible that the hormonal changes associated with pregnancy may play a role in stimulating replication of HPV and possibly making the virus more easily detectable. Interestingly, the higher prevalence of HPV positivity among obstetric patients has not been associated with a concomitant increase in the diagnosis of significant cytologic abnormalities during pregnancy (8,14). The clinical significance of increased detectability of HPV infection during pregnancy remains to be established, as does the practical utility of HPV testing within this population.

DIAGNOSIS

Cytologic Screening

In addition to HPV infection, the absence of regular cervical cytologic screening has emerged as a significant risk factor for cervical cancer (see Table 1). Since the initial description of cervical and vaginal cytologic screening in the 1940s, the Papanicolaou (Pap) smear has proven to be the most efficacious and cost-effective method of cancer screening. By increasing the detection of preinvasive and early invasive disease, cervical screening with the Pap smear has decreased both the incidence and mortality from cervical carcinoma (15). With the incorporation of cervical cytology into routine prenatal screening, clinicians are frequently presented with management decisions regarding cervical abnormalities during pregnancy.

In general, 1.3% to 2.2% of obstetric patients will have cervical cytologic abnormalities detected during pregnancy, although the exact incidence is highly dependent on the population screened and the referral base of the reporting institution (16,17). For example, abnormal cervical cytology has been reported in up to 8.5% of pregnant patients from a university-based population (18). The incidence of cervical carcinoma *in situ* (CIS) associated with pregnancy is somewhat lower. Wanless (19) reported an incidence of cervical CIS of 0.025%, while Hacker et al. (2) found an incidence of 0.13% (1 per 770 pregnancies) in a review of 14 series from the literature. Obstetric patients should receive cervical cytologic screening at their first prenatal visit; samples should be collected from both the ectocervix and endocervical canal. Recent studies of obstetric patients have shown that both clinically and statistically significant improvements in cytologic yield can be obtained by use of the Cytobrush (Medscand, Hollywood, Florida) to sample the endocervical canal, without an associated increase in adverse pregnancy outcome (20).

Natural History of Cervical Dysplasia

The behavior of preinvasive cervical lesions, or cervical intraepithelial neoplasia (CIN), has been studied extensively in the nonpregnant state. Although variable follow-up intervals have been reported, the approximate likelihood that a CIN 1 lesion will undergo spontaneous regression is 60%; 30% of such lesions will persist, 10% will progress to CIN 3, and 1% may progress to invasive carcinoma. Approximately one-third of high-grade lesions will regress spontaneously, while the majority will persist or progress (21).

Extrapolation of these numbers to the pregnant state must take into consideration the rate or risk of progression in relation to the length of a term gestation. In a prospective study using only cytology and colposcopy, Richart and Barron (22) followed 557 nonpregnant patients with cervical abnormalities to evaluate the transit time between different grades of preinvasive cervical neoplasia. Using life-table analysis, the mean transit time to CIS from very mild dysplasia was 85 months, from mild dysplasia 58 months, from moderate dysplasia 38 months, and from severe dysplasia 12 months. While these figures may not be directly applicable to the pregnant state, it is noteworthy that even the shortest progression interval is longer than the length of a term gestation.

Management of the Abnormal Pap Smear in Pregnancy

As for nonobstetric patients, colposcopy with directed biopsy has replaced iodine staining, random punch biopsies, and conization as the principal means of evaluating abnormal cervical cytology in pregnancy. Colposcopically directed biopsy is both safe and efficacious when performed during pregnancy. The diagnostic accuracy approaches that of cervical conization, with fewer complications (23–28). In reviewing 1064 colposcopic examinations during pregnancy, Hacker et al. (2) reported a diagnostic accuracy of 99.5%, with complications occurring in only 0.6% of cases. No cases of frankly invasive cervical carcinoma were missed using this approach. While biopsy of colposcopic abnormalities can be performed during all trimesters of pregnancy, many clinicians will defer biopsy until the second trimester when the risk of incidental spontaneous pregnancy loss is minimal. The risk of bleeding and premature rupture of membranes generally precludes the use of endocervical curettage during pregnancy (29).

All women with a cytologic cervical abnormality during pregnancy should undergo colposcopic examination. For women with a high-grade squamous intraepithelial lesion (HGSIL or CIN 2/3) or CIS on Pap smear, immediate colposcopic examination is indicated to exclude the presence of invasive carcinoma. Directed biopsies should be performed of the most suspicious areas to document the histologic severity of dysplasia and exclude the presence of early invasive disease. After documentation of HGSIL, close cytologic and colposcopic surveillance is indicated every 8 to 12 weeks, with additional biopsies if there is suspicion of disease progression (Fig. 1).

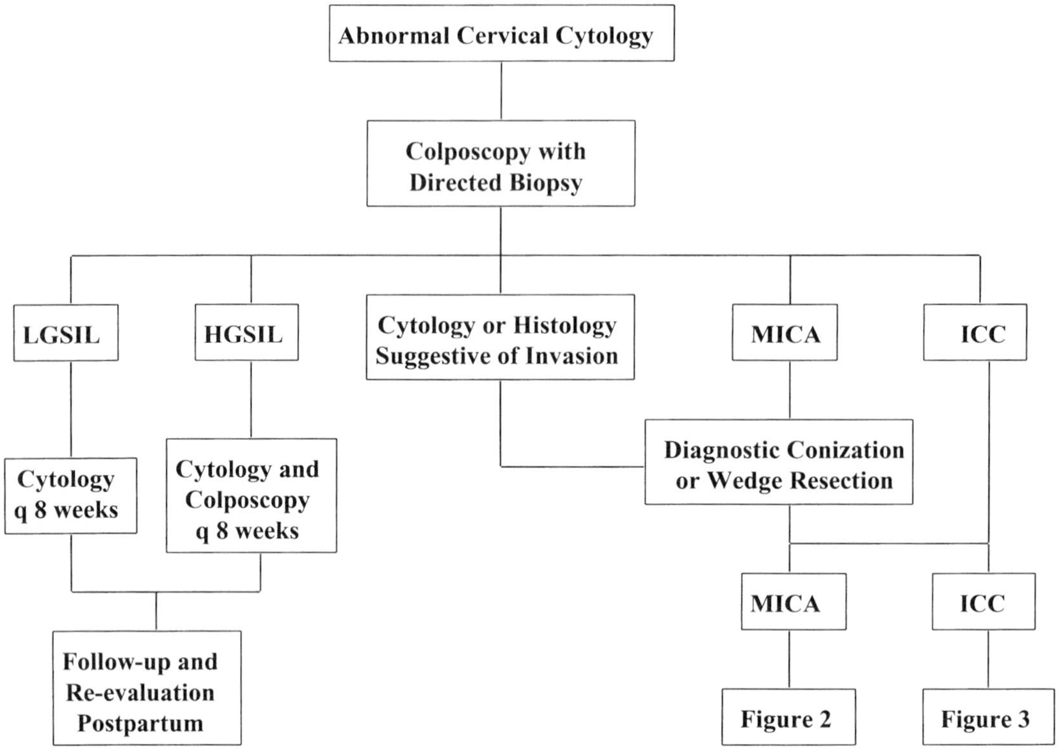

FIG. 1. Management of abnormal cervical cytology during pregnancy (LGSIL, low-grade squamous intraepithelial lesion; HGSIL, high-grade squamous intraepithelial lesion; MICA, microinvasive carcinoma [stage IA]; ICC, invasive cervical carcinoma).

With adequate surveillance and assurance that early invasive disease is not present, definitive therapy (ablation or excision) should be deferred until after delivery. Because of the possibility of spontaneous regression, all patients should be reevaluated with colposcopy and biopsy 8 to 12 weeks postpartum prior to the initiation of definitive treatment.

The management of patients with atypical squamous cells of undetermined significance (ASCUS) or a low-grade squamous intraepithelial lesion (LGSIL or CIN 1) is more controversial. Although some authors have suggested that initial colposcopic examination is unnecessary in these patients, our practice is to perform colposcopy on all patients with an abnormal cytologic result (30). In the setting of LGSIL on cervical cytology, the objective of colposcopy is to exclude HGSIL and early invasive carcinoma. HGSIL occurs in 10% of women reported as having LGSIL on Pap smear during pregnancy (30,31). Even if the colposcopic impression is consistent with LGSIL, colposcopically directed biopsies should be obtained from the most abnormal area, as 5% to 10% of such lesions will nevertheless show histologic evidence of HGSIL (31). Biopsy-confirmed LGSIL lesions can be followed safely through pregnancy without risk of progression to invasive cancer (30,32). These patients should have cervical cytology performed during each trimester and be reevaluated 8 to 12 weeks postpartum for definitive diagnosis and treatment, if necessary (see Fig. 1).

Several factors must be considered when colposcopy is performed during pregnancy. The vascularity of the cervix is normally increased in the gravid state. Coupled with an increase in active cervical metaplasia, this may produce a confusing angioarchitecture and cause a cervical lesion to appear to be a higher than actual grade. In addition, the traditional principles used to define a satisfactory colposcopic examination (visualization of each lesion, visualization of the entire transformation zone, obtaining a negative endocervical curettage, and concordant cytologic and histologic findings) are modified during pregnancy. Physiologic changes in the cervix that occur normally in pregnancy include stromal edema and progressive cervical eversion, which allow easier visualization of the transformation zone as pregnancy progresses. Consequently, if the initial examination is unsatisfactory, colposcopy should be repeated later in pregnancy when the likelihood of a satisfactory examination is increased.

Conization in Pregnancy

Indications for conization in the nongravid state are as follows:

- Unsatisfactory colposcopic examination
- HGSIL on endocervical curettage
- Histologic or colposcopic suspicion of microinvasive carcinoma
- Significant discrepancy (two or more grades) between cytology and histology
- Cytologic suspicion of adenocarcinoma *in situ*

While cervical conization offers excellent diagnostic accuracy, it has a significant complication rate, when performed during pregnancy. Consequently, traditional indications for the procedure are not directly applicable to the obstetric population. In contrast to the nonpregnant state, failure to visualize the entire transformation zone and an unsatisfactory colposcopic examination are not indications for conization in the absence of cytology suggestive of invasive disease. Conization is indicated in the presence of microinvasion on a colposcopically directed biopsy. Persistent cytologic evidence of invasive carcinoma in the absence of colposcopic confirmation is also an indication for conization in pregnancy. In general, diagnostic conization should only be considered when either biopsy or cytologic smear is suggestive of invasive carcinoma and a diagnosis of invasion will result in a modification of treatment recommendations, timing, or mode of delivery.

The increased uterine and cervical vascularity associated with pregnancy makes hemorrhage a significant risk of conization performed during pregnancy, with immediate excessive blood loss occurring in 8.9% of patients and delayed cervical hemorrhage complicating 3.3% of cases (33). The risk of excessive operative blood loss (exceeding 500 mL) is related to the trimester of pregnancy in which the conization is performed, ranging from negligible risk during the first trimester, to 5% in the second trimester, and 10% in the third trimester (34). Other maternal complications of cervical conization in pregnancy include lacerations of the cervix in patients undergoing subsequent vaginal delivery (7.2%), and cervical stenosis (2.2%) (34).

Fetal complications of cervical conization in pregnancy can be significant; therefore, the potential benefit of diagnostic clinical information to be gained from such a procedure must be considered carefully. Overall, spontaneous pregnancy loss follows cervical conization in 3.6% to 8.1% of patients; however, the risk is highest if conization is performed in the first trimester (17.7%) (35–37). Consequently, conization should be avoided in the first trimester. From an obstetric standpoint, the optimal time for cervical cone biopsy is either between 14 and 20 weeks' gestational age, or after fetal maturity has been reached. Conization should not be attempted within 4 weeks of the anticipated delivery date because of the potential risk of cervical laceration and excessive bleeding from the conization bed. While the incidence of premature delivery averages approximately 12%, successful delivery of a surviving infant can be expected in almost 90% of cases (25,34–36).

To minimize both maternal and fetal complications, most surgeons perform a more conservative conization than would necessarily be required in the nonpregnant state. Consequently, the risk of persistent dysplasia following conization in pregnancy is significantly higher than in nonpregnant counterparts. In the review by Hacker et al. (2) of women undergoing conization during pregnancy, residual CIS was detected in 43.4% of women undergoing postpartum hysterectomy or repeat conization. Thus, in most instances, conization performed during pregnancy should not be considered a therapeutic procedure.

Attempting to avoid the morbidity associated with formal cone biopsy, some authors have suggested that a wedge excision of the nonvisualized portion of the transformation zone may provide adequate diagnostic information (2,38). Loop electrosurgical excision procedures can also be performed safely during pregnancy; however, electrocautery artifact may make surgical margins or depth of invasion difficult to evaluate so that the traditional cold-knife approach may be preferred (39).

Glandular Lesions

Atypical glandular cells on a cytologic smear may present a difficult diagnostic problem. Decidual, trophoblastic, or Arias-Stella reaction cells may be present on the Pap smear and be misinterpreted as atypical glandular cells. In addition, HGSIL in the cervical canal may represent the shedding of atypical glandular cells. A particular problem associated with glandular abnormalities in pregnancy is the fact that these lesions are usually located high in the endocervical canal or deep within endocervical crypts, and are therefore less amenable to invasive biopsy procedures than squamous lesions located on the ectocervix. At a minimum, atypical glandular cells should be evaluated with colposcopy and biopsy, if indicated. Endocervical curettage should be avoided during pregnancy. Persistent atypical glandular cells without cytologic impression suspicious for malignancy can be followed expectantly with cytology and colposcopy every 8 weeks, with definitive evaluation delayed until postpartum. If the cytologic smear is highly suspicious for invasive adenocarcinoma and colposcopy is unrevealing, conization may be indicated.

SYMPTOMS OF INVASIVE CERVICAL CANCER

Symptoms of cervical carcinoma may be identical to those encountered during the course of an uncomplicated pregnancy (Table 2). Approximately 14.8% of patients with cervical carcinoma in pregnancy are asymptomatic at the time of diagnosis; however, the likelihood of making a diagnosis prior to the onset of symptoms is stage-dependent. Patients with stage I tumors are twice as likely to be asymptomatic at diagnosis as patients with more advanced disease (36% versus 18%) (40). Vaginal bleeding is by far the most common presenting complaint in obstetric or postpartum patients with cervical carcinoma, being present in 67.7% of all patients. Eighty percent of symptomatic patients complain of abnormal or postcoital bleeding (23,41–44). The extent of bleeding usually parallels tumor volume and may vary from scant postcoital spotting to hemorrhage of sufficient magnitude to require blood transfusion. Vaginal discharge may be interpreted as a normal physiologic change during pregnancy, but it is the presenting symptom in 13% of patients with cervical cancer. Pelvic pain is usually associated with advanced-stage disease and is an infrequent presenting symptom of cervical carcinoma associated with pregnancy (3.5% of patients).

Confusion between the symptoms of early cervical carcinoma and those of normal pregnancy frequently leads to a delay in diagnosis.

TABLE 2. *Symptoms of invasive cervical cancer in pregnancy*

Symptom	n	Percent
Asymptomatic	57/384	14.8
Abnormal bleeding	260/384	67.7
Vaginal discharge	37/284	13.0
Pain	6/171	3.5

Data from refs. 23, 41–44.

Hacker et al. (2) reported that when cervical cancer was associated with pregnancy, the average duration of symptoms prior to diagnosis was 4.5 months. In younger obstetric patients, the suspicion for malignancy is usually low, and diagnostic delays are especially common. In a report on 327 patients with invasive cervical carcinoma associated with pregnancy in Poland, Sablinska et al. (45) found that among women aged 20 to 29 years, only 14.3% were diagnosed prior to delivery, while 72.8% were diagnosed within the first postpartum year. Any pregnant patient presenting with symptomatic vaginal bleeding or discharge should be completely evaluated with cervical inspection, palpation, and cytology.

STAGING

The International Federation of Gynecology and Obstetrics (FIGO) staging system for the diagnosis and evaluation of cervical carcinoma is based on clinical evaluation (inspection, palpation, colposcopy), histologic examination of directed biopsy or conization specimens, and radiographic examination of the chest, kidneys, and skeleton (Table 3). Findings of computed tomography (CT), magnetic resonance (MR) imaging, lymphangiography, and laparotomy or laparoscopy should not be used to establish the clinical stage but may be useful in treatment planning.

Clinical staging begins with a thorough physical assessment and pelvic examination. Stage I neoplasms are clinically confined to the cervix. Microinvasive carcinoma (stage IA1) is defined as a tumor with stromal invasion no greater than 3 mm in depth beneath the basement membrane and no wider than 7 mm. Patients with stage IA1 are at very low risk of metastatic disease and may be treated more conservatively. Stage IA2 lesions invade to a depth of 3.1 to 5.0 mm and are no wider than 7 mm. The risk of pelvic lymph node metastases is approximately 6%, however, so that these patients require more aggressive therapy. Stage IB tumors are subclassified into stage IB1 (no greater than 4 cm in maximal diameter) and stage IB2 (greater than 4 cm in maximal diameter), reflecting the prognostic importance of tumor volume for macroscopic lesions limited to the cervix (46).

Careful palpation of the entire vagina is necessary to determine whether disease extends

TABLE 3. *International Federation of Gynecology and Obstetrics staging of cervical cancer*

Stage	Definition
0	Carcinoma *in situ,* intraepithelial carcinoma
I	Carcinoma strictly confined to the cervix
IA	Invasive cancer identified only microscopically. All gross lesions, even with superficial invasion, are stage IB cancers. Invasion is limited to measured stromal invasion with maximum depth of 5 mm and no wider than 7 mm
IA1	Stromal invasion no greater than 3 mm in depth and no wider than 7 mm
IA2	Stromal invasion greater than 3 mm but no greater than 5 mm, and no wider than 7 mm
IB	Clinical lesions confined to the cervix or preclinical lesions greater than stage IA
IB1	Clinical lesions no greater than 4 cm in maximal diameter
IB2	Clinical lesions greater than 4 cm in maximal diameter
II	Carcinoma extends beyond the cervix but has not extended to the pelvic wall. Carcinoma involves the vagina but not as far as the lower one-third
IIA	No obvious parametrial involvement
IIB	Obvious parametrial involvement
III	Carcinoma extends to the pelvic wall. Tumor involves the lower one-third of the vagina. All cases of hydronephrosis or nonfunctioning kidney are included unless known to be due to another cause
IIIA	No extension to the pelvic wall
IIIB	Extension to the pelvic wall, hydronephrosis, nonfunctioning kidney
IV	Carcinoma extends beyond the true pelvis or clinically involves the mucosa of the bladder or rectum. Bullous edema does not permit a case to be allocated to stage IV
IVA	Spread of growth to adjacent organs
IVB	Spread to distant organs

to the upper two-thirds of the vagina (stage IIA) or it also involves the lower one-third of the vagina (stage IIIA). Tumor extension into the parametrial tissue (stage IIB) or to the pelvic side wall (stage IIIB) is best appreciated on rectovaginal examination. Palpation of the parametrial and side wall tissues may be particularly challenging with advanced gestational age. Stage IV is assigned if disease involves the mucosa of the bladder or rectum (stage IVA) or extends outside of the true pelvis (stage IVB). A careful survey of inguinal and supraclavicular lymph nodes is mandatory. When there is doubt concerning which stage a tumor should be assigned, the lower stage is mandatory. Once a clinical stage has been determined and treatment initiated, subsequent findings on either extended clinical staging or surgical exploration should not alter the assigned stage.

A review of the published literature (1960 through 1981) found that the stage distribution for pregnant women with cervical carcinoma (stage IB, 42%; stage II, 33.2%; stages III and IV, 24.8%) was not significantly different from the stage distribution for nonpregnant women with cervical carcinoma (stage I, 38%; stage II, 32%; stages III and IV, 30%) (2,4). However, more contemporary series have found that the majority of patients with cervical carcinoma during pregnancy have stage I disease, with approximately 76% being stage IB (47–50). Compared to nonpregnant controls, women who were pregnant at the time of cervical cancer diagnosis are 3.1 times more likely to have stage I disease (51). This favorable stage distribution is likely related to both the incorporation of screening cytology into prenatal care and the association of early-stage disease with younger age (less 35 years) (5).

DIAGNOSTIC IMAGING

Diagnostic Imaging Techniques

The extent of the pretreatment radiographic evaluation is dictated by the clinical stage of disease, the estimated gestational age at the time of diagnosis, and the patient's wishes regarding continuation of the pregnancy. In circumstances in which the likelihood of extracervical disease is extremely low (stage IA or small stage IB lesions), pretreatment radiologic studies (chest x-ray, assessment of ureters) are not routinely necessary, as they are unlikely to affect therapeutic decisions. For patients with a larger volume of disease, a chest x-ray should be obtained to evaluate for pulmonary metastases. In addition, an accurate assessment of the renal collecting system and ureters is required. In nonpregnant patients, this is routinely accomplished with intravenous pyelogram (IVP) or CT with intravenous contrast. However, fetal radiation exposure during these procedures is not negligible and must be considered carefully if fetal viability is a possibility (52) (Table 4).

For pregnant patients with cervical carcinoma who choose to delay therapy or who have not yet decided the issue of fetal preservation, MR imaging is an appropriate substitute for IVP or CT for evaluation of the urinary system, and avoids exposing the fetus to ionizing radiation. MR imaging is capable of depicting pelvic anatomy in three imaging planes and is useful for calculating tumor volume and assessing spread to adjacent organs. The accuracy of MR imaging in assessing both pelvic and abdominal lymph node me-

TABLE 4. *Estimated fetal exposure to ionizing radiation from various diagnostic procedures*

Diagnostic procedure	Dose to uterus (mrad)
Chest radiograph	0.02–0.07
Intravenous pyelogram	686–1398
Barium enema	1945–3986
Upper GI series	56
Upper GI series with small bowel series	2123
KUB	122–245
Mammogram	7–20
CT scan: head	<50
CT scan: chest	<100
CT scan: abdomen	1700–2600
CT scan: pelvimetry	250
Bone scan	500

CT, computed tomography; GI, gastrointestinal; KUB, kidney, ureter, and bladder.
From ref. 52, with permission.

tastasis is similar to that of CT, and MR imaging is superior for visualizing nodal relationships to surrounding tissues, especially vessels (53,54). Ureteral dilatation is also detectable on MR imaging; however, the clinical significance of this finding must be interpreted within the context of the physiologic renal and ureteral dilatation of pregnancy. Upper urinary tract dilatation begins as early as the sixth or seventh week of gestation and may persist for 3 months after delivery. There is no evidence that the electromagnetic fields associated with MR imaging interfere with human development (33).

Effects of Diagnostic Imaging in Pregnancy

The effects of radiation from diagnostic procedures on the developing pregnancy become important considerations if treatment of cervical carcinoma is to be delayed until fetal viability has been reached. The periods of preimplantation and early implantation (10 days postconception) are the most sensitive to the lethal effects of *in utero* irradiation. However, embryos surviving radiation exposure during this period do not develop congenital abnormalities because of the pluripotential nature of the embryonic cells at this stage of development.

The period of organogenesis extends from postconceptional day 10 through 12 to 14 weeks' gestational age, and it is during this period that the fetus is at greatest risk for gross structural malformations from *in utero* irradiation. Using data based on Japanese atomic bomb survivors, Stovall et al. (55) suggested a dose threshold of 5 to 10 cGy that must be exceeded to significantly increase the risk of growth retardation, microcephaly, and severe mental retardation. Most organ systems become less susceptible to the effects of *in utero* irradiation after the period of organogenesis. However, central nervous system development continues throughout gestation, so that *in utero* irradiation exposure as late as 25 weeks' gestational age may result in significant abnormalities (mental retardation, microcephaly) (55). This stage of fetal development overlaps the period of organogenesis, extending from the eighth week of gestation until term. Radiation exposure during this period infrequently results in gross structural abnormalities; however, severe mental retardation, microcephaly, and growth retardation may be observed with doses greater than 50 cGy (55).

In general, current data suggest that for radiation doses less than 5 cGy, the risk of spontaneous abortion, growth retardation, or congenital malformation is minimal (56). Radiation exposure between 5 and 10 cGy may result in subtle pathologic effects on the fetus, but not gross malformations or growth retardation (57). It has been estimated that *in utero* radiation exposure of 1 cGy approximately doubles the incidence of childhood malignancies during the first 10 years of life (one-half being leukemias); however, the absolute risk of cancer induction remains quite low (58). Several authors have suggested that for radiation exposure in excess of 10 cGy during the first trimester, therapeutic pregnancy termination should be considered, as fetal radiation exposure between 10 and 50 cGy carries a significant risk of damage during the first trimester. Exposure to more than 50 cGy is associated with a high risk of fetal damage during all trimesters (57,59).

TREATMENT

Once the diagnosis of cervical cancer has been established, individual treatment recommendations are dependent on the stage of disease, gestational age at the time of diagnosis, and the desires of the mother regarding continuation of the pregnancy. Management decisions must take the following into consideration:

- Possible effects of pregnancy on the biology of cervical carcinoma
- Effects of mode of delivery on the biology of the disease
- Possible effects of cervical carcinoma on the health of the pregnancy and fetus
- Question of treatment delay until fetal maturity is achieved

Management of Microinvasive Carcinoma in Pregnancy

The diagnosis of microinvasive carcinoma of the cervix (stages IA1 or IA2) can only be reliably established by histologic examination of a sufficiently large, intact biopsy specimen (wedge resection or traditional conization) with clear surgical margins. The decision of when to institute treatment depends on the gestational age at the time of diagnosis and the mother's wishes regarding continuation of pregnancy (Fig. 2). There is no convincing evidence that the route of delivery influences the outcome for patients with microinvasive carcinoma, and intrapartum management should generally be dictated by obstetric indications. Vaginal delivery can usually be accomplished and definitive therapy delayed until 4 to 6 weeks after delivery. Patients with positive conization margins or an uncertain depth of invasion should be reevaluated with repeat conization prior to definitive therapy. For well documented stage IA1 lesions (clear conization margins, no lymph-vascular space invasion [LVSI]), conization alone is adequate treatment. Total hysterectomy may be performed if the patient has completed her childbearing. In the presence of LVSI, pelvic lymphadenectomy with or without modified radical hysterectomy is recommended. Patients with stage IA2 lesions should be treated with a modified radical hysterectomy with pelvic lymphadenectomy or radiation therapy.

If cesarean delivery is required for obstetric reasons or the patient desires immediate treatment, surgical therapy can be rendered concurrent with abdominal delivery (see Fig. 2). In choosing this therapeutic approach, however, clinicians must recognize that, while

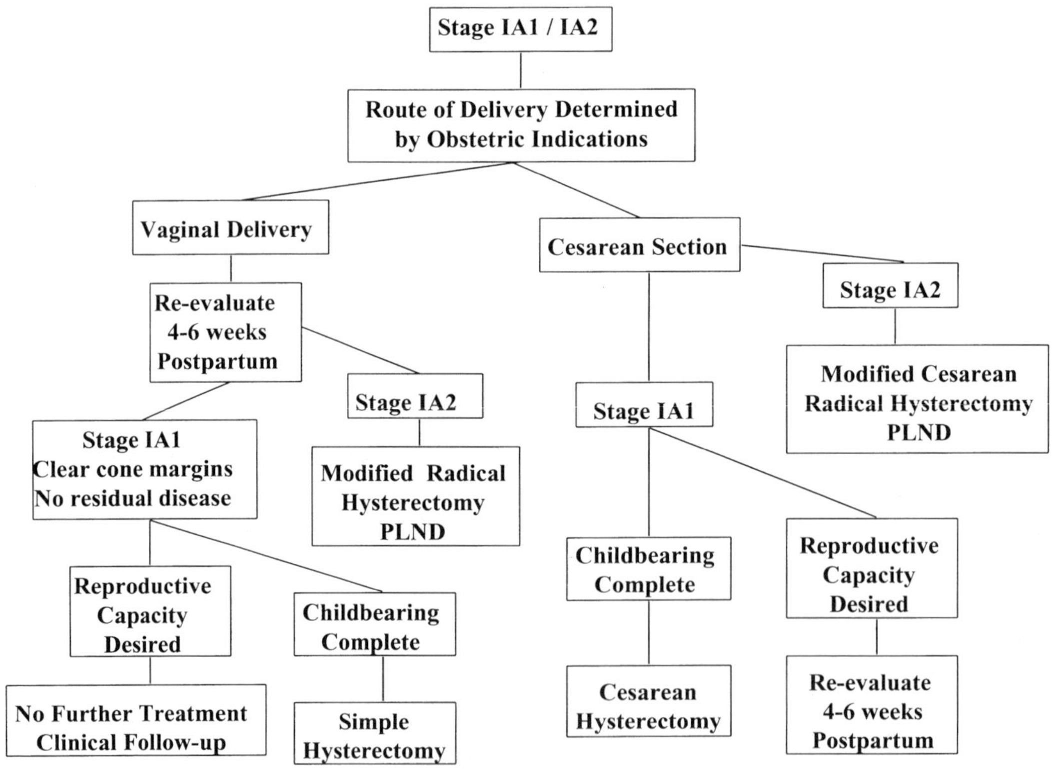

FIG. 2. Management of stage IA cervical cancer during pregnancy (PLND, pelvic lymphadenectomy).

generally safe, cesarean hysterectomy is associated with a higher risk of perioperative hemorrhage, infectious complications, and urinary tract injury than hysterectomy performed in the nongravid state (60).

Surgical Management: Stages IB to IIA

For a pregnant patient with stage IB or IIA disease, both radical surgery and radiation therapy offer similar cure rates (3,33). Survival rates following radical surgery for early-stage cervical cancer range from 64% to 100%, while primary radiation therapy is associated with long-term survival of 58% to 83% (39,43,49,50,61–65). Although selected series show a survival advantage for surgical therapy, selection bias with regard to tumor size and comorbid medical conditions must be considered in interpreting these results (49,66).

Our general preference is to recommend surgical therapy for obstetric patients with early-stage cervical carcinoma who are satisfactory operative candidates. Definitive surgery for stages IB or IIA disease consists of radical hysterectomy with bilateral pelvic (with or without paraaortic) lymphadenectomy. Advantages of the radical surgical approach include the provision of immediate treatment of the pelvic tumor, as well as the opportunity to perform a thorough pelvic and abdominal exploration, identifying patients with a disparity between the clinical and surgicopathologic stages. Based on surgical findings, patients can then be offered an individualized treatment plan based on their precise disease status. In young, reproductive-age patients, surgery permits conservation of the ovaries, which may be transposed out of subsequent radiation fields, and allows preservation of vaginal anatomy. Associated clinical conditions in which radical surgery is particularly preferable to radiation therapy include concomitant inflammatory bowel disease, previous radiation for other disease, and the presence of a simultaneous adnexal neoplasm.

Surgical therapy in pregnancy is feasible and safe, with acceptable associated morbidity. Most surgeons report that soft tissue edema associated with gestation results in more pronounced cleavage planes and facilitates the surgical dissection. Surgical tumor clearance and lymph node yield are comparable to radical hysterectomy performed in non-pregnant patients. In late pregnancy, clinical staging (pelvic examination) may be less accurate because of anatomic distortion created by the gravid uterus. In these cases, an intraoperative determination of operability should be made after evacuation of the uterus.

If the decision is made to proceed with therapy prior to 20 weeks' gestation, radical hysterectomy is performed with the fetus *in situ*. After 20 weeks, the uterus should be evacuated prior to hysterectomy (see "Treatment Delays" below). Comparing radical hysterectomy performed in the first and second trimesters (fetus *in situ)* with that performed in the third trimester in conjunction with cesarean delivery reveals that cesarean radical hysterectomy is associated with a higher blood loss (1750 mL versus 777 mL), a higher risk of requiring a blood transfusion (75% versus 54%), and a greater volume of blood transfusion (3.5 units versus 1.6 units) (50). Nevertheless, overall morbidity is acceptable. Incisional and fistulous (urinary and bowel) complications related to surgical management tend to occur early in the postoperative period and are usually amenable to surgical repair.

Radiation Therapy: Stages IIB to IV

Primary irradiation is the standard therapeutic approach for patients with stage IIB or greater cervical carcinoma. Concomitant cisplatin-based chemotherapy should also be considered. Patients with stage IB or IIA lesions who are poor operative candidates may also be treated by primary irradiation with curative intent. A standard contemporary treatment plan begins with the administration of whole-pelvic external-beam radiation to a dose of 4500 to 5000 cGy. In patients with radiographic evidence of paraaortic nodal involvement, the paraaortic fields are treated to a dose of 4500 cGy. Completion of external-beam therapy is followed by brachytherapy applications (usually two) to deliver a total dose of 8500 cGy to the central tumor mass and between 5000 to 6000 cGy to the pelvic side wall.

Radiation therapy for stage IB to IV carcinoma of the cervix may begin before or after delivery of the fetus, but generally therapy should be initiated as soon as possible in the presence of advanced disease (Fig. 3). If the diagnosis is made in the first or second trimester, treatment is initiated with whole-pelvic external-beam radiation with the fetus *in situ.* The exception may be if disease is so advanced that maternal survival is remote and fetal viability becomes of primary importance. Commonly, spontaneous termination of the pregnancy will occur prior to the administration of 4000 cGy of external-beam radiation. However, 27% of patients will not abort spontaneously and require surgical evacuation of the uterus (23). In patients who do experience spontaneous termination of pregnancy, the interval between onset of external radiotherapy and abortion is related to gestational age. Spontaneous abortion will occur an average of 32.7 days after beginning external-beam irradiation during the first trimester, while a mean of 43.9 days is required during the second trimester (44). If diagnosis is made in the third trimester, fetal viability is assessed and delivery accomplished by cesarean section with a vertical uterine corpus incision. Therapeutic radiation is then instituted by the second or third postpartum week.

The primary advantage of radiation therapy is that it can be used with curative intent for all

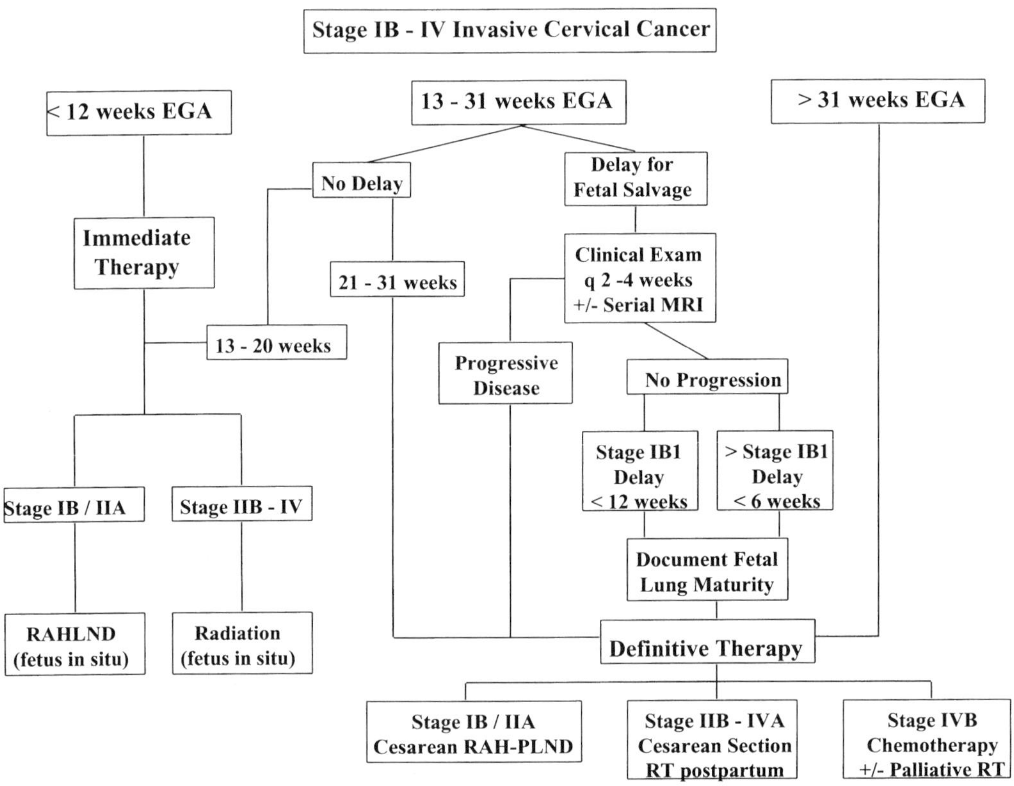

FIG. 3. Management of stages IB to IV cervical cancer during pregnancy (EGA, estimated gestational age; RAHLND, radical abdominal hysterectomy, pelvic lymphadenectomy; RT, radiation therapy; MRI, magnetic resonance imaging).

stages of disease and for most patients regardless of age, body habitus, or coexistent medical conditions. Ovarian function is lost in all patients undergoing therapeutic doses of radiation to the pelvis. Radiation therapy may also be complicated by vaginal fibrosis and associated sexual dysfunction. Chronic bowel (radiation enteritis, proctosigmoiditis) or bladder complications follow therapeutic doses of pelvic radiation in as many as 5% of patients. In contrast to surgical therapy, fistulous complications associated with radiation therapy tend to occur months to years after treatment and are less amenable to repair because of poor tissue vascularity and radiation fibrosis.

Patients with advanced metastatic disease (stage IVB) are usually treated with chemotherapy alone or in conjunction with palliative radiation therapy. These patients have a uniformly poor prognosis regardless of treatment modality.

SURVIVAL

Effect of Pregnancy on Invasive Cervical Cancer Survival

The physiologic immunosuppression of pregnancy has generated concern that the gravid state may have an adverse effect on the overall prognosis of concomitant invasive cervical cancer. Fortunately, studies controlling for the clinical stage of disease at diagnosis and other confounding variables have not substantiated this hypothesis (49,51). Van der Vange et al. (67) compared 44 women with pregnancy-associated cervical cancer to 44 control women matched for age, stage, tumor type, and treatment modality. The overall 5-year survival for pregnant patients was 80% compared to 82% for nonpregnant controls. Additionally, no differences in survival were detected between patients diagnosed during pregnancy and those diagnosed after delivery. In this series, both early- and late-complication rates were similar between the pregnant patients and nonpregnant controls. The authors concluded that pregnancy has no adverse effect on the prognosis of early-stage cervical carcinoma. Similarly, Zemlickis et al. (51) analyzed 40 women with pregnancy-associated cervical carcinoma and compared them to 89 controls matched for age and stage. They found no difference in the 30-year survival rates between the two groups. It is also noteworthy that after controlling for confounding variables, no effect on survival could be demonstrated for the trimester of diagnosis. Other investigators have confirmed that overall pregnancy does not have an adverse effect on the survival of patients with cervical carcinoma (49,68).

Effect of Gestational Age at Diagnosis on Survival

For pregnant patients with early-stage cervical carcinoma (stage I or II), gestational age at the time of diagnosis has no effect on survival, with 5-year survival rates ranging from 70% to 90% (49). Cervical cancer presenting during the third trimester or postpartum is frequently associated with a delay in diagnosis because of confusion between symptoms of cervical carcinoma and those of normal pregnancy. Advanced clinical stage is more likely in such cases, with correspondingly poor survival rates (2). After controlling for clinical stage, no independent adverse effect on survival can be demonstrated for the trimester of diagnosis (51).

Effects of Mode of Delivery on Survival

Controversy has surrounded the optimal method of delivery for women with cervical carcinoma associated with pregnancy. In patients with stage IB or IIA lesions, there are theoretic concerns over the risk of maternal hemorrhage and dissemination of disease associated with vaginal delivery, with case reports of recurrent cervical carcinoma presenting in the episiotomy site after vaginal delivery preceding definitive treatment (69). Despite these theoretic concerns, retrospective reviews have shown no association between the route of delivery and maternal survival in women with stage I cervical carcinoma (23,40,42,64). In satisfactory surgical candidates with early-stage cervical carcinoma, our general recommendation is for cesarean section and radical abdominal hysterectomy with pelvic lymphadenectomy. If patient is strongly desirous of vaginal delivery after discussion of the potential risk of metastases (and hemorrhage), cesarean delivery is reserved for obstetric indications. Successful vaginal delivery is then followed by radical abdominal hysterectomy or radiation therapy in the puerperium, depending on the extent of disease and the patient's wishes.

Among patients with advanced disease (stages III or IV), some investigators have found higher survival rates for patients undergoing vaginal delivery than for patients delivered by cesarean section (23,42,64). However, this is likely due to selection of patients with smaller lesions for vaginal delivery, so that equivalent survival rates can be expected for vaginal and abdominal delivery after controlling for tumor volume. Because large tumor mass poses a risk for both pelvic outlet obstruction and significant hemorrhage during labor, it is our practice to recommend abdominal delivery for pregnant patients with advanced cervical carcinoma.

Treatment Delays

In certain circumstances, the decision to institute immediate treatment or delay treatment in favor of fetal viability will be dictated by the clinical scenario: undesired pregnancy in the first or second trimester, fetal maturity attained prior to cancer diagnosis, or the presence of widely metastatic disease where a therapeutic delay will not worsen an already poor maternal prognosis. However, in the case of a desired but immature pregnancy, the question of delayed therapeutic intervention will undoubtedly arise.

The literature examining therapeutic delays of cervical cancer treatment during pregnancy consists largely of small case series of selected patients with early-stage disease (Table 5). In early reports, both radiation therapy and surgery were utilized effectively; however, in more contemporary series, radical surgery has been the therapeutic approach of choice. Boutselis (70) reported on five patients with stage IA cervical cancer diagnosed between 8 and 24 weeks' gestation. All patients underwent vaginal delivery prior to definitive therapy and were alive and free of disease 6 to 15 years after treatment. Lee et al. (40) reported on three patients with stage IB and five patients with stage II disease undergoing delays in therapy of up to 12 weeks without experiencing advancement of clinical stage during the waiting period. Similarly, Monk and Montz (50) described therapeutic delays of 10 to 16 weeks for three patients with stage IB cervical cancer diagnosed during the second

TABLE 5. *Therapy delays for cervical carcinoma during pregnancy*

Reference	Year	Stage	n	EGA (wk) at diagnosis	Delay (wk)	Fetal survival (%)	Treatment	Patient survival (%)
Prem et al. (44)	1966	I	9	20–34	11–17	100	RT	100
Boutselis (70)	1972	I	9	8–38	NS	NS	SRG	100
Thompson et al. (72)	1975	IA	7	10–33	5–28	86	SRG	100
Lee et al. (40)	1981	I–II	9	Third trimester	1–12	100	SRG or RT	—[a]
Greer et al. (48)	1989	IB	5	20–24	6–17	100	SRG	80
Monk and Montz (50)	1992	IA2	1	NS	23	100	SRG	100
		IB	6	19–39	1–16	100	SRG +/– RT	100
Sivanesaratnam et al.	1993	IA	1	24	12	100	SRG	100
(63)		IB	4	32–40	2–4	100	SRG	100
Duggan et al. (47)	1993	I	8	11–31	7–30	100	SRG	100
Sorosky et al. (71)	1995	I	8	0–34	8–40	100	SRG	100
Sood et al. (73)	1996	I	11	NS	3–32	100	SRG	100

EGA, estimated gestational age; NS, not stated; SRG, surgery; RT, radiation therapy.
[a]No progression of clinical stage during treatment delay.

trimester and delays of 3 weeks for three patients diagnosed during the third trimester. All patients had successful neonatal outcomes, and no apparent adverse effects on maternal survival were noted. Recently, Sorosky et al. (71) described eight patients with stage I cervical carcinoma during pregnancy who declined immediate therapy in order to improve fetal outcome. In this series, all lesions were smaller than 2.5 cm, and the mean diagnosis-to-treatment interval was 15.6 weeks. No clinical progression of disease was noted, and all patients were successfully delivered by cesarean radical hysterectomy. After a mean follow-up of 37 months, all patients remained alive and free of disease.

Other investigators have reported unfavorable outcomes associated with therapeutic delays. Dudan et al. (74) reported on eight patients diagnosed with cervical CIS or frank carcinoma experiencing apparent clinical progression of disease during delays of therapy ranging from 2 months to 6 years. However, it is unclear whether these delays were intentional and whether or not the patients were monitored closely.

Considering the majority of these reports, it appears that modest therapeutic delays in patients with early invasive carcinoma of the cervix are not detrimental to maternal outcome and can result in significant fetal salvage. However, the acceptable duration of delay is not entirely clear and should be mitigated by the clinical stage, gestational age at diagnosis, and histopathologic features. Stage IA1 tumors without LVSI diagnosed by an adequate conization specimen and with negative surgical margins may be managed expectantly during all trimesters until after delivery, at which time the patient is reevaluated. Patients with stage IA1 tumors and LVSI or stage IA2 disease diagnosed during the third trimester may delay therapy until fetal viability is achieved. Patients with these histologic features diagnosed during the first or second trimesters may consider either immediate treatment or therapeutic delay, depending on the patient's wishes. Therapeutic delay for these patients may carry some additional risk of disease progression; however, the degree of that risk is uncertain. Close clinical surveillance is mandatory if treatment is deferred until after delivery.

For patients diagnosed with stage IB1 tumors (less than 4 cm) during the second or third trimester, a delay in instituting therapy to improve fetal outcome is also a reasonable option based on the available, albeit limited, data. While delays of up to 29 weeks have been reported without an adverse effect on maternal survival, delays of this length should only be undertaken with caution and the mother's fully informed consent (71). In the absence of substantial objective data, limiting the interval between diagnosis and therapeutic intervention to not more than 12 weeks seems prudent for these patients. There is probably a greater risk of disease progression associated with delayed therapy for patients with larger-volume disease (stage IB2 and higher). In these patients, therapy should probably not be deferred for more than 6 weeks after diagnosis in order to maximize the chances for maternal survival (see Fig. 3). Patients choosing to delay therapy should be monitored closely for evidence of disease progression, with clinical evaluation performed by an experienced examiner at 2- to 4-week intervals until delivery. Serial MR imaging examinations have been used safely in pregnancy to monitor tumor volume in cervical cancer patients undergoing expectant management until fetal viability is achieved (71).

Neonatal outcome is closely linked to gestational age at the time of delivery. In reviewing 33,401 pregnancies, Copper et al. (75) calculated neonatal mortality in relation to gestational age. As can be seen from Table 6, a significant improvement in neonatal survival occurs between 25 and 26 weeks' gestation. Furthermore, a significant survival advantage can be achieved by prolonging pregnancy for even a few weeks beyond this critical juncture, as neonatal mortality decreases from 45.3% at 26 weeks to 9.4% at 30 weeks (75). Neonatal morbidity also depends on gestational age at delivery. At 26 weeks' gestation, the rates of respiratory

TABLE 6. *Predicted neonatal survival by gestational age*

Gestational age (wk)	Survival by gestational age (%)
22	0
23	1.8
24	9.9
25	15.5
26	54.7
27	67.0
28	77.4
29	85.2
30	90.6
31	94.2
32	96.5
33	97.9

From ref. 76, with permission.

distress syndrome, severe intraventricular hemorrhage, and neonatal sepsis are 92.6%, 29.6%, and 33.3%, decreasing to 54.7%, 1.9%, and 11.3%, respectively, at 30 weeks' gestational age (76). Therapy should only be delayed until there is documented fetal lung maturity. It is reasonable to perform amniocentesis for lung maturity assessment beginning at approximately 30 to 31 weeks. Subsequent taps can be performed weekly until a mature lung profile is obtained. In addition, betamethasone (Celestone) can be used to hasten the development of fetal lung maturity.

FOLLOW-UP GYNECOLOGIC CARE

Surveillance

Following definitive treatment for cervical carcinoma, patients should have a complete physical and pelvic examination every 3 months for 2 years, followed by semiannual examinations for an additional 3 years. Vaginal or cervical cytology should be performed at each examination. Approximately 80% of recurrences will present within 2 years of definitive therapy (4). For patients with advanced disease, a yearly chest x-ray is also advisable; however, the use of routine CT or MR imaging is of unproven benefit in the absence of clinical recurrence.

Hormone Replacement and Sexual Rehabilitation

For younger patients especially, cervical cancer treatment may result in premature loss of ovarian function, usually due to radiation therapy. Practical concerns related to premature menopause in young women include hot flashes, skin changes, vaginal dryness, and mood changes and also extend to the management of osteoporosis and cardiac risk factors. Estrogen replacement therapy is indicated for the majority of women suffering surgical or radiation-induced castration from cervical cancer treatment. Contraindications to estrogen replacement include active hepatic disease, a history of venous thrombosis, or a personal history of breast cancer. In women with the uterus *in situ,* hormone replacement therapy should consist of both conjugated estrogen and a progestational agent. Either a continuous or cyclic schedule of administration is suitable, depending on patient preference. Hypoestrogenic vaginal atrophy refractory to systemic hormone replacement can be treated with vaginal estrogen cream and a vaginal moisturizer (per vagina three times per week, regardless of sexual activity).

Sexual dysfunction following treatment for gynecologic cancer is common and includes inhibited sexual desire, excitement, and orgasm, as well as dyspareunia. Women undergoing therapy for cervical cancer are particularly prone to disturbances of the sexual-response cycle because of physiologic (loss of ovarian function) and anatomic (vaginal shortening or fibrosis) alterations, diminished body image, or disruption of the relationship with their sexual partner. The importance of addressing sexual function with patients and a willingness to refer them to an appropriate sexual counselor or therapist, if necessary, cannot be overemphasized. Surgical resection of the proximal vagina with radical hysterectomy can result in vaginal shortening and dyspareunia. While vaginal length will gradually increase with use, postoperative dyspareunia may be lessened and sensation enhanced by a change in coital position or the addition of lubrication. Vaginal fibrosis and stenosis are frequent complications of pelvic radiation therapy and can be treated with graduated vaginal dilators combined with topical estrogen cream and a vaginal lubricant. Severe cases may require surgical correction to produce a satisfactory vaginal capacity.

Fertility

Advances in reproductive technology have made it possible for women to explore the option of using their remaining reproductive capacity following treatment for gynecologic cancer. Standard treatment for cervical cancer other than stage IA1 involves loss of uterine reproductive function either because of radiation-induced fibrosis and atrophy or surgical extirpation. However, in reproductive-aged women undergoing radical hysterectomy for early-stage cervical cancer, grossly normal ovaries should be conserved, as the risk of occult metastasis is less than 1% (57). With intact ovarian function, a woman may undergo ovum harvesting and *in vitro* fertilization; the pregnancy is then carried in the uterus of a surrogate. The decision to transpose the ovaries out of the pelvis either at the time of radical hysterectomy in anticipation of adjuvant radiation therapy, or prior to primary irradiation, must be individualized. Even with ovarian transposition, ovarian failure occurs in 42% of patients receiving pelvic radiation therapy (77). Furthermore, approximately 20% of patients undergoing ovarian transposition at the time of radical hysterectomy will experience premature ovarian failure even without irradiation (77).

In an attempt to preserve fertility, some clinicians have advocated radical vaginal trachelectomy in conjunction with laparoscopic lymph node dissection as definitive treatment for early-stage cervical cancer (78,79). This technique is unstudied in the pregnant population and, if applicable, would probably be performed most successfully 4 to 6 weeks postpartum following either vaginal or cesarean delivery to allow uterine involution and restoration of anatomy. While it is technically feasible, no long-term follow-up data are yet available on patients undergoing this conservative procedure for early-stage cervical carcinoma. Therefore, radical vaginal trachelectomy and laparoscopic lymph node dissection must still be considered investigational.

SUMMARY

Despite an apparent increase in cervical cancer incidence among younger women, cervical neoplasia associated with pregnancy is still a relatively rare condition. Consequently, most institutions have not had sufficient experience with this condition to allow development of precise management protocols based on substantial objective data. Nevertheless, based on available data, some general management guidelines can be drawn. Management of CIN consists of almost exclusively expectant observation, with definitive therapy deferred until after delivery. Conization is reserved for rare cases in which microinvasive carcinoma is suspected or the diagnosis of invasive carcinoma will result in a change in the timing or route of delivery. Survival rates for pregnant patients with cervical cancer are comparable to those for nonpregnant women, when controlled for stage. Furthermore, delays in therapy in order to improve fetal salvage rates appear safe in selected circumstances for early-stage disease. However, such delays in therapy should only be undertaken with the fully informed consent of patients, and treatment should not be postponed beyond the time that fetal viability is reached, generally about 32 weeks. The diagnosis of cervical cancer in pregnancy presents a patient, her family, and the clinician with a complex array of decisions regarding diagnostic and treatment modalities, all of which must be carefully considered within the individual patient's social, religious, and ethical framework.

REFERENCES

1. Parker SL, Tong T, Bolden S, Wingo PA. Cancer statistics, 1997. *CA Cancer J Clin* 1997;47:5–27.
2. Hacker NF, Berek JS, Lagasse LD, Charles EH, Savage

EW, Moore JG. Carcinoma of the cervix associated with pregnancy. *Obstet Gynecol* 1982;59:735–746.
3. Shivvers SA, Miller DS. Preinvasive and invasive breast and cervical cancer prior to or during pregnancy. *Clin Perinatol* 1997;24:369–389.
4. Hatch KD. Cervical cancer. In: Berek JS, Hacker NF eds. *Practical gynecologic oncology*, 2nd ed. Baltimore: Williams & Wilkins, 1994:243–284.
5. Clark MA, Naahas W, Markert RJ, Dodson MG. Cervical cancer: women aged 35 and younger compared to women aged 36 and older. *Am J Clin Oncol* 1991;14: 352–356.
6. Cervical cancer. *National Institutes of Health Consensus Statement* 1996;14:1–38.
7. Brinton LA, Hoover RN. Epidemiology of gynecologic cancers. In: Hoskins WJ, Perez CA, Young RC, eds. *Principles and practice of gynecologic oncology*, 2nd ed. Philadelphia: Lippincott–Raven Publishers, 1997:3–30.
8. Fife KH, Katz BP, Roush J, Handy VD, Brown DR, Hansell R. Cancer-associated human papillomavirus types are selectively increased in the cervix of women in the first trimester of pregnancy. *Am J Obstet Gynecol* 1996;174:1487–1493.
9. Schneider A, Hotz M, Gissman L. Increased prevalence of human papillomavirus in the lower genital tract of pregnant women. *Int J Cancer* 1987;40:198–201.
10. Chang-Claude J, Schneider A, Smith E, Blettner M, Wahrendorf J, Turek L. Longitudinal study of the effects of pregnancy and other factors on detection of HPV. *Gynecol Oncol* 1996;60:355–362.
11. Rando RF, Lindheim S, Hasty L, Sedlacek TV, Woodland M, Eder C. Increased frequency of detection of human papillomavirus deoxyribonucleic acid in exfoliated cervical cells during pregnancy. *Am J Obstet Gynecol* 1989;161:50–55.
12. Weinberg ED. Pregnancy-associated depression of cell-mediated immunity. *Rev Infect Dis* 1984;6:814–831.
13. Gall SA. Maternal adjustments in the immune system in normal pregnancy. *Clin Obstet Gynecol* 1983;26: 521–536.
14. Malone JM, Sokol RJ, Ager JW. Pregnancy, human papillomavirus and cervical intraepithelial neoplasia. *Eur J Gynaecol Oncol* 1988;9:120–124.
15. Anderson GH, Boyes DA, Benedet JL, et al. Organisation and results of the cervical cytology screening programme in British Columbia, 1955-85. *BMJ* 1988;296: 976–978.
16. Lurain JR, Gallup DG. Management of abnormal Papanicolaou smears in pregnancy. *Obstet Gynecol* 1979; 53:484–488.
17. Abitol MM, Benjamin F, Gastillo N. Management of the abnormal cervical smear and carcinoma *in situ* of the cervix during pregnancy. *Am J Obstet Gynecol* 1973; 117:904–908.
18. Rivlin ME, Woodliff JM, Bowlin RB, et al. Comparison of Cytobrush and cotton swab for Papanicolaou smears in pregnancy. *J Reprod Med* 1993;38:147–150.
19. Wanless JF. Carcinoma of the cervix in pregnancy. *Am J Obstet Gynecol* 1971;110:173–177.
20. Paraiso MF, Brady K, Helmchen R, Roat TW. Evaluation of the endocervical Cytobrush and Cervex-Brush in pregnant women. *Obstet Gynecol* 1994;84:539–543.
21. Oster AG. Natural history of cervical intraepithelial neoplasia: a critical review. *Int J Gynecol Pathol* 1993; 12:186–192.
22. Richart RM, Barron BA. A follow-up study of patients with cervical dysplasia. *Am J Obstet Gynecol* 1969;105: 386–393.
23. Creasman WT, Rutledge FN, Fletcher GH. Carcinoma of the cervix associated with pregnancy. *Am J Obstet Gynecol* 1970;36:495–501.
24. DePetrillo AD, Townsend DE, Morrow CP, Lickrish GM, DiSaia PJ, Roy M. Colposcopic evaluation of the abnormal Papanicolaou test in pregnancy. *Am J Obstet Gynecol* 1975;121:441–445.
25. Fowler WC, Walton LA, Edelman DA. Cervical intraepithelial neoplasia during pregnancy. *South Med J* 1980;73:1180–1185.
26. Yoonessi M, Wieckowska W, Mariniello D, Antkowiak J. Cervical intra-epithelial neoplasia in pregnancy. *Int J Gynaecol Obstet* 1982;20:111–118.
27. Benedet JL, Selke PA, Nickerson KG. Colposcopic evaluation of abnormal Papanicolaou smears in pregnancy. *Am J Obstet Gynecol* 1987;157:932–937.
28. LaPolla JP, O'Neill C, Wetrich D. Colposcopic management of abnormal cervical cytology in pregnancy. *J Reprod Med* 1988;33:301–306.
29. Ostergard DR, Nieberg RK. Evaluation of abnormal cervical cytology during pregnancy with colposcopy. *Am J Obstet Gynecol* 1979;134:756–758.
30. Jain AG, Higgins RV, Boyle MJ. Management of low-grade squamous intraepithelial lesions during pregnancy. *Am J Obstet Gynecol* 1997;177:298–302.
31. Campion MJ, Sedlacek TV. Colposcopy in pregnancy. *Obstet Gynecol Clin North Am* 1993;20:153–163.
32. Patsner B. Management of low-grade cervical dysplasia during pregnancy. *South Med J* 1990;83:1405–1406.
33. Hannigan EV. Cervical cancer in pregnancy. *Clin Obstet Gynecol* 1990;33:837–845.
34. Averette HE, Nasser N, Yankow SL, Little WA. Cervical conization in pregnancy. *Am J Obstet Gynecol* 1970; 106:543–549.
35. Hannigan EV, Whitehouse HH, Atkinson WD, Becker SN. Cone biopsy during pregnancy. *Obstet Gynecol* 1982;60:450–455.
36. Daskal JL, Pitkin RM. Cone biopsy of the cervix during pregnancy. *Obstet Gynecol* 1968;32:1–5.
37. Nebel W, Shingleton HM, Swanton MC. Cold knife conization of the cervix uteri. *Surg Gynecol Obstet* 1967;125:780–784.
38. Hinde FC. Cervical biopsy in pregnancy. *J Obstet Gynaecol Br Commonwlth* 1964;71:707–711.
39. Robinson WR, Webb S, Tirpack J, Degefu S, O'Quinn AG. Management of cervical intraepithelial neoplasia during pregnancy with LOOP excision. *Gynecol Oncol* 1997;64:153–155.
40. Lee RB, Neglia W, Park RC. Cervical carcinoma in pregnancy. *Obstet Gynecol* 1981;58:584–589.
41. Williams TJ, Brack CB. Carcinoma of the cervix in pregnancy. *Cancer* 1964;17:1486–1491.
42. Bosch A, Marcial VA. Carcinoma of the uterine cervix associated with pregnancy. *Am J Roent Radium Ther Nucl Med* 1966;96:92–99.
43. Fogh I. Cancer colli uteri and pregnancy. *Cancer* 1972; 29:114–116.
44. Prem KA, Makowski EL, McKelvey JL. Carcinoma of the cervix associated with pregnancy. *Am J Obstet Gynecol* 1966;95:99–105.
45. Sablinska R. Tarlowska L, Stemachow J. Invasive carcinoma of the cervix associated with pregnancy: correla-

tion between patient age, advancement of cancer and gestation, and result of treatment. *Gynecol Oncol* 1977; 5:363–373.
46. Creasman WT. New gynecologic cancer staging. *Gynecol Oncol* 1995;58:157–158.
47. Duggan B, Muderspach LI, Roman LD, Curtin JP, d'Ablaing G, Morrow CP. Cervical cancer in pregnancy: reporting on planned delay in therapy. *Obstet Gynecol* 1993;82:598–602.
48. Greer BE, Easterling TR, McLennan DA, et al. Fetal and maternal considerations in the management of stage IB cervical cancer during pregnancy. *Gynecol Oncol* 1989;34:61–65.
49. Hopkins MP, Morley GW. The prognosis and management of cervical cancer associated with pregnancy. *Obstet Gynecol* 1992;80:9–13.
50. Monk BJ, Montz FJ. Invasive cervical cancer complicating intrauterine pregnancy: treatment with radical hysterectomy. *Obstet Gynecol* 1992;80:199–203.
51. Zemlickis D, Lishner M, Degendorfer D, Panzarella T, Sutcliff SB, Koren G. Maternal and fetal outcome after invasive cervical cancer in pregnancy. *J Clin Oncol* 1991;9:1956–1961.
52. Cunningham FG, MacDonald PC, Gant NF, Leveno JK, Gilstrap LC, eds. Imaging modalities during pregnancy. In: *Williams obstetrics,* 20th ed. Norwalk, CT: Appleton & Lange, 1996:1045–1058.
53. Waggenspack GA, Amparo EG, Hannigan EV. MR imaging of uterine cervical carcinoma. *J Comput Assist Tomogr* 1988;12:409–414.
54. Dooms GC, Hricak H, Crooks LE, Higgins CB. Magnetic resonance imaging of the lymph nodes: comparison with CT. *Radiology* 1984;153:719–728.
55. Stovall M, Blackwell CR, Cundiff J, et al. Fetal dose from radiotherapy with photon beams: report of AAPM radiation therapy committee task group no 36. *Med Phys* 1995;22:63–82.
56. Brent RL. The effect of embryonic and fetal exposure to x-ray, microwaves, and ultrasound: counseling the pregnant and nonpregnant patient about these risks. *Semin Oncol* 1989;16:347–368.
57. Shingleton HM, Orr JW. Cervical cancer complicating pregnancy. In: Shingleton HM, Orr JW, eds. *Cancer of the cervix.* Philadelphia: JB Lippincott Co, 1995:223–239.
58. Greer BE, Goff BA, Koh WJ, Petersdorf SH, Douglas JG. Cancer in the pregnant patient. In: Hoskins WJ, Perez CA, Young RC. eds. *Principles and practice of gynecologic oncology*, 2nd ed. Philadelphia: Lippincott-Raven Publishers, 1997:463–486.
59. Hall EJ. Effects of radiation on the embryo and fetus. In: Hall EJ, ed. *Radiobiology for the radiologist*, 4th ed. Philadelphia: JB Lippincott Co, 1994:363–393.
60. Park RC, Duff WP. Role of cesarean hysterectomy in modern obstetric practice. *Clin Obstet Gynecol* 1980; 23:601–620.
61. Sall S, Rini S, Pineda A. Surgical management of invasive carcinoma of the cervix in pregnancy. *Am J Obstet Gynecol* 1974;118:1–5.
62. Nisker JA, Shubat M. Stage IB cervical carcinoma and pregnancy: report of 49 cases. *Am J Obstet Gynecol* 1983;145:203–206.
63. Sivanesaratnam V, Jayalakshmi P, Loo C. Surgical management of early invasive cancer of the cervix associated with pregnancy. *Gynecol Oncol* 1993;48:68–75.
64. Waldrop GM, Palmer JP. Carcinoma of the cervix associated with pregnancy. *Am J Obstet Gynecol* 1963;86: 202–212.
65. Stander RW, Lein JN. Carcinoma of the cervix and pregnancy. *Am J Obstet Gynecol* 1960;79:164.
66. Jones WB, Shingleton HM, Russell A, et al. Cervical carcinoma and pregnancy: a National Patterns of Care study of the American College of Surgeons. *Cancer* 1996;77:1479–1488.
67. Van der Vange N, Weverling GJ, Ketting BW, Ankum WM, Samlal R, Lammes FB. The prognosis of cervical cancer associated with pregnancy: a matched cohort study. *Obstet Gynecol* 1995;85:1022–1026.
68. Baltzer J, Regenbrecht ME, Kopcke W, Zander J. Carcinoma of the cervix and pregnancy. *Int J Gynaecol Obstet* 1990;31:317–323.
69. Cliby WA, Dodson MK, Podratz KC. Cervical cancer complicated by pregnancy: episiotomy site recurrences following vaginal delivery. *Obstet Gynecol* 1994;84: 179–182.
70. Boutselis JG. Intraepithelial carcinoma of the cervix associated with pregnancy. *Obstet Gynecol* 1972;40: 657–666.
71. Sorosky JI, Squatrito R, Ndubisi BU, et al. Stage I squamous cell cervical carcinoma in pregnancy: planned delay in therapy awaiting fetal maturity. *Gynecol Oncol* 1995;59:207–210.
72. Thompson JD, Caputo TA, Franklin EW, Dake E. The surgical management of invasive cancer of the cervix in pregnancy. *Am J Obstet Gynecol* 1975;121:853–859.
73. Sood AK, Sorosky JI, Krogman S, Anderson B, Benda J, Buller RE. Surgical management of cervical cancer complicating pregnancy: a case-control study. *Gynecol Oncol* 1996;63:294–298.
74. Dudan RC, Yon JL, Ford JH, Averette HE. Carcinoma of the cervix and pregnancy. *Gynecol Oncol* 1973;1: 283–289.
75. Copper RL, Goldenberg RL, Creasy RK, et al. A multicenter study of preterm birth weight and gestational age-specific mortality. *Am J Obstet Gynecol* 1993;168:78–84.
76. Robertson PA, Sniderman SH, Laros RK, et al. Neonatal morbidity according to gestational age and birth weight from five tertiary centers in the United States, 1983 through 1986. *Am J Obstet Gynecol* 1992;166: 1629–1641.
77. Morrow CP, Curtin JP, eds. Surgery for cervical neoplasia. In: *Gynecologic cancer surgery*. New York: Churchill Livingstone, 1996:451–568.
78. Roy M, Plante M, Renaud MC, Tetu B. Vaginal radical hysterectomy versus abdominal radical hysterectomy in the treatment of early-stage cervical cancer. *Gynecol Oncol* 1996;62:336–339.
79. Childers JM, Hatch K, Surwit EA. The role of laparoscopic lymphadenectomy in the management of cervical carcinoma. *Gynecol Oncol* 1992;47:38–43.

9

Leukemia in Pregnancy

Joanna Brell and *Matt Kalaycio

Department of Oncology, Moll Cancer Center, Fairview Hospital, Cleveland, Ohio 44111;
**Department of Hematology and Medical Oncology, Cleveland Clinic Foundation, Cleveland, Ohio 44195*

Acute and chronic leukemias are uncommon diseases of reproductive-age women. However, few are curable but all are treatable. The treatment is often complex; some leukemias are treated for years with standard chemotherapy, and others must be approached with allogeneic bone marrow transplantation. Patients must survive infection, hemorrhage, the adverse effects of treatment, and the possibility of resistant or relapsing disease before issues of reproductive health can be considered. The addition of a pregnancy to these issues further complicates a grave situation. Despite the often physically demanding therapy, reproductive-age patients have successfully delivered healthy offspring conceived before, during, or after chemotherapy for leukemia.

REVIEW OF LEUKEMIA

Incidence

The categories of leukemia include the following:

- Acute myelogenous leukemia (AML)
- Acute lymphocytic leukemia (ALL)
- Chronic myelogenous leukemia (CML)
- Chronic lymphocytic leukemia (CLL)

These leukemias differ by the leukocyte lineage involved and the level of maturation of the cell line. The incidence and prognosis for each leukemia classification is distinct. Overall, however, the leukemias account for less than 3% of all malignancies in the United States but are the leading cause of cancer deaths among people younger than 35 years (1). In 1997, there were approximately 28,300 cases of all leukemias in the United States, with the number of deaths from disease estimated at 21,310 (75%) of those diagnosed. AML accounts for 9200 (32.5%) of total cases and is the most common acute leukemia (AL) in reproductive-age women (2). The risk for AML increases with older age; the median age at diagnosis is 65 years. Though it is uncommon, AML develops in younger adults with an estimated incidence of 0.5 cases per 100,000 population (3). This rate rises to only 1 in 100,000 at age 40, but after age 75, 15 in 100,000 people acquire AML (1). ALL most commonly occurs in children younger than 10 years or in adults older than 70 years; ALL accounts for approximately 15% of adult leukemia (3).

The chronic leukemias (CLs) are more common in older patients (1). The incidence of CML is increased with advancing age; the median age of onset occurs in the sixth decade (3). Of the total number of cases of leukemia in the United States, 7400 (25%) are CLL (2), which is most commonly seen in older men and is rare in patients younger than 30 years (3).

For women aged 18 to 35 years, the incidence of any type of leukemia is approximately 1 in 100,000. Malignancy is somewhat unique in women of reproductive age. In Sweden, malignancies and live births were analyzed over a 30-year period in approximately 2.3 million women aged 15 to 44 years, with several findings (4). First, not many cancers were discovered in this age group; there were 32,848 (1.4%) cases of malignancy. Second, only 1.3% of malignancies occurred during the 9-month gestational period, while 4.3% were diagnosed in the year following delivery (lactation period). The authors found fewer malignancies than expected in this population. In addition, they believe there may be a delay in the diagnosis of cancers in early pregnancy compared to the third trimester or the lactation period (4). For example, 55 patients with breast cancer were diagnosed during pregnancy, and 248 patients were observed in the lactation period. This does not rule out the possibility of physiologic dysregulations during pregnancy that could make one more prone to carcinogenesis, but does give evidence against an increased incidence of malignancies during gestation. This delay could be related to difficulty in assessing abnormal tissue conditions during pregnancy, especially with breast cancer, or perhaps due to a reluctance to suggest an aggressive workup with the potential for adverse effects during pregnancy. In addition, these numbers do not reflect the therapeutic abortions that were most likely performed during the first trimester when the malignancy was diagnosed (4).

Etiology

In general, the cause of leukemia is unknown. There are, however, several known predisposing factors associated with AL. Exposure to ionizing radiation, seen in Japanese atomic bomb survivors, increases the incidence of leukemia several years after exposure (5). Excessive medical radiation exposure for diagnosis (i.e., thorium dioxide [Thoratrast] contrast agent) and treatment (i.e., pelvic irradiation) can also increase the risk of acquiring AL. There is still much speculation regarding the risk to neonates exposed to maternal radiation *in utero.* An increased risk of AL has been suggested with occupational exposure of workers in the nuclear industry, fallout from nuclear weapons testing sites, environmental or background exposure to compounds such as radon, and cigarette smoking. Chemicals such as benzene, ethylene oxide, and styrene are causative agents. Only one virus, human T-cell lymphotrophic virus 1, has been implicated in the pathogenesis of leukemia; this subtype is rarely seen in the United States (5).

There is no evidence implicating pregnancy as a cause of leukemia, nor have there been any studies implicating increased estrogen, progesterone, or corticosteroids, with the exception of one report (6). In this case, a 28-year-old women was diagnosed with acute promyelocytic leukemia with 90% bone marrow myeloblasts at 32 weeks' gestation. She received platelets, four units of red blood cells, and intravenous antibiotics, and approximately 4 days after admission, she delivered a normal neonate by cesarean section. Twelve days after delivery, her peripheral blood counts normalized, and a repeat bone marrow biopsy showed only 2% myeloblasts (normal); the patient began breast-feeding the infant. Her disease relapsed approximately 2 months later, with 90% myeloblasts in the bone marrow and extensive leukemic infiltrates in both breasts. Of the few other reports of spontaneous remission of AL reported by Antunez et al. (6), most were preceded by life-threatening infections, which may correlate with endogenous steroid levels. Maternal levels of progesterone, 17α-hydroxyprogesterone, estradiol, estriol, estrone, estetrol, and deoxycorticosterone peak as a pregnancy progresses to the end of the third trimester and fall precipitously after delivery (7). Estrogen receptors on myeloblasts have been demonstrated in 18 (78%) of 23 patients with AL (8), but clinical correlations have not been elucidated (9). As outlined above, there is no information to indicate that AL occurs more often in younger women regardless of parity or hormonal status.

Diagnosis

Suspicion for AL occurs when there is an abnormality in the peripheral blood cell count (or complete blood cell count [CBC]) in one or more of the three cellular blood components: white cells, hemoglobin, or platelets. Leukemic blasts are immature hematologic cells of the bone marrow that cannot function as normal myelocytes or lymphocytes. They also interfere with normal hematopoiesis. Patients present with bone marrow failure: anemia, neutropenia, or thrombocytopenia. The diagnosis of AL is made by detecting 30% or more blasts either circulating in the peripheral blood or found in a bone marrow aspirate. Cytogenetics and immunophenotyping help classify the leukemia and complement bone marrow morphologic assessment with histochemical staining.

The diagnosis of CLs does not require bone marrow examination. CML typically presents with a left-shifted mature leukocytosis with varying degrees of basophilia and circulating blast cells. Leukocyte alkaline phosphatase scores are generally low, which helps differentiate CML from leukemoid reactions. Splenomegaly is common and may be massive. The diagnosis is made by demonstrating the chromosome rearrangement t(9;22), or the Philadelphia chromosome, on karyotypic analysis of blood or marrow. Alternatively, in the absence of a Philadelphia chromosome, the diagnosis may be made by demonstrating the chimeric products (*bcr/abl*) of the translocation by molecular techniques on peripheral blood.

Lymphocytosis of at least 5000/μl is required to make a diagnosis of CLL. The lymphocytes appear mature, and smudge cells are often noted on the peripheral blood smear. The diagnosis is usually confirmed by demonstrating coexpression of CD5 (a T-cell marker) with CD19 (a B-cell marker) by immunophenotypic analysis of blood or bone marrow.

Prognosis

Unfortunately, the prognosis for leukemia in general is quite poor. In ALL and AML, survival depends on eradication of myeloblasts and lymphoblasts (less than 5% blasts on bone marrow aspirate only), a normal CBC, and excellent patient performance status after initial chemotherapy. This situation is termed a *complete response* (CR) and must be achieved if long-term survival is the goal. For all adult patients regardless of age, the CR rate to induction chemotherapy with cytarabine (Cytosar-U) and an anthracycline is now 50% to 80% for AML (10) and 70% to 80% for ALL (1); four decades ago a CR occurred only episodically. Among patients older than 55 years, there are essentially no long-term survivors of AML. The prognosis for ALL dramatically worsens in patients older than 10 years; therefore, the relative prognosis in pregnant women with ALL is quite poor, compared to the results in children, but in AML the reproductive-age range includes most long-term survivors. Adverse prognostic factors for both types of AL influence prognosis and treatment options (Table 1). CR

TABLE 1. *Poor prognostic factors for overall survival in acute leukemia*

Factors	AML	ALL
Age	>55–60 yr	>10 yr
White blood cell count	No impact	>30,000/μL
Cytogenetics	All abnormalities except for t(8;21), inv(16), and t(15;17)	t(9;22) or any translocation of chromosome 11
Prior hematologic disorder	Especially MDS or secondary leukemia	Transformation from CML
Time to achieve complete response	No impact	>4–5 wk
Immunophenotype	CD34+	Precursor B cell

AML, acute myelogenous leukemia; ALL, acute lymphocytic leukemia; CML, chronic myelogenous leukemia; MDS, myelodysplastic syndrome.

rates for ALL and AML are the same in pregnant patients and in nonpregnant patients (11).

Prognostic factors for the CLs have also been described. High percentages of circulating myeloid blast cells and basophils connote a poorer prognosis in CML, as does massive splenomegaly. Cytogenetic abnormalities in addition to t(9;22) or the absence of a detectable *bcr/abl* rearrangement also portend a worse prognosis.

Several systems have been devised to classify CLL into prognostic categories. In general, however, worse prognosis is indicated by increasing bulk of disease at diagnosis. Diffuse marrow infiltration with subsequent cytopenias and constitutional symptoms generally indicates worse or progressing disease. Abnormal cytogenetics and high β_2-microglobulin levels also portend poorer-risk disease. A rapid lymphocyte doubling time also suggests more aggressive disease.

Treatment

The following sections provide an overview of treatment for the leukemias (Table 2).

Acute Myelogenous Leukemia

There are two necessary phases of treatment for AML: induction and postremission therapy. Induction chemotherapy is critical for decreasing the tumor burden and promoting normal marrow function. The standard therapy is commonly referred to as "7 and 3," consisting of 7 days of continuous infusion cytarabine, 100 mg/m^2 per day, and 3 days of idarubicin hydrochloride (Idamycin), 12 mg/m^2 per day, or daunorubicin hydrochloride (Cerubidine), 45 mg/m^2 per day, as bolus injections. The goal is to eradicate all leukemic blasts, restore hematopoiesis, and recover from chemotherapy toxicity; this state is referred to as a CR and is required to obtain long-term cure. The majority of patients achieve a CR (10). Remissions after induction treatment are short-lived, and postremission therapy must be employed to eliminate microscopic leukemia and obtain a 5-year overall survival of 20% to 25% for all AML patients (1).

Two options are available for postremission therapy for patients in CR. One alternative is high-dose cytarabine for approximately two cycles if the patient has good-risk disease (see Table 1); still, the majority of patients die

TABLE 2. *Chemotherapeutic agents most commonly used for the treatment of acute and chronic leukemia*

Name	Half-life	Major toxicities
Cytarabine (Cytosar-U)	2 h	Myelosuppression, mucositis, cerebellar dysfunction, conjunctivitis, skin
All-*trans*-retinoic acid (tretinoin)	40 min	Fever with respiratory distress and edema
Daunorubicin HCl (Cerubidine)	1–3 h	Myelosuppression, cardiotoxicity, cerebellar/cerebral toxicity, intrahepatic cholestasis, mucositis, nausea/emesis, alopecia
Idarubicin HCl (Idamycin)	11 h	Similar to daunorubicin
Chlorambucil (Leukeran)	1.5 h	Myelosuppression, infertility
Cyclophosphamide	3–10 h	Myelosuppression, hemorrhagic cystitis, SIADH
Etoposide (VePesid)	5–10 h	Leukopenia, mucositis, alopecia
Hydroxyurea (Hydrea)	~4 h	Myelosuppression, N&V, skin changes
Interferon alfa	4–9 h	Fever, fatigue, malaise, anorexia
L-Asparaginase (Elspar)	14–22 h	Hypersensitivity reaction, pancreatitis, decreased vitamin K–dependent coagulation factors, decreased proteins
Methotrexate	2–10 h	Myelosuppression, mucositis, nephrotoxicity, hepatotoxicity
Mercaptopurine (Purinethol)	50–90 min	Myelosuppression, stomatitis, hepatic cholestasis
Thioguanine	90 min	Myelosuppression, stomatitis, hepatic cholestasis
Vincristine sulfate	50–155 min	Peripheral neuropathy, SIADH

SIADH, syndrome of inappropriate antidiuretic hormone.

from recurrent disease. The other option is myeloablative chemotherapy with allogeneic bone marrow transplantation (BMT) for patients with poor-risk disease who are younger than 60 years and have a matched related donor. This is the only curative regimen for the majority of young women with AML; however, there is a matched sibling marrow donor for only 30% of all eligible patients. For poor-risk patients, the estimated 5-year disease-free survival is 20% to 35% after BMT. Graft-versus-host disease, infection, and chemotherapy toxicity are the leading causes of death in these patients. BMT-preparative regimens leave the majority of patients infertile; there are no reports of pregnant patients who have undergone BMT.

Acute Promyelocytic Leukemia

Acute promyelocytic leukemia (APL) (or FAB-M3 by the French-American-British classification), a subtype of AML, has a unique biology and treatment. APL accounts for 10% of all AML but appears to occur more commonly in younger reproductive-age adults (1). In APL, genetic material is translocated between chromosomes 15 and 17, creating a chimeric gene that transcribes the PML-RAR alpha (promyelocytic leukemia–retinoic acid receptor) fusion protein. Approximately 80% to 100% of patients with APL have identifiable levels of this protein (12). Phenotypically, there is an arrest of maturation at the promyelocyte stage; these early myeloid cells contain numerous cytoplasmic granules with substances that can generate a life-threatening consumptive coagulopathy or disseminated intravascular coagulopathy. Regardless, the 5-year overall survival at 35% to 45% has been somewhat better in APL patients than in those with other AML subtypes (13).

All-*trans*-retinoic acid (ATRA), a vitamin A derivative, is thought to block transcription of the PML-RAR alpha protein, with resultant differentiation of the APL cells, maturation, often a peripheral leukocytosis, and then cell death. In a randomized trial, induction with ATRA prolonged disease-free survival, compared to induction chemotherapy with cytarabine and daunorubicin (14). In Europe, a trial of ATRA induction followed by three cycles of cytarabine and daunorubicin versus cytarabine and daunorubicin alone was closed prematurely when event-free survival was significantly better in the ATRA arm (15). The adverse events seen with most cytotoxic chemotherapies, such as bone marrow aplasia, do not generally occur with ATRA, although in approximately 25% to 30% of patients a syndrome known as the retinoic acid syndrome (RAS) will occur (16). RAS can cause up to 10% to 15% mortality and is most similar to a capillary leak state with pleural effusions and pulmonary infiltrates, hypotension, peripheral edema, and fever. The risk of RAS most often increases with a rising white blood cell count (WBC), and it has been recommended to start steroids prophylactically if the total WBC is more than 5000 to 10,000/μl or if the WBC is found to be rising rapidly. Administering steroids when symptoms, such as dyspnea or mild weight gain, first appear may markedly decrease the severity of RAS, irrespective of the total WBC. Once symptoms have progressed, acute respiratory failure rapidly develops in many patients.

Another approach advocates the addition of cytarabine and daunorubicin to ATRA to manage a high initial or rising WBC and help prevent RAS (16). Though the induction CR rate is close to 90% with ATRA, these are not durable responses (12). Postremission chemotherapy with cytarabine and daunorubicin after induction with ATRA is required for disease-free survival (14).

Mortality in untreated APL patients is almost always from hemorrhage; this risk is maintained during treatment until the coagulopathy diminishes and the platelet count increases. Preliminary results of a randomized trial of induction with ATRA followed by chemotherapy versus ATRA given concurrently with chemotherapy were recently disclosed. The CR rate and disease-free survival were higher if ATRA and chemotherapy were received concomitantly; most patients would benefit from this schedule (17).

Myelodysplastic Syndrome

Myelodysplastic syndrome (MDS) consists of five categories of disorders with varying degrees of dysplastic hematopoiesis, trilineage dysplasia, and progression into AML. Most often, MDS is indolent but unrelenting; either death from the complications of prolonged pancytopenia occurs, or the disease state is transformed into AL that is rarely responsive to therapy. MDS has been called preleukemia. This is definitely a condition of the elderly, although 10% of patients are younger than 40 years or have cytogenetic changes induced by chemotherapy or irradiation for other conditions. Diagnosis requires anemia, often macrocytic, or other cytopenias with classification based on bone marrow biopsy morphology (i.e., presence of ringed sideroblasts or myeloblasts). Treatment ranges from supportive care only to myeloablative chemotherapy with BMT; in young women the only curative therapy is BMT.

Siddiqui et al. (18) described five women diagnosed with MDS during pregnancy (Table 3). Obviously, there are too few cases to construct conclusions. No causal relationship between MDS and pregnancy can be established, just as with the other forms of AL. This is one entity in the differential diagnosis of anemia in any person, including vitamin B_{12} and folate deficiency. If these levels are in the normal range, a bone marrow biopsy may be necessary to exclude the diagnosis.

Chronic Myelogenous Leukemia

CML was originally thought to be incurable, progressing from a peripheral leukocytosis, to severe marrow dysfunction, to AL unresponsive to all therapies. Therapy with agents such as hydroxyurea (Hydrea) and busulfan (Myleran), leukapheresis, and splenectomy can control hematologic parameters for a finite time, but all patients eventually progress into AL when so treated.

Since the 1970s, it has been known that CML is associated with a reciprocal translocation between chromosomes 9 and 22; the resultant fusion gene *bcr/abl* encodes a protein that alters cellular tyrosine kinase and subsequently increases cellular proliferation (19). Interferon alfa-2b (IFN alfa), through not well explained mechanisms, has activity

TABLE 3. *Myelodysplasia associated with pregnancy*

Maternal age (yr)	Week of gestation	Initial CBC	Class; course or treatment	Pregnancy outcome	Maternal outcome
22	16	Hgb 7.7 g/dL WBC 1200/μL PLT 62,000/μL	RAEB; septic endometritis	Therapeutic abortion	AML by 4th month; expired 2 yr
31	12	Hgb 7.0 g/dL WBC 2000/μL PLT 14,000/μL	RA; no CBC changes after abortion	Therapeutic abortion	Expired 1 mo after MRD-BMT
32	20	Hgb 5.9 g/dL WBC < 500/μL PLT 61,000/μL	RA; transfusional support	Healthy, term infant	Increased PLT postpartum; in 5th month AML; expired
31	30 (history of anemia)	Hgb 8.5 g/dL WBC 4400/μL PLT 264,000/μL	RAEB; no treatment	Infant with Down syndrome at 36 wk	AML by 24th month; no CR; expired
31	Details unknown	Hgb 8.0 g/dL WBC 4200/μL PLT 250,000/μL	Details unknown	Low-birthweight infant	RA 3 yr postpartum; AML; expired

AML, acute myelogenous leukemia; BMT, bone marrow transplantation; CBC, complete blood cell count; CR, complete response; Hgb, hemoglobin; MDR, matched related donor; PLT, platelet count; RA, refractory anemia; RAEB, refractory anemia with excess blasts; RAEBT, refractory anemia with excess blasts in transformation; RARS, refractory anemia with ringed sideroblasts.

Modified from ref. 18.

against CML, as evidenced by cytogenetic responses. Cytogenetic responses—eradication of some or all of the cells with t(9;22)—have been achieved with IFN alfa when other therapies have failed (20). Suppression of the *bcr/abl* gene appears necessary to delay progression to AL, as demonstrated in a randomized trial of IFN alfa versus hydroxyurea (21). Patients treated with IFN alfa who achieved a cytogenetic response had better survival than those who did not, but all IFN-treated patients, regardless of response, had a statistically significant improvement in survival, as the time to progression was prolonged (21). The adverse effects of IFN alfa can be dose-limiting: viral-like syndrome with fevers, depression, and severe fatigue. Many patients cannot tolerate long-term use.

Importantly, cure has been reported with myeloablative chemotherapy and allogeneic BMT in chronic-phase CML. Allogeneic BMT can induce cure in close to 50% of patients, especially if BMT occurs within the first year of diagnosis before there is any evidence of disease progression from the chronic or early phase, and if prior busulfan therapy was avoided (22). All other medications can be employed while the patient is being assessed for BMT; some patients may not need any form of therapy prior to BMT. In patients unable to undergo BMT, treatment is usually administered for symptom control.

Acute Lymphocytic Leukemia

In adults, ALL does not respond as favorably to chemotherapy as it does in children. The CR rates are comparable, both in the range of 80% to 95%, but most adults experience relapse and 5-year overall survival is 20% to 30% (1). Five-year pediatric overall survival is approximately 70%. The treatment for all ages involves four phases: induction, consolidation, maintenance, and central ner-

TABLE 4. *Regimen for the treatment of acute lymphoblastic leukemia (ALL) in adults*

Induction chemotherapy	
Daunorubicin HCl (Cerubidine)	Days 1–3
Vincristine sulfate	Days 1, 8, 15, 22
Prednisone	Days 1–28
L-Asparaginase (Elspar)	Days 17–28
Repeat for a 2-wk course if residual ALL found on bone marrow biopsy performed on day 28	
Central nervous system prophylaxis	
Methotrexate	Once a week intrathecally for 6 wk
Cranial radiation	10 fractions over 12–14 d
Consolidation chemotherapy	
When complete response achieved, alternate courses of regimens A and B for eight cycles; regimen C is ninth cycle	
Regimen A	
Daunorubicin	Day 1, 2
Vincristine	Day 1, 8
Prednisone	Day 1–14
L-Asparaginase	Day 2,3,7,9,11,14
Regimen B	
Teniposide (Vumon)	Day 1, 4, 8, 11
Cytarabine (Cytosar-U)	Day 1, 4, 8, 11
Regimen C	
Methotrexate	Day 1–2 over 42 h
Leucovorin/calcium	Day 2–5 start after methotrexate
Maintenance chemotherapy	
Methotrexate	Once a week PO for 30 mo
Mercaptopurine/(Purinethol)	Once a day PO for 30 mo

Modified from Linker CA, Levitt LJ, O'Donnell M, et al. Improved results of treatment of adult acute lymphoblastic leukemia. *Blood* 1991;78:2814.

vous system prophylaxis. Multiple cytotoxic agents are utilized, including vincristine sulfate, steroids, anthracyclines, asparaginase (Elspar), cytarabine, methotrexate, and mercaptopurine (Purinethol) in various schedules. Treatment regimens are lengthy and differ only by the timing of medication administration with minor changes in doses (Table 4). The folate antimetabolites are not employed until consolidation or maintenance therapy and can usually be held until the second trimester. Allogeneic BMT is necessary for cure in patients younger than 55 years with poor-risk disease (see Table 1) or upon relapse.

Chronic Lymphocytic Leukemia

Unlike the ALs and CML, CLL is not generally considered curable. Treatment then is palliative, since no therapy has been shown to improve survival. Many patients have no complaints at diagnosis and have only peripheral lymphadenopathy or splenomegaly as their presenting feature. There are staging systems correlating with disease progression (23), and treatment is not advocated in the early, asymptomatic stages, as the course of the disease is varied and there are no data supporting improvement in survival with early intervention (24). When therapy is indicated, first-line interventions usually include either chlorambucil (Leukeran) or a purine analog, such as fludarabine phosphate (Fludara). The disease may be controllable for many years.

HEMATOLOGIC FUNCTION IN PREGNANCY

Normal Hematologic Changes with Pregnancy

Several discrete alterations occur in hematologic function with pregnancy. There is an approximately 50% increase in plasma volume with only a 20% to 50% rise in red cell mass. These changes result in a normocytic anemia with a new normal hemoglobin of 10 to 12 g/dL (25). Hematopoiesis can be severely impaired if iron and folic acid stores are not supplemented in advance. The normocytic anemia often becomes microcytic, as iron metabolism cannot always keep pace with fetal demand, even with supplementation. A macrocytic anemia in pregnancy is uncommon and should be further investigated.

Leukocytosis develops during pregnancy, probably due to increased levels of endogenous steroids. This increase in the WBC may mimic a reaction to infection (25), and any questions regarding the etiology of the leukocytosis should be addressed. By the third trimester, the WBC may reach as high as 12,000/μL and reach 20,000 to 30,000/μL during labor (26).

Usually, there are no perturbations in the platelet count during pregnancy, but not uncommonly platelet counts in the low normal range are seen during gestation (gestational thrombocytopenia) (22). Immune thrombocytopenic purpura is seen more often in young women; any platelet count that acutely decreases or is less than 50,000/μL must be examined.

Screening for Leukemia

Many women would unnecessarily be screened to find the relatively small number of hematologic malignancies. ALs are rarely found in an asymptomatic patient. The CBC does not always illuminate bone marrow dysfunction until the disease is more advanced. The CLs can be discovered with a routine physical examination and CBC. Abnormalities in the CBC are the most frequent indicator of AL, and the CBC constitutes the best form of surveillance whenever it is ordered in a healthy individual. However, for all age groups, there is no documented beneficial screening program for leukemia.

DIAGNOSIS DURING PREGNANCY

Prenatal Care

Prenatal care is an excellent medical monitoring program for young women. Prenatal care involves a CBC at the patient's first presentation; any abnormalities that deviate from expected hematopoietic alterations should be further investigated. Chronic conditions previously unknown to a patient, such as a thalassemia or sickle cell trait, are sometimes discovered during the prenatal evaluation. Nutritional supplements such as iron and folic acid are prescribed. According to the guidelines established by the American Academy of Pediatrics and the American College of Obstetricians and Gynecologists in 1992, a repeat hemoglobin/hematocrit (with automation, an entire CBC is easier to obtain than any of its parts) should be performed at approximately 26 to 28 weeks' gestation and again at 32 to 36 weeks, with further testing according to any abnormal results (27). Because the physiologic hematologic changes of pregnancy are well recognized, any perturbations outside of these variations in the CBC should be assessed.

The symptoms of leukemia are protean and nonspecific: fatigue, shortness of breath, fever or chills, and malaise. Usual signs may include an increase in bleeding, bruising, or infections that points to hematologic dysfunction; often there is the development of a new form of anemia. Pregnant patients are instructed to seek medical attention with any of these problems; the symptoms of AL will only worsen with time. Diagnosing any form of malignancy during pregnancy can be difficult, as constitutional symptoms are often attributed to a normal pregnancy.

Diagnostic Workup

If there is suspicion of marrow dysfunction based on the peripheral blood smear or if circulating leukemic blast cells are found, then a bone marrow biopsy and aspirate must be performed. This procedure can safely be performed on patients at any gestational age; only local anesthetic is employed, and pregnant patients can maintain a lateral decubitus position for the estimated 20-minute procedure.

Because frequent blood draws are necessary in treating AL, as are chemotherapy infusions, transfusions, and antibiotics, a multilumen central venous catheter is generally required. Either a general surgeon or an interventional radiologist can perform the procedure. Fluoroscopy is often used for guidance during placement but can be eliminated or utilized sparingly with pelvic shielding. Interventional radiology also has ultrasound readily available for assistance during the procedure. Another requisite pretreatment measurement is evaluation of the left ventricular ejection fraction (LVEF). As the anthracyclines are cardiotoxic, baseline LVEF should be documented. Multiple-gated acquisition (MUGA) angiocardiographic scans are a simple way to obtain this information, but an echocardiogram can obtain a good estimate of LVEF and circumvent the issue of radiation exposure. Only rarely would computed tomography (CT) of the abdomen and pelvis be desired to assess lymphadenopathy in ALL. CT scans of the abdomen and pelvis are not critical for prognosis or therapy and can therefore be deleted. In summary, there is little potential for fetal harm in the maternal diagnostic workup for AL and preparation for treatment.

TREATMENT OF LEUKEMIA DURING PREGNANCY

Overview

Being faced with a life-threatening illness simultaneously with pregnancy is a most formidable challenge for an individual. Conclusions regarding treatment must be reached by the consensus of a patient and her physician. All risks, benefits, and alternatives for the patient and fetus should be discussed in detail. The patient must understand that no outcome can be guaranteed, but the known information in the literature should be presented to her in a comprehensive manner. No one should attempt to underestimate the complexity of the decision regarding treatment and continuing the pregnancy.

The available data in the literature to discuss with patients come primarily from retrospective case reports. Fortunately, in the last two decades, the treatment of leukemia has undergone many improvements in type of therapy administered and supportive care of pancytopenia. Unfortunately, it is nearly impossible to interpret some of the data on maternal–fetal outcome in light of today's practices. For instance, antimetabolites are not used as commonly now for induction therapy of AL; these agents are known to be teratogenic, so their exclusion from chemotherapeutic regimens may decrease the malformation rate.

Combination chemotherapy has been utilized since the mid-1970s. Only recently was the combination of cytarabine and an anthracycline established as the most efficacious regimen for AML. New drug developments in the late 1980s have changed the way in which AL is managed: Improved antiemetics, antibiotics, and hematopoietic growth factors (i.e., granulocyte colony-stimulating factor) have helped make treatment safer and more tolerable for patients. Better blood banking, especially with platelet products, has decreased bleeding complications. These advances in supportive care expanded treatment options to include high-dose chemotherapy with allogeneic BMT and were critical for the improvement in CR and survival rates in all AL patients. Table 5 illustrates some of the nonchemotherapeutic agents often used to treat leukemia.

Pharmacokinetics with Pregnancy

Specific maternal modifications occur during pregnancy that affect the metabolism of drugs (28):

- Increased plasma volume, which can increase the volume for drug dilution
- Decreased albumin and increased plasma proteins from estrogen, which can alter ratios of free and bound drugs
- Increased renal blood flow and glomerular filtration rate, which influence excretion of drugs

TABLE 5. *Agents used as supportive care in the management of acute leukemia*

Classification of agents	Examples
Antibiotics	Aminoglycosides Penicillins Cephalosporins Fluoroquinolones Sulfonamides
Antifungals	Amphotericin B (Fungizone) Fluconazole (Diflucan)
Antivirals	Acyclovir (Zovirax) Ganciclovir Sodium (Cytovene)
Antiemetics	Ondansetron HCl (Zofran) Granisetron HCl (Kytril) Dexamethasone Lorazepam (Ativan)
Blood products	Red blood cells Platelets Cryoprecipitate Fresh frozen plasma Immunoglobulin
Hematopoietic growth factors	Filgrastim (Neupogen) Sargramostim
Miscellaneous	Allopurinol Acetaminophen Diphenhydramine HCl (Benadryl)

The majority of patients require most of these agents; all patients utilize antiemetics and blood products. These agents do have teratogenic effects that are impossible to delineate from those of cytotoxic chemotherapy; the exact combinations of drugs that produce adverse effects are unknown.

- Increased activity of hepatic mixed function oxidases, which directly changes metabolism
- Decreased gastric emptying, which interferes with drug absorption

Fetal pharmacokinetics are not as well known; the fetal liver and kidneys do develop some metabolic function *in utero,* but this has not been qualified or quantified. The length of exposure to possible teratogens is always an important factor; metabolites of maternal medications can be eliminated by the fetus into the amniotic fluid, with subsequent fetal ingestion, gastrointestinal absorption, and elimination continuing the cycle (28). For example, metabolites of cocaine and morphine have been found in the meconium of rats and offspring of substance-abusing mothers (29). Depending on the efficacy of these processes and the types of drugs and their metabolites, there may be increased or decreased fetal exposure to these medications.

It is not known whether the amniotic fluid functions as a third-space compartment, and there is no information available on how this could affect the dosing of medications during pregnancy. There is no evidence to suggest that doses of chemotherapeutic agents should be altered. Given the poor overall survival of patients with AL and the severe toxicity from treatment, dose reductions have been attempted anecdotally, with no real diminution of adverse effects but with decreased therapeutic responses. The current treatment schedules for AML have been carefully studied, with promotion of the regimens that offer the best response rates (30,31). Dose reduction can worsen the prognosis of a patient in the reproductive-age group.

Administration of chemotherapy and supportive medications to patients physiologically stressed from pregnancy, as well as from leukemia, has not been well studied. Evidence is lacking for changes in dosing. As will be discussed, most agents do not have to be substituted or withheld. There are no studies assessing maternal–fetal pharmacokinetics with antitumor drugs, and there is no evidence to suggest that adjustments in dosing are necessary to account for the new metabolic function in the mother.

Placental Function

The placenta separates maternal and fetal circulatory systems and is the regulator for all transport between the two systems. Transfer of any maternally derived molecules must take place across the placental membrane, composed of fetal tissue (32). Maternal arterial blood is driven by the blood pressure into the intervillous spaces. Fetal blood is confined across the placental membrane to the villous vascular system. Substances cross by simple diffusion, facilitated diffusion, active transport, and pinocytosis. Placental membrane interruptions can occur, especially as gestational period advances, because the placental membrane thins over time. Additionally, the fetal capillary system becomes progressively better exposed to the intervillous spaces. There is a long list of substances that can easily transfer across this membrane, including most nutrients, waste products, proteins such as IgG antibodies, some hormones, viruses, and water-soluble vitamins (32). Substances that are lipid-soluble, not extensively plasma protein–bound, nonionized, or of low molecular weight can cross; most chemotherapeutic agents have these characteristics that facilitate passage (28).

Theoretically, most agents seem capable of crossing the placenta, but only two reports show placental transfer of doxorubicin hydrochloride in humans (33,34). A 28-year-old woman with a peripheral T-cell non-Hodgkin's lymphoma received 900 cGy of radiation to a symptomatic mediastinal mass at 25 weeks' gestation and then doxorubicin, 45 mg/m^2, during week 31. A prechemotherapy ultrasound showed normal fetal heart rate, but the repeat ultrasound performed 36 hours after chemotherapy was consistent with fetal demise. The placenta examination showed infarcted regions and thrombosis of the chorionic blood vessels. No doxorubicin was noted in the fetal tissues, but a probable, newly identified doxorubicin metabolite was found in the fetal spleen. However, given the condition of the placental vessels, it is unlikely that doxorubicin itself could be the causative agent of the fetal death (33). The role of radiation therapy in this situation, with an estimated 9 to 16 cGy exposure to the uterus, is unknown.

D'Incalci et al. (34) treated a woman at 17 weeks' gestation for Hodgkin's disease with doxorubicin, 86 mg/m^2 total dose. Approximately 15 hours later, the patient underwent a therapeutic abortion. Fetal tissues, murine tissue as control, and maternal plasma samples were assessed by liquid chromatography. No doxorubicin or metabolites were found in fetal brain, intestine, or gastrocnemius muscle; the heart was not available for testing. Doxorubicin was present in fetal liver, lung, and kidney in higher concentrations than was detected in maternal plasma. Fetal liver and mouse liver with doxorubicin added were positive, but no doxorubicin was found in the amniotic fluid or murine liver without the addition of doxorubicin. In another case, a 30-year-old woman with ALL received doxorubicin, 45 mg/m^2, at 34 weeks' gestation and spontaneously went into labor 48 hours later. Assessment of the placenta found doxorubicin levels in the placenta distal to the umbilical cord, as well as in the proximal placenta. No levels were detected in the cord blood, but minor levels were found in the cord tissue (33).

At the time of delivery for a woman with APL, ATRA levels were measured in her venous blood and in the neonate's umbilical artery and vein and peripherally. Maternal ATRA levels were detectable at 2 and 4 hours after the last dose; no neonatal levels were found at 2 or 4 hours (35).

Roboz et al. (36) reported on a 26-year-old woman with a metastatic granular myoblastoma during week 20 of gestation who received doxorubicin, 30 mg/m^2, each day for 3 days. Assessment of amniotic fluid was performed at 4 hours and then 16 hours after the day 1 treatment. No doxorubicin or metabolite levels were detected (39). D'Incalci et al. (34) speculated that there is rapid passage of doxorubicin out of the amniotic fluid, which may be due in part to the drug's predilection for accumulating in tissue compartments. If this is the case, absence of the drug in the amniotic fluid would not exclude fetal tissue involvement.

D'Incalci et al. (37) have published the only report on cyclophosphamide maternal–fetal transfer. They measured drug levels in the amniotic fluid 1 hour after the second cycle of cyclophosphamide, 400 mg/m^2, was administered to the mother; fetal amniotic fluid levels of 2.1 μg/mL were obtained, thought to be 25% of the maternal serum levels at 1 hour. The authors speculated about the activity and efficiency of the fetal hepatic monooxygenase P-450 system and activation of cyclophosphamide. However, there are no studies on this issue to date.

There are conflicting data regarding the passage of chemotherapeutic agents, but it is assumed that almost all drugs do cross the placental barrier and that other factors, such as fetal metabolism, may be the major determinant of teratogenicity.

Teratogenicity of Chemotherapeutic Agents

Chemotherapeutic agents cause cell death through several different mechanisms. Cells that divide quickly are optimal targets for most chemotherapeutic agents, which interrupt normal cell division. Some agents are cell cycle- or phase-specific and kill cells more efficiently in particular phases of the cellular life cycle, especially the S phase (38). Chemotherapy does not differentiate between normal and malignant cells. The most commonly affected nonmalignant tissues are those that are actively being replaced with new cells, such as bone marrow, epithelial linings of the gastrointestinal and urogenital tracts, and skin, especially hair.

Fetal cells are also undergoing rapid growth with multiple cell divisions during the first trimester, mainly during organogenesis. When exposure to chemotherapy occurs during the first few weeks of gestation, the most likely result will be fetal death due to the immaturity of all fetal tissues. During organogenesis, drug-induced teratogenesis may manifest itself with major or minor abnormalities of organ systems without fetal death. After this period, cell division is not as rapid, and the rate of cell injury from chemotherapy as expressed by congenital malformations is at baseline (11), with a background rate of malformations at 3% (39).

Doll et al. (28) reported on 139 cancer patients given various chemotherapies during the first trimester; the rate of fetal malformations was 17%. In 45 of these patients exposed to two or more agents simultaneously, 16% had infants with malformations. When patients receiving folate antagonists and radiation therapy in the first trimester were not considered, the malformation rate dropped to 6%; only in the treatment of ALL are the folate antagonists widely utilized. Additionally, 150 patients first exposed to chemotherapy from the second trimester to delivery had a 1.3% rate of malformations (28). Table 6 summarizes many of the malformations reported in neonates whose mothers were treated for leukemia.

There have been many reports in the literature, mainly in the 1980s, of maternal–fetal

TABLE 6. *Fetal malformations or complications (excluding low birthweight) listed by exposure during gestation to chemotherapeutic agents for acute leukemia*

Trimester exposed	Chemotherapy	Sex; delivery (wk)	Birthweight (g)	Malformation/ complication	Reference
First	Ara-C	Male; term	2863	Right hand and bilateral lower limb defects	44
First	Ara-C, 6-TG	Male; 38	2210	Distal limb defect	45
First	Ara-C, dauno	Unknown	Unknown	Seizures, respiratory distress syndrome (recovered with normal development)	11
First	Ara-C, CTX, MTX, 6-MP, steroids, VCR	Male; 34	1000	Panycytopenia (resolved by death at age 21 d from sepsis)	55
First	CTX, steroids	Female	1490	Normal	82
		Male; 37	1300	Malformations; low IQ; thyroid cancer age 16; neuroblastoma age 14	
Second	Ara-C, dauno, VCR	Male; unknown	2430	Leukopenia, transient	96
Second	Ara-C, dauno, 6-TG	Male; 34	3840	Sixth digit on right foot; family history polydactyly	58
Second	Ara-C, dauno	Female; 29	1350	Growth retardation; prematurity	96
Second	CTX, dauno, L-ASP, 6-MP, MTX, steroids, VCR	Female; 31	2380	Hydrops fetalis; transient bone marrow hypoplasia	68
Second	Ara-C, dauno, VP-16	Female; 32	1460	Anemia, required ventilation; neutropenic sepsis (recovered)	69
Second	Ara-C, doxo, 6-TG, VCR	Female; 29	1000	Urgent c-section after fetal distress; meningeal hemorrhage; hyaline membrane disease	57
Third	Ara-C, dauno, 6-TG	Male; 29	1000	Unilateral adherence of iris to cornea	82
Third	Ara-C, dauno, steroids, hydrea, 6-TG, VCR	Male; 34	2130	Growth retardation through 13 mo; perinatal electrolyte abnormalities	70

Ara-c, cytarabine; C-section, cesarean section; CTX, cyclophosphamide; dauno, daunorubicin; doxo, doxorubicin; hydrea, hydroxyurea; L-ASP, L-asparaginase; 6-MP, mercaptopurine; MTX, methorexate; 6-TG, thioguanine; VCR, vincristine; VP-16, etoposide.

outcomes after chemotherapy given during gestation. These reports are listed case by case and are usually few in number. Hematologic malignancies including leukemias have been reported with solid tumors. In 1989, Caligiuri and Mayer (11) published a report of 72 women who were newly diagnosed with leukemia during pregnancy from 1975 to 1988. Prior to 1988, they estimated that more than 350 pregnant patients with leukemia were recorded, beginning in 1845. These cases were retrospectively reported; oncologic protocols almost universally exclude pregnant patients. A Registry of Pregnancies Exposed to Chemotherapeutic Agents has been established at the University of Pittsburgh. All clinicians who care for women receiving cancer chemotherapy during pregnancy should report their experiences to this database. For details or a patient abstract form, clinicians should contact Dr. John Mulvihill at the University of Pittsburgh (phone: 412-624-9951; fax: 412-624-3020; e-mail: jjm@helix.hgen.pitt.edu).

Many case series have examined the same patients. As one would expect, the true incidence and course of pregnancy and leukemia are unknown because there is some inherent bias in reporting cases. Usually, the most interesting cases are presented, while unremarkable outcomes are not publicized. Fetal outcome secondary to chemotherapy exposure is the issue most closely attended to in most of these cases, but there is no mention of other teratogenics, such as antibiotics, that may have been received by the patients. Nor are the reports controlled for malformations that may be more related to family history (i.e., cleft lip, polydactyly). Other well known factors that influence teratogenicity are drug dose, length of exposure, interactions among multiple medications, and genetic predisposition—features not accounted for in most reports.

No specific malformations have been connected to any chemotherapy used in AL, except for aminopterin, an antimetabolite used in the past to induce abortions (40). Aminopterin has been reported to cause death in all fetuses of less than 40 days' gestation (41). There exists an aminopterin syndrome with many malformations, especially in skeletal formation. The most frequently observed deformity is cranial dysostosis, and hypertelorism, micrognathia, and limb malformations may also occur (28). This agent is not commonly used in the United States. A similar antimetabolite, methotrexate, is now used in treatment of ALL and other malignancies. Like all of the folate antimetabolites developed after aminopterin, methotrexate is approached with more caution and not recommended for use in the first trimester. Methotrexate is administered in the consolidation phase of ALL but can be withheld until the organogenesis phase has ended, or substituted with another agent but are not associated with a particular constellation of abnormalities.

Hydroxyurea, mercaptopurine, thioguanine, and cytarabine are widely utilized in the treatment of leukemia. With the exception of the folate antagonists, teratogenesis cannot be accurately attributed to one agent when combination chemotherapy is administered with various antiemetics, antibiotics, antifungals, antivirals, premedications, and blood products in a pregnant, neutropenic patient with AL. Preclinical studies may suggest possible teratogenicity, but animal studies cannot consistently predict human reactions (e.g., salicylic acid and thalidomide).

Adverse Effects of Chemotherapy

Malformations

Mutations of chromosomes affecting certain genes, environmental toxins, ionizing radiation, and infections all cause congenital malformations, but defining the specific cause in a particular case is difficult (41). Two chromosomal anomalies in phenotypically normal infants after maternal chemotherapy have been described (42). One infant had trisomy C syndrome after maternal exposure to cytarabine and thioguanine (43). In the other case, an ALL patient was administered daunorubicin, vincristine, prednisolone, and asparaginase followed by cyclophosphamide, cytarabine, and mercaptopurine (44). She also underwent prophylactic whole-brain irradiation and intrathecal methotrexate. Her maintenance therapy consisted of methotrexate and mercaptopurine. Chemotherapy was initiated at 22 weeks' gestation; she delivered a healthy female infant at 40 weeks. Cytogenetic analysis of the neonate's lymphocytes was performed, and though the karyotype was (46,XX), several chromatid breaks or gaps and one ring chromosome were found. These changes are most commonly seen in patients after receiving chemotherapy or radiation therapy; the implications of this finding are unknown. Although these changes may last for several years, it is not known whether or not the alterations persist long enough for a malignancy to develop or for the infant to pass these changes on to her progeny.

Acute Leukemia

Ebert et al. (42) updated all reported cases of ALL, AML, or CML in conjunction with pregnancy from 1983 to 1995, presenting the latest account of AL patients. Of the 96 patients recorded, only two received single-agent chemotherapy. Radiation therapy was added to the regimen of seven patients. It is all but impossible to delineate the drugs, the combination of drugs, or other factors that lead to malformation or fetal death (5%). A total of 12 neonates were affected: two therapeutic abortions, one spontaneous abortion, two stillbirths, one infant with abnormal chromosomal karyotype, and eight with congenital abnormalities. Points of issue from this data set include (a) the implication of cytarabine as the agent most often seen with these abnormalities (9 of 12 cases) and (b) the majority (7 of 8) cases of congenital abnormality were exposed in the first trimester. Eighty-two percent of these pregnancies resulted in the live birth of neonates who subsequently underwent normal development, 10% of progeny suffered abnormal development, and another 8% were stillborn or deceased from elective abortion, spontaneous abortion, or maternal demise (42).

It is difficult at best to assess definitively the teratogenicity of cytarabine, an important antileukemic agent. Reports of cytarabine's being utilized as a single agent or with an anthracycline in pregnant women are scarce. Wagner et al. (45) treated a patient for ALL, with relapse of disease on maintenance therapy, who acquired a second CR. She was on maintenance treatment with cytarabine when she conceived. It was suspected that her three cytarabine cycles coincided with normal limb bud development, as her infant had a malformed right hand and bilateral femur, tibiofibular, and foot defects. In addition, bilateral external ear abnormalities were present (45).

Another woman with AML conceived while receiving cytarabine subcutaneously and oral thioguanine twice a day and continued this regimen until her term delivery. The neonate had upper and lower distal limb abnormalities, especially of his hands. The patient was continued on the same medications and again conceived 2 to 4 weeks after her last dose of maintenance therapy. This infant had no abnormalities; both infants were developing normally (46).

Caligiuri and Mayer (11) reported on an additional 30 leukemic patients treated with cytarabine as a single or combination agent. Eighteen of these patients gave birth to normal offspring, and five pregnancies ended in elective abortions. Another AML patient was 20 weeks pregnant when treated with cytarabine and daunorubicin; she was then given mitoxantrone hydrochloride (Novantrone) and cytarabine as a second induction. Her consolidation consisted of one cycle of cytarabine and idarubicin at approximately weeks 29 to 30; 2 days after discharge she complained of no fetal movement for several hours and delivered a stillborn but phenotypically normal infant (47). The authors speculated that the idarubicin might have been important in causing fetal death; however, this and all the above cases illustrate the point that many factors—leukemia, current combination chemotherapy, and a recent history of cytotoxic drug treatment—are at work in producing malformations.

The anthracyclines, another class of agents active against leukemia, have been evaluated in combination when utilized in pregnant patients with leukemia by Turchi and Villasis (48). Among 20 AL patients treated during pregnancy, no malformations occurred. There was one maternal–fetal death, one therapeutic abortion, one spontaneous abortion, and four neonatal problems (marrow hypoplasia, pneumothorax, sepsis, and polycythemia) that entirely resolved (48). In the case involving infant polycythemia, the maternal course was complicated by relapsed null-cell ALL after conception while on maintenance folate antimetabolites, reinduction chemotherapy, pulmonary infiltrates requiring mechanical ventilation, and prolonged bone marrow aplasia. The infant, born at 36 weeks' gestation, weighed 2400 g, and the polycythemia resolved with normal marrow function (49).

Caligiuri and Mayer (11) compiled 72 cases of new-onset leukemia diagnosed with or during pregnancy from 1975 to 1988 in the English literature. AML was found in 44 patients, ALL in 20, CML in five (four in chronic phase), and hairy cell leukemia in one patient; two cases were not specified. They reported on 58 patients who were administered chemotherapy while pregnant; only eight patients were not given cytarabine, an anthracycline, or both. Fetal results of chemotherapy given for AL based on trimester of first exposure are found in Table 7. As the date of the first exposure to chemotherapy moved from first to third trimester, the number of spontaneous abortions and stillbirths decreased, with most neonates normal regardless of premature or term birth. Surprisingly, there were no first trimester exposures resulting in congenital defects. There were no perinatal deaths; overall fetal survival was 84% (49 of 58) (11).

Catanzarite and Ferguson (50) reviewed records regarding pregnancy and AL from 1972 to 1982 in the English, French, and German literature, including a few cases previously reported. They assembled outcome data on 39 fetuses first exposed to chemotherapy during gestation, ranging from conception to the third trimester. A total of 31 patients received induction chemotherapy for ALL (n=7) or AML (n=24) during their pregnancy; eight patients conceived on maintenance therapy. Twenty infants were delivered at term, while 12 were premature. There were three therapeutic abortions, two perinatal deaths (at 21 days and 3 months, both from infection with no evidence of leukemia), and two intrauterine deaths (at 24 and 30 weeks) for a long-term fetal survival of 32 of 39 (82%). No malformations were recorded (50).

Zuazu et al. (51) appealed for information on pregnant patients with hematologic malignancies in Spain; they received results by mailed questionnaires on 56 pregnancies in 48 women, 22 of whom were with leukemia patients. Twelve cases of AML, ALL, or CML were diagnosed during pregnancy, and two patients became pregnant while receiving chemotherapy for CML and AML. Both latter patients had treatment discontinued after the first month and gave birth to 2200-g normal infants at 34 and 36 weeks. There were three elective abortions performed for the other 12 patients; one spontaneous abortion occurred 20 days af-

TABLE 7. *Fetal results of chemotherapy given for acute leukemia by trimester of first exposure*

Trimester exposed	Elective abortion	Spontaneous abortion/stillbirth	Premature, normal	Full-term, normal	Full-term, low weight	Malformations
First	2	1/2	6	1	1	0
Second	0	1/3	10	7	1	1[a]
Third	0	0/0	10	13	0	1[b]
Total	2	2/5	26	21	2	2

[a]Polydactyly as seen in other family members (Volkenandt M, Buchner T, Hiddeman W, van de Loo J. Acute leukaemia during pregnancy. *Lancet* 1988;1:1404).
[b]Adherence of iris to cornea, diagnosed at age 2 years (93).
Data from ref. 11, with permission.

ter chemotherapy given in week 11, one spontaneous abortion 3 weeks after chemotherapy given at week 12, one maternal–fetal death after therapy given at 22 weeks, and one intrauterine demise during chemotherapy given at week 29. The other five patients delivered normal infants; two had low birthweight but were progressing normally on follow-up. Obviously, there is some bias on the part of the respondents; all responses were generated from only 10 hospitals, and the sample size was quite small. Overall fetal survival was only 50% (7 of 14) (51). There are also reports with smaller series of patients, which adds to the anecdotal evidence (66,67).

The majority of patients and neonates survive gestation, labor, and delivery without major complication. Though more malformations occur with chemotherapy exposure in the first trimester, most infants do not suffer untoward outcomes, even with early exposure. Ascertaining the relative contribution of chemotherapy to teratogenesis in these cases is not currently possible.

Acute Promyelocytic Leukemia

APL was treated with chemotherapy alone before the introduction of ATRA. In 1995, Hoffman et al. (52) published a case report and a review of the English literature that compiled 24 cases of APL coinciding with pregnancy. Ten of these patients received an anthracycline with or without cytarabine or another agent for induction therapy, without ATRA. Three fetuses were exposed in the first trimester, with one spontaneous abortion, and five were exposed in the second trimester; the seven live neonates were normal. Two patients were treated in the third trimester, with one intrauterine death at 29 weeks' gestation.

Requena et al. (53) described two patients with APL treated with cytarabine, thioguanine, daunomycin (daunorubicin), and mitoxantrone during the second trimester. Both women delivered normal neonates, though one infant was intubated for a total of 7 minutes (52). Takatsuki et al. (54) evaluated two patients with APL who were both given a non-ATRA containing regimen that resulted in 440 mg total daunorubicin for each. One patient received the chemotherapy at 14 weeks, when she presented with APL and disseminated intravascular coagulopathy (DIC); intrauterine fetal death occurred at 19 weeks. The fetus had a hypoplastic bone marrow and severe anemia. The other patient also had DIC at time of diagnosis; she started chemotherapy at 29 weeks' gestation. Her infant was delivered at 35 weeks without any abnormalities or complications. These cases appear similar, with differing responses to daunorubicin, emphasizing again the variables in teratogenicity (54). In another instance, a women conceived while receiving cytarabine and daunorubicin for APL; at approximately 5 weeks, she had cytarabine and thioguanine. All chemotherapy was discontinued at this time, and the fetus was delivered at term. This neonate required immediate intubation for respiratory distress; it was severely brachycephalic and had other craniofacial abnormalities, as well as hypoplastic thumbs and absent radii bilaterally with only four digits per hand. The infant's motor development was slightly retarded, with normal development in all other categories (55).

The advent of ATRA brought unknown risks to pregnant patients with APL. Another vitamin A derivative, 13-*cis*-retinoic acid, causes a specific retinoic embryopathy, when taken in the first trimester (41). Therefore, ATRA would be suspected of causing a similar set of deformities. Because patients can be critically ill with DIC when diagnosed with APL, treatment should not be delayed for delivery.

Three patients described by Hoffman et al. (52) received ATRA between gestational weeks 30 and 32; they delivered a total of four normal but premature neonates. One patient was diagnosed with relapsed APL in the first trimester and was treated with ATRA. Her infant was premature, but healthy at 15 months of age. Another six pregnant patients who received ATRA are reported in the current English literature and their fetal outcomes are listed in Table 8. No cases of retinoid embryopathy have been reported.

TABLE 8. *Pregnancy outcomes of 11 patients with acute promyelocytic leukemia who received therapy with all-trans-retinoic acid during gestation*

Reference	Year	Week treated	Response	Other agents administered	DIC	Week delivered; outcome
Harrison et al. (56)	1994	26, for 30 d	CR	None	Yes	30; normal but cardiac arrest (recovered)
Stenloft et al. (57)	1994	23, for 35 d	CR	None	Yes; clinically mild but excess perinatal hemorrhage	32; normal twins
Tsuda et al. (58)	1994	28, for 4 wk	CR	None	No	29; normal
Nakamura et al. (59)	1995	30, for 2 wk	CR	Daunorubicin, steroids day of delivery	Yes	32; fetal distress, normal
Simone et al. (60)	1995	6, for 4 wk	CR but relapsed at 30 wk	Prednisone	Yes	32, normal but RDS (resolved)
Wantanabe et al. (61)	1995	28, for 30 d	CR		Yes	32; normal
Lin et al. (62)	1996	14, for 60 d	CR	rhG-CSF, rhEPO	No; Jehovah's Witness	40; normal
Lipovsky et al. (63)	1996	34, for 4 wk	CR	None	Yes; received blood products	38; normal
Sham (64)	1996	29, for 1 d; labor began 24–36 h later	NR	None	No; no bleeding complications	Postnatal death; bilateral renal agenesis before APL diagnosed
Incerpi et al. (65)	1997	24, until delivery	CR	Daunorubicin, IV heparin	Yes; received multiple blood products	33; small intracranial hemorrhages by imaging
Terada et al. (35)	1997	30, for 38 d	CR	None	No	33; atrial arrhythmia 2 d before, 1 day after birth; otherwise normal

CR, complete remission; DIC, disseminated intravascular coagulation; IV, intravenous; NR, no response; rhEPO, recombinant erythroporetin; rhG-CSF, recombinant granulocyte-colony stimulating factor; RSD, respiratory distress syndrome.

Chronic Myelogenous Leukemia

Unlike the ALs, CLs often do not require immediate therapy. With the delay in the institution of therapy, many pregnancies can be completed without additional complications. Sometimes, however, therapy is needed urgently to control symptoms and signs of disease.

There are only a few cases of hydroxyurea use during pregnancy. However, most patients conceived while receiving treatment, and their fetuses were exposed to the drug throughout gestation (Table 9). Other therapies such as leukapheresis or splenectomy may be employed without consideration of teratogenic consequences.

Treatment with IFN alfa may rarely be necessary during gestation. Although the exact mechanisms of action may not be known, this cytokine does not work by interfering directly with deoxyribonucleic acid synthesis; therefore, one would expect fewer teratogenic effects. In pregnant murine model, IFN alfa produces adverse effects not seen in nonpregnant mice, such as hypersplenism, neutropenia, thrombocytopenia, and spontaneous abortions (68). In humans, the first report of a

TABLE 9. *Use of hydroxyurea during pregnancy*

Reference	Diagnosis (mo before pregnancy)	Gestational age at diagnosis	Use of hydroxyurea	Pregnancy outcome	
				Delivery (wk)	Fetal status; weight (g)
Patel, et al. (115)	7	12–14 weeks	Conception until term	36	normal; 2670
Delmer, et al. (119)	12	Unknown	Conception until term	26	Eclampsia: stillborn; phenotype normal
	8	Unknown	Conception until term	40	Normal; 3200
Jackson, et al. (116)	11	11 wk	Conception until term	37	Normal; 2850
Terian, et al. (117)	48	Unknown	Conception until 37 wk[a]	38	Normal; 3100
Fitzgerald, McCann (118)	6	HU stopped 6 wk before β-hCG positive	mid-2nd trimester[b] until 1 mo before term	Term	Normal; 3400

[a]Patient also received 1.5 Gy to spleen at approximately 16 wk.
[b]Patient underwent leukapheresis during first trimester.
β-hCG, human chorionic gonadotropin; HU, hydroxyurea.

patient conceiving while receiving IFN alfa for CML was published in 1991. IFN alfa, 4 million U subcutaneously every other day, controlled her blood counts, and she delivered a healthy infant at term (69). Subsequently, Baer et al. (70) reported on two other patients with CML: one patient receiving IFN alfa at conception and the other starting treatment at 2 months' gestation. The pregnancies were without complication, and the offspring were healthy, delivered at term. Another patient conceived during month 32 of IFN alfa therapy. Her dosage had to be decreased from 6 million U per day to 3 million U; in the third trimester, the dose was administered every other day because of excessive myelosuppression. Regardless, she delivered a healthy term infant (71). Yet another patient had been on IFN alfa for approximately 2 years when she became pregnant. She tolerated continued therapy and delivered a normal term infant (72). Haggstrom et al. (73) examined two women, both diagnosed with CML in week 13 of pregnancy with elevated WBC and platelet counts. IFN alfa was administered three times per week at a dose of 8 million U. Healthy term infants were delivered without complication. These neonates had less than 1 U/mL of IFN alfa in their serum, compared with the mothers who had 20.8 U/mL and 58 U/mL in their serum samples. Breast milk levels of IFN were found to be greater than the neonates' levels at 1.4 U/mL and 6 U/mL (73). There are no cases of neonates who were breast-fed while their mothers received IFN alfa.

No publications of adverse fetal effects have been found in the literature. While CML in pregnant patients is uncommon, the incidence may increase, as with CLL, as childbirth is progressively delayed until later years. Cytotoxic chemotherapy can usually be delayed until delivery if a patient remains in the chronic phase. Patients in accelerated-phase CML should proceed immediately to high-dose chemotherapy; variables include the time required to prepare for bone marrow transplant (BMT), the need for standard-dose chemotherapy in the interval, and gestational age of the fetus.

Chronic Lymphocytic Leukemia and Hairy Cell Leukemia

CLL is so rarely diagnosed in reproductive-age women that only one case has been reported. Because of the indolent course of the disease, this patient was not treated. However, she did receive multiple antibiotics and blood products during her pregnancy. She delivered a healthy near-term infant. The placenta contained mature lymphocytes in the intervillous spaces but otherwise was normal (74).

Usually, a chronic condition of older men, hairy cell leukemia (HCL) is highly responsive to purine analogs such as cladribine (Leustatin). HCL has been observed in several pregnant patients (70,75,76). In one instance, treatment was deferred until after delivery, but the patient required a splenectomy at 16 weeks; the pregnancy then continued without complication (75). Two patients received IFN alfa for HCL in the second and third trimesters of pregnancy. No adverse effects were reported, and both offspring were healthy (70).

Bone Marrow Suppression

Other conditions, such as pancytopenia, can be present in neonates exposed during gestation to chemotherapeutic agents. One would assume marrow suppression from maternal chemotherapy, implying that chemotherapy is crossing the placenta. One report involved seven infants whose mothers received chemotherapy in the second or third trimester. Two neonates were neutropenic after cytarabine, one neutropenic after an anthracycline (unspecified), and four others were leukopenic after receiving cyclophosphamide, mercaptopurine, methotrexate, and vincristine (50).

Okun et al. (77) reported on an infant with myelosuppression after maternal treatment for ALL. The patient received therapy from 12.5 to 27.5 weeks' gestation that included prednisone, vincristine, cyclophosphamide, daunorubicin, asparaginase, intrathecal methotrexate, whole-brain irradiation, and mercaptopurine maintenance. At the time of her uncomplicated delivery at 31 weeks, maternal counts had been within normal range for 2 weeks, but the neonate was born with pancytopenia (platelet count, 5,000/μL) and heart failure from anemia. A bone marrow biopsy on day 2 of life revealed no megakaryocytes and decreased myeloid and erythroid precursors. The biopsy was repeated on day 9, with normal megakaryocyte, myeloid, and erythroid maturation. Peripheral blood counts on day 21 showed a WBC of 5700/μL, hemoglobin of 7.6 g/dL, and platelets 275,000/μL (77).

Another fetus was subjected to cytarabine, daunorubicin, and etoposide (VePesid) at 29 weeks and again at 34 weeks for maternal AML. Eleven days after the second course, fetal distress was noted, and an emergency cesarean section was performed, with a maternal absolute neutrophil count (ANC) of 800/μL. The neonate suffered from anemia, leukopenia, and neutropenia; she required red cell transfusion and granulocyte colony-stimulating factor (G-CSF) for neutropenic sepsis. By day 4 of life, the counts were improving, and 1 year later she was developing normally without hematologic sequelae (78).

In another case, an infant was delivered to a mother with AML after two induction courses of chemotherapy starting at 27 weeks' gestation. Labor began in week 31 while the mother was pancytopenic, with a total WBC of 100/μL. The neonate's hematocrit was 22% to 25%, with multiple serum electrolyte abnormalities, which were corrected. The remainder of the CBC was within normal limits, and the hematocrit normalized after several months (79).

Neonatal myelosuppression and even complete marrow suppression may be an adverse effect of maternal chemotherapy, but as in preceding cases, there is full recovery with vigorous supportive care. Transfusions are well tolerated by neonates. Despite passage of chemotherapy to the fetus, the ability for postnatal hematopoiesis is not compromised. Not all neonates born during maternal myelosuppression have pancytopenia. In 1987, Meador et al. (80) chronicled four cases in which the CBCs of the neonates were normal after birth. One case concerned a patient treated for ALL who delivered with a total WBC of 100/μL, expiring in the postpartum period with normal peripheral blood counts (78). Another patient with AL vaginally delivered a neonate with a normal CBC while she was pancytopenic with a WBC of 200/μL cells and platelet count of 58,000/μL after transfusion

(81). In the other two cases, patients with Ewing's sarcoma and Hodgkin's disease also delivered neonates with normal counts and without complications (80).

However, significant mortality and morbidity are associated with fetal anemia, as seen with hydrops fetalis and nonimmune etiologies of anemia (82). A sinusoidal fetal heart rate pattern, defined as "a pattern of regular variability resembling a sine wave," with an amplitude of 5 to 30 or 40 beats per minute has been thought to correlate with impending fetal demise in 50% to 70% of cases, most often from life-threatening anemia (82,83). Perhaps anemia-induced hypoxia interferes with the fetal cardiac autonomic nervous system, causing the vacillations seen with a sinusoidal pattern (82). There is a case of a 22-year-old woman diagnosed at 20 weeks' gestation with AML accompanied by severe anemia (84). She was treated with daunorubicin and cytarabine without a CR and was then reinduced with mitoxantrone, cytarabine, etoposide, and G-CSF at 31 weeks' gestation. Bone marrow biopsy at week 35 revealed no leukemia with unremarkable peripheral blood counts. The fetus tolerated this regimen without difficulty until after the second cycle of chemotherapy, when an intermittent sinusoidal heart rate pattern was noted during scheduled fetal monitoring. A week later, extreme fetal distress occurred, and a 1046-g neonate with pancytopenia was delivered by cesarean section; the hemoglobin was 5.4 g/dL. Treatment included blood transfusion and intravenous antibiotics; the infant's peripheral blood counts were improving at day 9 of life and normal by discharge at approximately 8 weeks (84).

Thus, no strong correlation has been shown between maternal and fetal blood counts. The threat of neonatal thrombocytopenia, in addition to many other obstetric factors, may alter the method of delivery. Assessing prenatal fetal blood counts could definitively answer the question of cytopenias, so that delivery can be planned at the optimal time for mother and fetus. Morishita et al. (85) followed a 23-year-old woman found to have AML at 23 weeks' gestation. She was treated with a cytarabine analog, daunorubicin, mercaptopurine, and prednisone at weeks 24 and 29 of gestation; bone marrow biopsy confirmed CR at 32 weeks. At 31 weeks, ultrasound-guided transabdominal cordocentesis disclosed a fetal WBC of 3800/μL, hemoglobin of 10.9 g/dL, and platelet count of 190,000/μL. These counts were repeated at 33 weeks and 5 days, with a slight trilineage increase in counts; the next day the signs and symptoms of premature placental separation occurred, and an emergency cesarean section was performed. The neonate had Apgar scores of 1 at 1 minute, improving to 8 at 5 minutes. At day 10 of life, the neonate had a decreased hemoglobin of 8.9 g/dL and received a transfusion of red blood cells. There was no report of any other hematologic difficulties at 5 months of age (85).

Low Birthweight

As progress has been made in neonatal intensive care, the overall survival of premature, low-birthweight, and critically ill neonates has improved. Low-birthweight infants weigh less than 2500 g by World Health Organization standards. The survival rate of infants weighing only 1000 to 1500 g is excellent, with approximately 90% overall survival in neonates weighing 1500 g at birth (86). In the United States, approximately 7% of all infants born each year are considered to be at low birthweight, although low birthweight accounted for 67% of neonatal deaths two to three decades ago (87). Women and Infants Hospital of Rhode Island noted 62 neonatal deaths in 5429 live births in 1972 that involved neonates weighing 2500 g or less. The number decreased to 58 deaths in 6309 live births in 1982 (86).

Low-birthweight infants have increased susceptibility to many acute problems in the first few days of life. They are at a higher risk for intraventricular hemorrhage (mainly as a result of trauma at birth or hypotension), respiratory distress syndrome if lung development is incomplete at birth, hyperbilirubinemia, and infections (86). Neurologic development in low-birthweight neonates can be impeded, and those with extreme low birthweight have a 9% to 18% chance of severe handicaps; cerebral palsy and seizure disorders are most often encountered. Developmental delays in other fields, such as academic success, are difficult to assess independent of other issues, such as environmental factors (87).

Mechanisms of Low Birthweight. Intrauterine growth restriction (IUGR) occurs in approximately 30% of all low-birthweight infants, and there are many possible causes (88). There are several possible mechanisms by which infants born to mothers treated for AL may weigh less than 2500 g at birth. One factor could be related to placental function; perhaps the leukemia or the treatment could induce infarction of placental vessels (88). DIC can also damage these blood vessels (50). Leukemic infiltrates, as will be discussed, have been found in the placenta (89,90), which could inhibit blood flow. Maternal issues must also be considered, such as infections associated with neutropenia, poor nutritional intake, and altered metabolism. The correlation between inadequate diet and fetal size was established during wartime when large populations in Holland and Russia had caloric restrictions because of World War II food shortages (88). Maternal anemia may result in less oxygen transferred to the placental circulation, leading to IUGR (50). In patients with CML and CLL, large spleen size can mechanically prevent uterine expansion.

INTERACTIONS AMONG PREGNANCY, LEUKEMIA, AND MATERNAL–FETAL OUTCOME

Impact of Pregnancy on Leukemia

Pregnancy has not been shown to have any effect on the development, response to treatment, duration of response, or overall survival in AL (11,50). The CR rates appreciated by Reynoso et al. (91) of 76% to 77% in both pregnant AML and ALL patients is consistent with responses in nonpregnant patients for the 1980s. AL is fatal if untreated. In all patients, untreated AL has an overall survival (OS) from 2 to 3 weeks to 2 to 3 months (1), with death most commonly the result of infection or hemorrhage.

There is a maternal–fetal risk with delaying treatment until after delivery. Patients diagnosed with AL who did not receive any treatment before labor and delivery had an approximately 60% perinatal mortality rate in the 1960s to 1970s (92), an often quoted but now outdated statistic. However, the majority of maternal deaths associated with labor and delivery appear to occur in women with either untreated AL or with disease unresponsive to therapy (50).

In the early stages of CML (chronic phase) and CLL, treatment is not always indicated, and if adequate hematologic parameters are maintained without significant hemorrhage or infection, uncomplicated gestation and delivery can occur before any therapy needs to be instituted. Cytoreduction can episodically be achieved with leukapheresis, as needed. ALs, however, are more aggressive, and patients require therapy for disease control almost immediately upon diagnosis.

There are a few reports of pregnant patients not receiving chemotherapy for AL. In some of these patients, leukemia was diagnosed at delivery or in the last few weeks of gestation, and labor was quickly induced before the beginning of treatment (91). With a total of seven cases, Catanzarite and Ferguson (50) illustrated the range of fetal outcomes when maternal AL is not treated:

- Diagnosis close to delivery, induced or spontaneous, at 37, 40, 41, or 42 weeks: all healthy infants
- Diagnosis at 14 weeks: chemotherapy given, then elective abortion with retained placenta and maternal death from hemorrhage
- Diagnosis at 28 weeks: intrauterine death, then maternal demise from intracerebral hemorrhage in week 30
- Diagnosis 1 month prior to conception: DIC at 34 weeks with fetal demise within 24 hours

Maternal outcomes were poor: One patient survived 11 months, another was last evaluated at discharge with persistent leukemia, and the other five patients expired 33 days or less after diagnosis, mainly from postpartum hemorrhage and infection (50). These examples illustrate the need for early intervention against AL. Pregnant patients require the same aggressive approach as nonpregnant AL patients to increase the chances of a CR or possible cure.

Impact of Leukemia on Labor, Delivery, and the Perinatal Period

Bleeding is uncommonly problematic, even though many patients have thrombocytopenia, hypofibrinogenemia, and/or DIC. Nonmalignant thrombocytopenia has been assessed in pregnant women by Burrows and Kelton (93). Admissions to the obstetric unit were monitored for 1 year; 1357 patients had uncomplicated pregnancies without any comorbid conditions, and 111 (8.2%) of these women had incidental platelet counts less than 150,000/μL. Only 4.3% of neonates born to these mothers were thrombocytopenic, and all but 12 were delivered by vaginal birth. These neonates had no hemorrhagic complications (93). Uterine (myometrium) contractions are an important method of thrombostasis for normal placental tissue, provided that there is no injury (94). Patients undergoing physiologic labor and delivery have a mechanism for control of bleeding in place that supersedes thrombostasis and coagulation. With planned cesarean section, these contractions do not occur to the same degree, and the risk of bleeding is higher because there are fewer platelets available for hemostasis. An uncomplicated vaginal delivery results in approximately 500 to 700 mL of blood loss; abnormal hemorrhage is most likely to occur in the 1 hour after placental discharge (95). Hemostasis of the episiotomy incision is almost always easily obtained. No evidence is available to suggest that a cesarean section is necessary for incidental, low-normal platelet counts.

In immune thrombocytopenic purpura (ITP), the most common cause of thrombocytopenia in reproductive-age women, IgG antibodies destroy maternal platelets, and some of these antibodies can cross the placenta, with the development of thrombocytopenia in 44% to 70% of infants (96). It has been thought that mothers with low platelet counts should not undergo vaginal delivery, as the infant may bleed, especially intracranially, from the trauma of labor and delivery. However, the relationship between maternal and fetal platelet counts may not be reliable (97). Kagan and Laros (96) studied 15 pregnant ITP patients, 12 of whom were taking steroids during pregnancy. There were 13 live births, and 54% of these neonates were thrombocytopenic, with no sequelae. One intrauterine death occurred when the patient discontinued all medication; at 39 weeks she was found to have a platelet count of 4000/μL and fetal demise. Autopsy of the fetus revealed subgaleal hemorrhage. The other death was secondary to sepsis. Three neonates had platelet counts less than 100,000/μL (7000, 13,000, and 83,000/μL) and no hemorrhagic complications. The thrombocytopenic mothers did not have an increased incidence of bleeding. Eight of them had vaginal deliveries and the other five underwent cesarean section for the standard obstetrical reason (96).

Patients with leukemia may have other coagulation abnormalities that may increase the risk of bleeding compared to the risk in ITP patients. Thus, direct comparisons of thrombocytopenia from immunologic causes with that from known marrow suppression cannot easily be made. However, one could extrapolate the data obtained from patients with ITP to suggest that low platelet counts are well tolerated in vaginal deliveries and that even leukemia patients can deliver safely with platelet counts less than 100,000/μL, provided that other coagulation parameters are within normal limits. Except for an extenuating circumstance, leukemia patients and their offspring are not at any higher risk for bleeding complications with a vaginal delivery.

Severe infection or sepsis causes major morbidity and mortality in leukemia patients. Chemotherapy can induce neutropenia; therefore, chemotherapy should be scheduled to allow patients to deliver after chemotherapy-induced leukopenia has resolved. However, chemotherapy itself can cause a chronic leukopenia in recovered patients, or the leukemia itself can be the cause of neutropenia, leaving patients with a less than preferred WBC count. In the report by Juarez et al. (98), 4 of 10 patients had postpartum infections: Staphylococcus aureus skin infection, perirectal abscess, pneumonia, and an episiotomy wound infection with perineal necrosis and sepsis. This last patient was severely ill and recovered; the other patients expired within weeks to months from the sequelae of these infectious events. One patient who conceived on maintenance therapy for ALL expired at 5 months' gestation from *Pseudomonas* pneumonia. Death from any infection occurs in nonpregnant AML patients at an estimated mean incidence of 14% to 15% (99). Life-threatening but usually successfully treated infections are prevalent in many leukemia patients.

Passage of Metastatic Disease to Fetus

Maternal cancer can metastasize to the placenta and occasionally to the fetus, although few cases are reported in the literature. In 1981, Read and Platzer (89) reported on 44 cases compiled since 1866, and Dildy et al. (90) published an updated list of 53 cases in 1989. Among these 53 cases, there were eight cases of either leukemia or lymphoma in the placental tissue, and in four instances there was evidence of fetal involvement (90). Read and Platzer (89) found six cases of AL involving the placenta or fetus: three patients with AML and no fetal disease (fetus not assessed in one instance), one with ALL and no fetal involvement, and two with ALL in whom the placenta not examined but ALL was found in the fetus.

Five more cases of AL with placental involvement were added to the literature by Honore and Brown (100) in 1990. One patient was diagnosed with AML at 16 weeks' gestation; at the same time ultrasound of the uterus was consistent with a missed abortion. Pathologic examination of the uterine contents revealed a partial hydatidiform mole and many leukemic cells in the intervillous tissue without villous invasion. A 32-year-old woman was diagnosed with monocytic AML 1 day after the delivery of a healthy male infant; at 20 months of age, the child was diagnosed with monocytic AML. The histochemical staining and immunophenotyping of the mother and child's leukemic cells were identical. Additionally, the child's bone marrow cytogenetic karyotype was 40% 46, XY, but the remaining 60% was 46,XX and presumably derived from his mother. The child had no other cytogenetic anomalies, and both patients were in complete remission when last assessed. The authors speculated that the leukemia was transmitted via the placenta; the infant's early immune system could not recognize the mother's cell as foreign because he had inherited her HLA type with expression of the same antigens (101). The other two known cases of maternal transmission of AL were reported in 1958 and 1964 (90), before instruments to demonstrate clonality were available. Both cases involved ALL, with infant death in less then 1 year (50). Possible mechanisms for the development of maternal–fetal AL include the following:

- Direct maternal metastases through the placenta
- Transfer of a population of cells that is dormant but somehow becomes activated in the infant to become leukemic disease at a later time, appearing as *de novo* leukemia
- Genetic alterations from chemotherapy exposure or from inherent familial mutations that lead to the development of AL

One could assume that the strength of the fetal/infant immune system plays a role in the development of AL. There is recorded ultrastructural demonstration of villous syncytiotrophoblasts phagocytosing nucleated cells thought to be of maternal origin (102). With implantation of the embryo, syncytiotrophoblasts have been known to phagocytose maternal cells, possibly using the maternal cell products as nutrients, but this phenomenon has not been demonstrated later in pregnancy (102). If the involved cells are maternal leukemic blasts as speculated, this could explain the discrepancy in the number of placentas with maternal metastatic disease but without transfer of the malignancy to the fetus.

Long-term Follow-up of Progeny after *in Utero* Exposure to Chemotherapy

Most neonates born to mothers with leukemia have no abnormalities at birth or through the first postnatal year, with practically all offspring maintaining normal growth and development for the first few years of life. Several authors have examined these offspring as they mature to ascertain whether there are any late developmental consequences from *in utero* exposure to maternal therapy.

Aviles and Niz (103) followed 17 children from 1963 to 1981 after their birth to mothers with AL; there were five maternal–fetal deaths in the original study group and 20 births with three neonatal deaths. Ten of the surviving offspring were exposed to chemotherapy in the first trimester; eight of these were exposed to doxorubicin. Their ages ranged at the time of last report from 4 to 22 years. They were compared to their siblings and a normal control group of similar age. These 17 children all had normal growth patterns. Bone marrow biopsies were all unremarkable with normal cytogenetics. There was no increase in infection rate. Two neonates were born with pancytopenia: Both recovered their counts, although one expired from sepsis on day 21 with a normal CBC. Neurologic development was unaltered, no teachers reported unusual behavior, and their mean intelligence quotient scores ranged from 115 to 123, as did their siblings' and the control group's scores. The oldest child conceived and gave birth to a normal 3200-g infant. In this cohort, there were virtually no abnormal consequences from maternal therapy (104). Aviles et al. (104) added another six leukemia patients to this group: All had normal progeny after chemotherapy, and one-half of these patients received treatment during the first trimester. The median age of the offspring was 15 years (range, 8 to 19 years), and their development and health have been unremarkable.

Reynoso et al. (91) with the Toronto Leukemia Study Group followed seven offspring for 1 to 17 years after birth. All but one mother received chemotherapy during gestation; she was diagnosed at 38 weeks' gestation with ALL and delivered by cesarean section before treatment. There was one set of fraternal twins. The only perinatal complication was mild thrombocytopenia in one neonate; birthweights ranged from 1000 to 3420 g. Two congenital malformations were noted. The first was diagnosed at age 2 years in a male infant exposed to chemotherapy in the third trimester (adherence of iris to cornea), and the second was apparent at birth in the male twin. He had a club hand (absent thumb, hyperflexion of wrist, paraxial hemimelia), an anomalous inferior vena cava, esophageal atresia, undescended testes bilaterally, and duplication of the renal collecting system bilaterally. He had no chromosomal abnormalities of his peripheral blood. At 11 years of age, he was found to have learning difficulties with a low intelligence quotient. He had a large neuroblastoma of the adrenal gland diagnosed at age 14, and at age 16 was diagnosed with metastatic papillary thyroid carcinoma. After treatments at age 17 years, he had no evidence of disease at last report. His twin sister developed normally without any complications, and none of the other six offspring have any developmental difficulties (91). There are no other reports of mental developmental delay after *in utero* exposure to chemotherapy.

In 1989, Garber (105) published 64 cases of children exposed *in utero* to chemotherapy for all types of malignancies, but few details of these cases were provided. There were two reports of retarded growth at 14 months in two children. Two additional children were noted to have malformations: one with an imperforate anus and rectovaginal fistula and the other with distal limb defects (46,106).

IMPACT ON FUTURE PREGNANCY AND GYNECOLOGIC HEALTH

Breast-feeding

One could assume that most drugs or their metabolites are excreted in the breast milk. Demonstrations of cyclophosphamide, methotrexate, hydroxyurea, cisplatin, and doxorubicin in breast milk have been published. One patient with APL who received mitoxantrone and etoposide had breast milk drug levels assessed after her third postremission treatment. The etoposide levels were apparent immediately after administration, becoming undetectable by 24 hours. The mitoxantrone remained present in the breast milk at approximately 18 ng/mL at chemotherapy day 28 (107).

An infant being breast-fed by a mother receiving cytotoxic agents would be ingesting a small but measurable amount of these agents and their metabolites, possibly negating some of the numerous advantages to feeding with breast milk. Though not proven, theoretically adverse effects from these medications could be seen in infants who may also have been exposed to chemotherapy *in utero;* chromosomal alterations of uncertain significance may also occur with long-term exposure. Given the paucity of knowledge on this subject, unnecessary exposure of neonates to cytotoxic chemicals should be avoided whenever possible.

Fertility and Sterility

There are more long-term survivors of childhood cancers and more young women with significant remission after AL. Survivor issues now include fertility after treatment.

Specific chemotherapeutic agents have been implicated as definite or probable causes of infertility: chlorambucil, busulfan, doxorubicin, and cytarabine. These agents and others promote atrophy of follicles with ovarian fibrosis, perhaps in a dose-dependent manner. Less estradiol is produced, and amenorrhea occurs (38). It has been incidentally noted that women treated in their early 20s have a higher probability of regaining ovarian function, compared to those treated in later life. Otherwise, there are no further indicators of retaining fertility; some patients will regain ovarian function with time. In the literature, there are reports of patients who have successfully conceived (or fathered offspring) after treatment. As noted in the previous section, there are basically no short-term or long-term sequelae for these children.

Eight patients who responded to Zuazu et al.'s (51) questionnaire conceived after antileukemia therapy. The median time to conception after treatment was 5 years (range, 2 months to 8 years). Patients experienced a range of therapies, from splenic radiation, cytarabine with an anthracycline, and thioguanine or busulfan in seven patients (51). Although few cases are represented here, some patients experienced rapid recovery of ovulation.

More recently, findings on offspring of patients who had AL were published from Japan (108). In this account, 1136 men and women were identified as greater than 5-year survivors, and 43 of them produced progeny after their first remission. In these patients, there were eight sets of siblings, one elective abortion, and four spontaneous abortions. The resulting 46 children were born without malformations or developmental problems from ages 3 months to 15 years. Only 4% of these survivors reproduced; the number of patients who were unable to conceive, did not attempt to become pregnant, or were too old to have reproductive capacity conserved after treatment is not known (108).

The offspring of patients able to conceive after treatment for childhood malignancy have not been at any greater risk of acquiring a malignancy. Li et al. (109) studied 146 male and female adult patients who were at least

5-year survivors of their childhood cancers. There were 286 pregnancies with 242 live births; cousins of the offspring, as well as statistics from the general population, were utilized for comparison. Nineteen pregnancies ended in elective abortions, with 25 spontaneous abortions and one stillbirth. Malignancy developed in only two offspring (0.8%): bilateral hereditary retinoblastoma and AML. Hodgkin's disease developed in one child in the control group. The rate of survival to age 10 years (96%), malformations (four fatal, four major, 16 minor), and fetal deaths after the first trimester (less than 4%) were all consistent with the general population and/or the control group (109). One group has recorded a 9% incidence of minor congenital malformations in the offspring of pediatric ALL survivors, compared to 4% to 15% in the general population (110).

The offspring of patients with AL, both adult and pediatric, do not appear to be at any increased risk for malformations or developmental delays.

Genetic Counseling

There is no known inheritance pattern for ALs, and population studies over the years have yielded few cases to assess. There are reports of several relatives in a family being afflicted (111). Gunz et al. (112) assessed the relatives of approximately 900 leukemia patients and concluded that first-degree relatives had a fourfold increase in their risk for disease. Siblings of pediatric cancer patients are known to be particularly at risk for malignancies, probably due to a higher frequency of inherited conditions in pediatric malignancies (113, but this does not appear to hold true for the siblings of adult leukemia patients.

In reports by Gunz et al. (112) and Eriksson and Bergstrom (114), CLL has the strongest evidence for a familial relationship. However, there is not enough evidence to have leukemia patients or their offspring undergo genetic assessment, and as specified earlier, there is no role for screening any type of leukemia.

SUMMARY

Regardless of parity, standard induction chemotherapy for AML and ALL will result in a 60% to 85% CR rate. Other information regarding the treatment of AL concurrent with pregnancy is anecdotal; with this in mind, some inferences can be loosely drawn, based on the available information.

It is in the best interest of the fetus not to be exposed to chemotherapy during the first trimester, as the malformation rate from all therapy, including radiation therapy, is approximately 17%. If folate antagonists, such as methotrexate, and radiation therapy can be avoided in the first trimester, the fetal malformation rate is closer to 6%, only double the background rate of 3%. The rate of spontaneous abortions, stillbirths, and maternal–fetal demise is approximately 20% to 40%, depending on the medications given and the timing of administration. These estimated rates are based on AL treatments from the 1980s, not from the 1990s.

Cytarabine, a deoxycytidine antimetabolite, and an anthracycline are most often dispensed as antileukemia therapy in patients with AML and appear to be correlated with more adverse outcomes when given in the first trimester. There is no detectable increase in malformation rates of fetuses exposed to antineoplastics after the first trimester.

Withholding treatment in AL is usually fatal to the patient and fetus. Delaying treatment until the second trimester or until delivery may decrease the chances of long-term remission for the mother, make labor and delivery more hazardous, and cause harm to the fetus due to maternal infection or anemia.

When the decision to treat is made, patients should be treated in the same aggressive manner as nonpregnant patients are treated. Attentive supervision of fetal status will be necessary from an obstetrician experienced with high-risk pregnancies. Close to one-half of the progeny of treated leukemics have low birthweight, but in virtually all children studied, development appears to proceed normally without sequelae. In almost every report, greater than 80% of offspring survived and matured appropriately. With vigilant monitoring, delivery of a healthy infant can occur without compromising maternal care.

REFERENCES

1. Scheinberg DA, Maslak P, Weiss M. Acute leukemias. In: DeVita VT, Hellman S, Rosenberg SA, eds. *Cancer: principles and practice of oncology*, 5th ed. Philadelphia: Lippincott–Raven Publishers, 1997:2293.
2. Parker SL, Tong T, Bolden S, Wingo PA. Cancer statistics, 1997. *CA Cancer J Clin* 1997;47:5.
3. Groves DF, Linet MS, Devesa SD. Epidemiology of leukemia: overview and patterns of occurrence. In: Henderson ES, Lister TA, Greaves MF, eds. *Leukemia*, 6th ed. Philadelphia: WB Saunders, 1996:145.
4. Lambe M, Ekbom A. Cancer coinciding with childbearing: delayed diagnosis during pregnancy? *BMJ* 1995;311:1607.
5. Cartwright RA, Staines A. Acute leukemias. *Baillieres Clin Haematol* 1992;5:1.
6. Atunez de Mayolo J, Ahn YS, Temple D, Harrington WJ. Spontaneous remission of acute leukemia after the termination of pregnancy. *Cancer* 1989;63:1621.
7. Lui JH, Kebar RW. Endocrinology of pregnancy. In: Creasy RK, Resnik R, eds. *Maternal–fetal medicine,* principle and practice, 4th ed. Philadelphia: WB Saunders, 1999:382.
8. Larocca LM, Piantelli M, Leone G, et al. Type II oestrogen binding sites in acute lymphoid and myeloid leukaemias: growth inhibitory effect of oestrogen and flavonoids. *Br J Haematol* 1990;75:489.
9. Lippman M. Steroid hormone receptors in human malignancy. *Life Sci* 1976;18:143.
10. Stone RM, Mayer RJ. The approach to the elderly patient with acute myeloid leukemia. *Hematol Oncol Clin North Am* 1993;7:65.
11. Caligiuri MA, Mayer RJ. Pregnancy and leukemia. *Semin Oncol* 1989;16:388.
12. Warrell RP, Frankel SR, Miller WH, et al. Differentiation therapy of acute promyelocytic leukemia with tretinoin (all-*trans*-retinoic acid). *N Engl J Med* 1991; 324:1385.
13. Cunningham I, Gee TS, Reich LM, Kempin SJ, Naval AN, Clarkson BD. Acute promyelocytic leukemia: treatment results during a decade at Memorial Hospital. *Blood* 1989;73:116.
14. Tallman MS, Anderson JW, Schiffer CA, et al. All-*trans*-retinoic acid in acute promyelocytic leukemia. *N Engl J Med* 1997;337:1021.
15. Fenaux P, LeDeley MC, Castaigne S, et al. Effect of all-*trans* retinoic acid in newly diagnosed promyelocytic leukemia: results of a multicenter randomized trial. *Blood* 1993;82:3241.
16. Frankel SR, Eardley A, Lawrence G, Weiss M, Warrell RP. The retinoic acid syndrome. *Ann Intern Med* 1992;117:292.
17. Fenaux P, Chastang C, Sanz M, et al. ATRA followed by chemotherapy (CT) vs. ATRA plus CT and the role of maintenance therapy in newly diagnosed acute promyelocytic leukemia (APL): first interim results of APL 93 trial. *Blood* 1997;90:122a(abst).
18. Siddiqui T, Elfenbein GJ, Noyes WD, Moreb JS, Oblon D, Weiner RS. Myelodysplastic syndromes presenting in pregnancy. *Cancer* 1990;66:377.
19. Barnett MJ, Eaves CJ. Chronic myeloid leukemia. In: Henderson ES, Lister TA, Greaves MF, eds. *Leukemia*, 6th ed. Philadelphia: WB Saunders, 1996: 535.
20. Enright H, McGlave PB. Biology and treatment of chronic myelogenous leukemia. *Oncology* 1997;11: 1295.
21. Italian Cooperative Study Group on Chronic Myeloid Leukemia. Interferon alfa-2a as compared with conventional chemotherapy for the treatment of chronic myeloid leukemia. *N Engl J Med* 1994;330:280.
22. Goldman JM, Szydlo R, Horowitz MM, et al. Choice of pretransplant treatment and timing of transplants for chronic myelogenous leukemia for chronic phase. *Blood* 1993;82:2235.
23. Rai KR, Sawitsky A, Cronkite EP, et al. Clinical staging of chronic lymphocytic leukemia. *Blood* 1975;24: 219.
24. Cheson BD, Bennett JM, Rai KR, et al. Guidelines for clinical protocols for chronic lymphocytic leukemia: recommendations of the National Cancer Institute-sponsored working group. *Am J Hematol* 1988;29: 152.
25. Duffy TP. Hematologic aspects of pregnancy. In: Hoffman R, Benz EJ, Shattil SJ, Furie B, Cohen HJ, Silberstein LE, eds. *Hematology*, 2nd ed. New York: Churchill Livingstone, 1995:2117.
26. Peck TM, Arias F. Hematologic changes associated with pregnancy. *Clin Obstet Gynecol* 1979;22:785.
27. American Academy of Pediatrics and American College of Obstetricians and Gynecologists. *Guidlelines for perinatal care,* 4th ed. Elk Grove Village, IL, 1997:67.
28. Doll DC, Ringenberg QS, Yarbro JW. Antineoplastic agents and pregnancy. *Semin Oncol* 1989;16:337.
29. Ostrea EM, Brady MJ, Parks PM, Asenio DC, Naluz A. Drug screening of meconium in infants of drug-dependent mothers: an alternative to urine testing. *J Pediatr* 1989;155:474.
30. Rai KR, Holland JF, Glidewell OJ, et al. Treatment of acute myelocytic leukemia: a study by cancer and leukemia group B. *Blood* 1981;58:1203.
31. Mayer RJ. Current chemotherapeutic treatment approaches to the management of previously untreated adults with *de novo* acute myelogenous leukemia. *Semin Oncol* 1987;14:384.
32. Moore KL. *The developing human, clinically oriented embryology*, 4th ed. Philadelphia: WB Saunders, 1988:38.
33. Karp GI, von Oeyen P, Valone F, et al. Doxorubicin in pregnancy: possible transplacental passage. *Cancer Treat Rep* 1983;67:773.
34. D'Incalci M, Broggini M, Buscaglia M, Pardi G. Placental passage of doxorubicin [Letter]. *Lancet* 1983;1: 75.
35. Terada Y, Shindo Y, Endoh A, Wantanabe M, Fukaya T, Yajima A. Fetal arrhythmia during treatment of pregnancy-associated acute promyelocytic leukemia with all-*trans* retinoic acid and favorable outcome. *Leukemia* 1997;11:454.
36. Roboz J, Gleicher N, Wu K, Chahinian P, Kerenyi T, Holland J. Does doxorubicin cross the placenta? *Lancet* 1979;2:1382.

37. D'Incalci M, Sessa C, Colombo N, de Palo G, Semprini AE, Pardi G. Transplacental passage of cyclophosphamide. *Cancer Treat Rep* 1982;66:1681.
38. Collins JM. Pharmacokinetics and clinical monitoring. In: Chabner BA, Longo DL, eds. *Cancer chemotherapy and biotherapy:* principle and practice, 2nd ed. Philadelphia: Lippincott–Raven Publishers, 1996:17.
39. Kalter H, Warkany J. Congenital malformations: etiologic factors and their role in prevention (first of two parts). *N Engl J Med* 1983:308:424.
40. Briggs GG, Freeman RK, Yaffe SJ, eds. *Drugs in pregnancy and lactation, a reference guide to fetal and neonatal risk*, 4th ed. Baltimore: Williams & Wilkins, 1994.
41. Jones KL. Effects of therapeutic, diagnostic, and environmental agents. In: Creasy RK, Resnik R, eds. *Maternal–fetal medicine:* principle and practice, 4th ed. Philadelphia: WB Saunders, 1999:132.
42. Ebert U, Loffler H, Kirch W. Cytotoxic therapy and pregnancy. *Pharmacol Ther* 1997;74:207.
43. Maurer LH, Forcier RJ, McIntyre OR, Benirschke K. Fetal group C trisomy after cytosine arabinoside and thioguanine. *Ann Intern Med* 1971;75:809.
44. Schleuning M, Clemm C. Chromosomal aberrations in a newborn whose mother received cytotoxic treatment during pregnancy. *N Engl J Med* 1987;317:1666.
45. Wagner VM, Hill JS, Weaver D, Baehner RL. Congenital abnormalities in baby born to cytarabine-treated mother. *Lancet* 1980;2:98.
46. Schafer AI. Teratogenetic effects of antileukemic chemotherapy. *Arch Intern Med* 1981;141:514.
47. Reynoso EE, Huerta F. Acute leukemia and pregnancy: fatal fetal outcome after exposure to idarubicin during the second trimester. *Acta Oncol* 1994;33: 709.
48. Turchi JJ, Villasis C. Anthracyclines in the treatment of malignancy in pregnancy. *Cancer* 1988;61:435.
49. Dara P, Slater LM, Armentrout SA. Successful pregnancy during chemotherapy for acute leukemia. *Cancer* 1981;47:845.
50. Catanzarite VA, Ferguson JE. Acute leukemia and pregnancy: a review of management and outcome, 1972–1982. *Obstet Gynecol Surv* 1984;39:663.
51. Zuazu J, Julia A, Sierra J, et al. Pregnancy outcome in hematologic malignancies. *Cancer* 1991;67:703.
52. Hoffman MA, Wiernik PH, Kleiner GJ. Acute promyelocytic leukemia and pregnancy: a case report. *Cancer* 1995;76:2237.
53. Requena A, Velasco JG, Pinilla J, Gonzalez-Gonzalez A. Acute leukemia during pregnancy: obstetric management and perinatal outcome of two cases. *Eur J Obstet Gynecol Reprod Biol* 1995;63:139.
54. Takatsuki H, Abe Y, Goto T, et al. [Two cases of acute promyelocytic leukemia in pregnancy and the effect of anthracyclines on fetal development]. *Rinsho Ketsueki* 1992;33:1736(abst).
55. Artlich A, Moller J, Tschakaloff, Schwinger E, Kruse K, Gortner L. Teratogenic effects in a case of maternal treatment for acute myelocytic leukaemia—neonatal and infantile course. *Eur J Pediatr* 1994;153:488.
56. Harrison P, Chipping P, Fothergill GA. Successful use of all-*trans* retinoic acid in acute promyelocytic leukemia presenting during the second trimester of pregnancy. *Br J Haematol* 1994;86:681.
57. Stenloft J, Nielson L, Hvidman LE. All-*trans* retinoic acid in acute promyelocytic anemia in late pregnancy. *Leukemia* 1994;8:1585.
58. Tsuda H, Doi H, Inada T, Shirono K. [Successful treatment of acute promyelocytic leukemia in a pregnant women by using all-*trans* retinoic acid]. *Rinsho Ketsueki* 1994;35;719(abst).
59. Nakamura K, Dan K, Iwakiri R, Gomi S, Nomura T. Successful treatment of acute promyelocytic leukemia in pregnancy with all-*trans* retinoic acid. *Ann Hematol* 1995;71:263.
60. Simone MD, Stasi R, Venditti A, et al. All-*trans* retinoic acid (ATRA) administration during pregnancy in relapsed acute promyelocytic leukemia. *Leukemia* 1995;9: 1412.
61. Watanabe R, Okamoto S, Moriki T, Kizaki M, Kawai M, Ikeda Y. Treatment of acute promyelocytic leukemia with all-*trans* retinoic acid during the first trimester of pregnancy. *Am J Hematol* 1995;48:210.
62. Lin C, Huang M, Liu H, Chang IY, Tsai C. Successful treatment of acute promyelocytic leukemia in a pregnant Jehovah's Witness with all-*trans* retinoic acid, rhG-CSF, and erythropoietin. *Am J Hematol* 1996; 51:251.
63. Lipovsky MM, Biesma DH, Christiaens GC, Petersen EJ. Successful treatment of acute promyelocytic leukemia with all-trans-retinoic-acid during late pregnancy. *Br J Haematol* 1996;94:699.
64. Sham RL. All-*trans* retinoic acid-induced labor in a patient with acute promyelocytic leukemia. *Am J Hematol* 1996;53:145.
65. Incerpi MH, Miller DA, Posen R, Byrne JD. All-*trans* retinoic acid for the treatment of acute promyelocytic leukemia in pregnancy. *Obstet Gynecol* 1997;89:826.
66. Pizzuto J, Aviles A, Noriega L, Niz J, Morales M, Romero F. Treatment of acute leukemia during pregnancy: presentation of nine cases. *Cancer Treat Rep* 1980;64:679.
67. Volkenandt M, Buchner T, Hiddemann W, van de Loo J. Acute leukaemia during pregnancy [Letter]. *Lancet* 1987;2:1521.
68. Vassiliadis S, Athanassakis I. Type II interferon may be a potentially hazardous therapeutic agent during pregnancy [Letter]. *Br J Haemetol* 1992;82:782.
69. Baer MR. Normal full-term pregnancy in a patient with chronic myelogenous leukemia treated with alpha-interferon [Letter]. *Am J Hematol* 1991;37:66.
70. Baer MR, Ozer H, Foon KA. Interferon-alpha therapy during pregnancy in chronic myelogenous leukaemia and hairy cell leukaemia. *Br J Haematol* 1992;81:167.
71. Delmer A, Rio B, Bauduer F, Ajchenbaum F, Marie JP, Zittoun R. Pregnancy during myelosuppressive treatment for chronic myelogenous leukaemia [Letter]. *Br J Haemetol* 1992;82:783.
72. Reichel RP, Linkesch W, Schetitska D. Therapy with recombinant interferon alpha-2c during unexpected pregnancy in a patient with chronic myeloid leukaemia. *Br J Haematol* 1992;82:472.
73. Haggstrom J, Adriansson T, Hybbinette T, Harnby E, Thorbert G. Two cases of CML treated with alpha-interferon during second and third trimester of pregnancy with analysis of the drug in the new-born immediately postpartum. *Eur J Haematol* 1996;57:101.
74. Chrisomalis L, Baxi LV, Heller D. Chronic lymphocytic leukemia in pregnancy. *Am J Obstet Gynecol* 1996;175:1381.

75. Alothman A, Sparling TG. Managing hairy cell leukemia in pregnancy [Letter]. *Ann Intern Med* 1994; 120:1048.
76. Williams JK. Hairy cell leukemia in pregnancy: a case report. *Am J Obstet Gynecol* 1987;156:210.
77. Okun DB, Groncy PK, Sieger L, Tanaka KR. Acute leukemia in pregnancy: transient myelosuppression after combination chemotherapy in the mother. *Med Pediatr Oncol* 1979;7:315.
78. Murray NA, Acolet D, Deane M, Price J, Roberts IAG. Fetal marrow suppression after maternal chemotherapy for leukaemia. *Arch Dis Child Fetal Neonatal Ed* 1994;71:F209–210.
79. Doney KC, Kraemer KG, Shephard TH. Combination chemotherapy for acute myelocytic leukemia during pregnancy: three case reports. *Cancer Treat Rep* 1979; 63:369.
80. Meador JM, Armentrout SA, Slater LM. Third trimester chemotherapy and neonatal hematopoiesis. *Cancer Chemother Pharmacol* 1987;19:177.
81. Dietz KA, Gee TS. Case report of 6 women diagnosed with acute leukemia during pregnancy. *Oncology Nursing Society* 1983:51(abst).
82. Elliot JP. Massive fetomaternal hemorrhage treated by fetal intravascular transfusion. *Obstet Gynecol* 1991; 78:520.
83. Young BK, Katz M, Wilson SJ. Sinusoidal fetal heart rate. *Am J Obstet Gynecol* 1980;136:587.
84. Hsu KF, Chang CH, Chou CY. Sinusoidal fetal heart rate pattern during chemothrapy in a pregnant woman with acute myelogenous leukemia. *J Formos Med Assoc* 1995;94:562.
85. Morishita S, Imai A, Kawabata I, Tamaya T. Acute myelogenous leukemia in pregnancy: fetal blood sampling and early effects of chemotherapy. *Int J Gynaecol Obstet* 1994;44:273.
86. Kashore WJ, Stern L. Neonatal problems of the preterm baby. *Clin Obstet Gynecol* 1984;11:391.
87. McCormick MC. The contribution of low birth weight to infant mortality and childhood morbidity. *N Engl J Med* 1985;312:82.
88. Creasy RK, Resnik R. Intrauterine growth restriction. In: Creasy RK, Resnik R, eds. *Maternal–fetal medicine:* principle and practice, 4th ed. Philadelphia: WB Saunders, 1999:569.
89. Read EJ, Platzer PB. Placental metastasis from maternal carcinoma of the lung. *Obstet Gynecol* 1981;58:387.
90. Dildy GA, Moise KJ, Carpenter RJ, Klima T. Maternal malignancy metastatic to the products of conception: a review. *Obstet Gynecol Surv* 1989;44:535.
91. Reynoso EE, Sheperd FA, Messner HA, Farquharson HA, Garvey MB, Baker MA. Acute leukemia during pregnancy: the Toronto Leukemia Study Group experience with long-term follow-up of children exposed *in utero* to chemotherapeutic agents. *J Clin Oncol* 1987; 5:1098.
92. Lilleyman JS, Hill AS, Anderton KJ. Consequences of acute myelogenous leukemia in early pregnancy. *Cancer* 1977;40:1300.
93. Burrows RF, Kelton JG. Incidentally detected thrombocytopenia in healthy mothers and their infants. *N Engl J Med* 1988;319:142.
94. Heys RF. Childbearing and idiopathic thrombocytopenic purpura. *J Obstet Gynaecol Br Commonwlth* 1966;73:205.
95. Zlatnick FJ. The puerperium: normal and abnormal. In: Scott JR, DiSaia PJ, Hammond CB, Spellacy WN, eds. *Danforth's Obstetrics and Gynecology*, 6th ed. Philadelphia: JB Lippincott Co, 1990:189.
96. Kagan R, Laros RK. Immune thrombocytopenia. *Clin Obstet Gynecol* 1983;26:537–546.
97. Cines DB, Dusak B, Tomaski A, Mennuti M, Schreiber AD. Immune thrombocytopenic purpura and pregnancy. *N Engl J Med* 1982;306:826.
98. Juarez S, Cuadrado Pastor JM, Feliu J, Gonzalez Baron M, Ordonez A, Montero JM. Association of leukemia and pregnancy: clinical and obstetric aspects. *Am J Clin Oncol* 1988;11:159.
99. Bassan R. The management of infections in patients with leukemia. In: Henderson ES, Lister TA, Greaves MF, eds. *Leukemia*, 6th ed. Philadelphia: WB Saunders, 1996:257.
100. Honore LH, Brown LB. Intervillous placental metastasis with maternal myeloid leukemia. *Arch Pathol Lab Med* 1990;114:450.
101. Osada S, Horibe K, Oiwa K, et al. A case of infantile acute monocytic leukemia caused by vertical transmission of the mother's leukemic cells. *Cancer* 1190;65: 1146.
102. Wang T, Hamann W, Hartage R. Structural aspects of a placenta from a case of maternal acute lymphocytic leukemia. *Placenta* 1983;4:185.
103. Aviles A, Niz J. Long-term follow-up of children born to mothers with acute leukemia during pregnancy. *Med Pediatr Oncol* 1988;16:3.
104. Aviles A, Diaz-Maqueo JC, Talavera A, Guzman R, Garcia EL. Growth and development of children of mothers treated with chemotherapy during pregnancy: current status of 43 children. *Am J Hematol* 1991;36: 243.
105. Garber JE. Long-term follow-up of children exposed *in utero* to antineoplastic agents. *Semin Oncol* 1989; 16:437.
106. Murray CL, Reichert JA, Anderson J, Twiggs LB. Multimodal cancer therapy for breast cancer in the first trimester of pregnancy: a case report. *JAMA* 1984;252: 2607.
107. Azuno Y, Kaku K, Fujita N, Kaneko T, Matsumoto N. Mitoxantrone and etoposide in breast milk. *Am J Hematol* 1995;48:131.
108. Kawamura S, Suzuki Y, Tamai Y, et al. Pregnancy outcome among long-term survivors with acute leukemia. *Int J Hematol* 1995;62:157.
109. Li FP, Fine W, Jaffe N, Holmes GE, Holmes FF. Offspring of patients treated for cancer in childhood. *J Natl Cancer Inst* 1979;62:1193.
110. Green DM, Hall B, Zevon MA. Pregnancy outcome after treatment for acute lymphoblastic leukemia during childhood or adolescence. *Cancer* 1989;64:2335.
111. Rigby PG, Pratt PT, Rosenlof RC, Lemon HM. Genetic relationships in familial leukemia and lymphoma. *Arch Intern Med* 1968;121:67.
112. Gunz FW, Gunz JP, Veale AMO, et al. Familial leukemia: a study of 909 families. *Scand J Haematol* 1975;15:117.
113. Green DM. Childhood cancer in siblings. *Pediatr Hematol Oncol* 1986;3:229.
114. Eriksson M, Bergstrom I. Familial malignant blood disease in the country of Jamtland, Sweden. *Eur J Haematol* 1987;38:241.
115. Patel M, Dukes IAF, Hull JC. Use of hydroxyurea in

chronic myeloid leukemia during pregnancy: a case report. *Am J Obstet Gynecol* 1991;165:565.
116. Jackson N, Shukri A, Ali K. Hydroxyurea treatment for chronic myeloid leukaemia during pregnancy. *Br J Haematol* 1993;85:203.
117. Terian G, Tchernia G, Papiernik E, Elefant E. Hydroxyurea and pregnancy [Letter]. *Am J Obstet Gynecol* 1992;166:1868.
118. Fitzgerald JM, McCann SR. The combination of hydroxyurea and leucapheresis in the treatment of chronic myeloid leukaemia in pregnancy. *Clin Lab Haematol* 1993;15:63.
119. Delmer A, Rio B, Bauduer F, Ajchenbaum F, Marie JP, Zittoun R. Pregnancy during myelosuppressive treatment for chronic myelogenous leukemia. *Br J Haematol* 1992;82:783.

10

Lymphoma in Pregnancy

Brad Pohlman, *Janice A. Lyons, and *Roger M. Macklis

*Department of Hematology and Medical Oncology; *Department of Radiation Oncology, Cleveland Clinic Foundation, Cleveland, Ohio 44195*

No situation in the practice of medicine is as potentially difficult or emotional as that of a pregnant woman with cancer. Although diagnostic and therapeutic interventions are potentially deleterious to both the fetus and mother, one would ideally like to maintain the pregnancy and deliver a healthy infant and yet still administer standard treatment to the mother to optimize her chance for cure. Management of these patients must include consideration of the disease presentation, the impact of pregnancy on lymphoma and lymphoma on pregnancy, the outcome of both pregnancy and lymphoma, and the effects of diagnostic procedures and treatment on the fetus and its future children, as well as the gynecologic health of the mother and her future children.

INCIDENCE OF LYMPHOMA AND PREGNANCY

Lymphoma, including both Hodgkin's disease (HD) and non-Hodgkin's lymphoma (NHL), is the fourth most frequent cancer diagnosis among pregnant women behind cancers of the breast, cervix, and ovary (1). Exact figures on the coincidence of HD and pregnancy are not available. Prior estimates have ranged from 1 in 1000 to 1 in 6000 deliveries (1–3). According to the American Cancer Society (ACS), approximately 3400 women in the United States will be diagnosed with HD, and approximately 700 will die from it in 1998 (4). The median age of HD at diagnosis is 33 years, and approximately 65% of newly diagnosed women are of childbearing age (5). In the United States, the incidence of HD in women aged 15 to 44 years is 2 to 6 in 100,000 (5). According to the latest data from the U.S. Census Bureau, approximately 4000 to 11,000 births occur per 100,000 women per year (depending on maternal age) (6). Together, these figures predict that HD may be associated with as many as 1 of every 1000 to 3000 births. Since most of these women will be cured of their disease, will remain fertile, and will potentially become pregnant again, the number of women with persistent or relapsed HD or simply a history of HD in association with pregnancy may be higher.

Estimates of the incidence of NHL in association with pregnancy are not available, although the number is certainly less than in HD. The ACS estimates that approximately 24,300 women in the United States will be diagnosed with NHL, and 11,900 women will die from it in 1998 (4). However, the median age of patients with newly diagnosed NHL is 65 years, and less than 20% of women are of childbearing age (5). Nevertheless, NHL is the fifth leading cause of cancer death in the United States among women aged 15 to 34 (5). The incidence of NHL among women age 15 to 45 increases from approximately 1 to 8 per 100,000 (5). In conjunction with the United States census data, a diagnosis of

NHL may be expected to occur in up to 1 in 5000 deliveries.

The incidence of HD in the United States has remained relatively stable during the past two decades; however, the incidence of NHL has increased more than 50% during this period (5). Since the 1970s, the annual age-adjusted incidence of NHL in women has increased by 3% per year. During this same period, the incidence of human immunodeficiency virus (HIV) infection among women has also increased. HIV infection, however, is responsible for only a small percentage of the increased incidence of NHL. Regardless of the reason for the increase, the coincident occurrence of both NHL (with or without HIV infection) and pregnancy will undoubtedly continue to increase.

IMPACT OF PREGNANCY ON LYMPHOMA AND LYMPHOMA ON PREGNANCY

Hodgkin's Disease

The presentation of HD in pregnant women does not differ significantly from that in nonpregnant women (7–9). One study noted a slightly higher proportion of advanced stage among pregnant compared to nonpregnant women (7). These authors speculated that this difference might be due to masking of early signs by the pregnancy. In a large population-based study from Sweden, investigators reported a lower than expected incidence of HD during pregnancy and a greater than expected incidence of HD during the first 6 months postpartum (9). They speculated that the diagnosis of HD might be delayed until the postpartum period.

Fetal and placental involvement by HD is rare. Only one case of placental involvement with HD and delivery of a normal fetus, and one case of probable transmission of HD from the mother to fetus have been reported (10).

Several older studies, which predate modern treatment modalities, suggested that HD has no biologic effect on pregnancy and similarly that pregnancy has no biologic effect on the course of HD (11,12). In a series of 84 pregnant women with HD, pregnancy had no influence on the lymphoma outcome; specifically, response rate and median duration of survival seemed identical to that of nonpregnant patients with the same lymphoma (11). Both studies also demonstrated no difference in survival among women who had a therapeutic abortion compared to women who did not have one. These patients also did not have an increased risk of spontaneous abortion (12). More recent studies have come to the same conclusion (7,10,13,14).

In a large recent study, investigators at the Hospital for Sick Children and Princess Margaret Hospital in Toronto reviewed their records from 1958 to 1984 and identified 48 women with 50 pregnancies and HD (8). For each pregnant woman, they identified three nonpregnant controls of similar age, stage, and year of diagnosis. Twelve women were diagnosed with HD before conception, 10 during pregnancy, and 27 after delivery or pregnancy termination. Of the 22 women diagnosed before or during the pregnancy, 16 received radiation while pregnant, one received chemotherapy during the first trimester, and five received combination chemotherapy and radiotherapy while pregnant. No statistically significant difference in stage at diagnosis, maternal outcome, or pregnancy outcome was identified between any of these subgroups and the similar control group.

Ebert et al. (15) identified 24 cases in the literature between 1983 and 1995, in which women with HD received chemotherapy while pregnant. Two women who received chemotherapy (mechlorethamine, vincristine [Oncovin], procarbazine, and prednisone [MOPP] and MOPP without mechlorethamine) and one who received cyclophosphamide plus radiation therapy during the first trimester had therapeutic abortions; all three fetuses had multiple anomalies. One woman had a therapeutic abortion 15 hours after receiving the first dose of doxorubicin hydrochloride (Adriamycin), bleomycin, vinblastine, and dacarbazine (ABVD) at gestational week 15. Two women had spontaneous abortions after receiving chemotherapy—one received MOPP and the other received vinblastine, and procarbazine—beginning in the first trimester; one fetus had multiple anomalies. One woman received MOPP during the first trimester; the infant died 4 hours after birth with hydrocephalus. One mother received single-agent cyclophosphamide beginning in the first trimester; the infant was born with multiple anomalies. Another woman received vinblastine, vincristine, and procarbazine beginning in gestational week 25; the infant was born with an atrial septum defect and died 2 days after delivery. In contrast, 15 other women received cyclophosphamide, vincristine (Oncovin), procarbazine, and prednisone (COPP) (n=1), MOPP (n=4), ABVD (n=7), or MOPP/ABVD (n=3) beginning in the first (n=5), second (n=8), and third (n=2) trimesters. All 15 infants were normal and remain healthy a median of 9 (range, 0 to 17) years after delivery.

In another recent report, investigators from Stanford University described the outcome of 17 pregnancies associated with HD between 1987 and 1993 (16). The diagnosis was made 2 to 10 weeks after the onset of signs and/or symptoms at a median of 24 (range, 4 to 30) weeks' gestation. Only three patients were diagnosed during the first trimester. Three women had therapeutic abortions at 4, 8, and 17 weeks' gestation, and one woman had a spontaneous abortion at 8 weeks (all prior to initiation of therapy). At least three other women delivered prior to initiation of therapy. Patients received radiation therapy (n=6), chemotherapy (n=4), or combined-modality therapy (n=5), although the timing was not stated, except for the seven who specifically received chemotherapy after abortion or delivery. Excluding spontaneous or therapeutic abortions, no congenital anomalies were noted at delivery, and all children were reported to be healthy at the time of last follow-up, although three infants had longer hospital stays due to premature delivery. One mother who received MOPP chemotherapy after delivery died of HD, and one mother who had a therapeutic abortion at 8 weeks' gestation is alive with the disease. With a median follow-up of 35 (range, 6 to 79) months, 15 of the 17 mothers remain in complete remission.

Finally, Sutcliffe (17) recently reported on three women, ages 23 to 27 years, who were diagnosed with stage II nodular sclerosis HD at 21 to 23 weeks' gestation. All three received ABVD chemotherapy during the second and third trimesters of pregnancy. In addition, two received mantle-field radiation therapy following delivery. All three delivered healthy infants between 32 and 35 weeks' gestation. Chromosome analysis of all three children was normal. The three children and their mothers remain healthy 1+, 5+, and 7+ years later.

Non-Hodgkin's Lymphoma

NHL associated with pregnancy is most commonly of an aggressive histology and advanced stage (18–19). In a recent review, diffuse large cell, Burkitt's, and lymphoblastic lymphomas accounted for 60%, 27%, and 8% of cases, respectively; no women had low-grade or indolent lymphoma (19). Furthermore, 67% of patients had stage IV, 12% had stage III, 5% had stage II, and 16% had stage I disease. The aggressive histology and advanced stage in these patients may simply reflect the histology and stage that generally affects young women of childbearing age. Alternatively, advanced-stage disease may be due to delayed diagnosis.

In fact, patients with NHL during pregnancy often have unusual manifestations, and their diagnosis is frequently delayed. One review of the literature, which included 37 cases of NHL during pregnancy, noted that patients often presented with unusual symptoms and organ involvement (20) (Table 1). Twenty-eight of 37 patients presented with extranodal involvement other than bone marrow. The initial diagnosis was correct in only 16 of 37 cases. The correct diagnosis was made a median of 17 (range, 1 to 365) days after presentation and was delayed more than 3 weeks in 40% and more than 3 months in 20% of patients.

An unexpectedly high incidence of breast, uterine, cervical, and ovarian involvement has been noted in pregnant women (19,30,33,38,

TABLE 1. *Abnormal presentations of non-Hodgkin's lymphoma (NHL) in pregnancy*

Case	Year (ref)	Symptoms	Organ system	Days to Dx	Initial Dx
1	1985 (21)	35 yo, 32 wk; tumorous enlargement of rt tonsil	Tonsil	1	NHL
2	1985 (21)	35 yo, 37 wk; rt axillary node enlarged	Lymphatics	1	NHL
3	1976 (22)	18 yo, 26 wk; c/o sternal swelling	Breast, mediastinum	1	NHL
4	1988 (23)	23 yo, 30 wk; c/o increased abd girth; ascites; dyspnea; adnexal mass	Ovary	1	NHL
5	1990 (24)	33 yo, 34 wk; c/o claudication and pain in rt lower limb; muscular weakness; mass in rt hip; splenomegaly via ultrasonogram; BM bx = lymphoma	Bony pelvis	1	NHL
6	1981 (25)	41 yo, 12 wk; vaginal bleeding × 30 d, lg mass in rt iliac fossa	Uterus, cervix	1	NHL
7	1989 (26)	28 yo, 14 wk; tonsillar enlargement and pouch of Douglas and contiguous w/ cervix	Tonsils	1	NHL
8	1983 (27)	30 yo, 28 wk; present w/ lt abducens palsy, diplopia and rt abd pain, fever, sweats, and nausea	CNS, eye, bone marrow	1	NHL
9	1980 (28)	34 yo, 24 wk; lt axillary node enlarged; endoscopy revealed infiltration to stomach	Lymphatics, stomach	1	NHL
10	1967 (29)	36 yo, pp breast swelling and nodularity; bx performed	Breast	1	NHL
11	1976 (30)	18 yo, 10 wk; amenorrhea and abdominal swelling; dehydrated with profuse sweating; afebrile and mental confusion	Ovary, stomach	2	Malaria, dehydration
12	1980 (31)	26 yo, 21.5 wk; severe respiratory distress; superior vena cava syndrome (neck swelling) = mediastinal mass	Trachea, major vessels, thyroid	2	NHL
13	1963 (32)	19 yo, 21.5 wk; c/o a painless marble-sized nodule in episiotomy scar with gradual increase in size, w/ later breast involvement	Perineum, breast	6	Inclusion cyst
14	1974 (33)	24 yo, 20 wk; c/o n/v and diarrhea; 5-cm nontender firm mass on chest wall above rt breast	Mediastinum, chest wall	7	Pregnancy, gastroenteritis
15	1985 (21)	26 yo, 27 wk; signs of obstructive jaundice	Stomach, duodenum, hepatic portal system	14	Obstructive jaundice
16	1985 (34)	22 yo, 18 wk; c/o dyspnea, acute onset substernal chest pain	Mediastinum	14	NHL
17	1966 (35)	26 yo, 24 wk; dyspnea on exertion, cough, SOB, treated for URI × 2 wk w/o improvement, CXR = mediastinal mass	Mediastinum	14	URI
18	1991 (36)	34 yo, 20.5 wk; tachypnea, dyspnea on exertion, nonproductive cough, and mediastinal mass	Mediastinum	14	NHL
19	1966 (37)	36 yo, 32 wk; c/o breast tumors; died 9 d pp (pp Dx)	Breast, CNS, uterus	17	Lactation
20	1985 (21)	29 yo, 38 wk; GI bleeding; endoscopy 3 d pp = ulcerative tumor of stomach	Stomach, pancreas, omentum, mediastinum	17	Upper GI bleeding
21	1967 (29)	15 yo, 28 wk; c/o painless breast enlargement, increased dental looseness w/ maxillary osteolytic tumors, abdominal mass and axillary node enlargement	Breast, bone, lymphatics	21	Abnormal lactation

22	1980 (38)	17 yo, 15 wk; c/o bluish discoloration and bilateral enlargement of breasts; later had gingival and rectal bleeding; wt loss, good appetite	Breast, abd mass	21	Mastitis, pregnancy
23	1977 (39)	33 yo, 16 wk; c/o groin and axillary node enlargement; respiratory distress	Lymphatics	23	NHL
24	1963 (32)	21 yo, 32 wk; c/o pain in rt inguinal region; disturbed rt leg function; palpable pubic ramus mass	Bony pelvis	24	Pregnancy
25	1989 (26)	30 yo, 37 wk; rt cervical node enlargement (neck node)	Lymphatics, mediastinum	28	Generalized lymphadenopathy
26	1980 (40)	24 yo, 24 wk; dry cough and dyspnea at rest; 4 wk prior to admission treated for URI; acute arrest	Mediastinum, bone marrow	28	URI
27	1972 (41)	32 yo, 28 wk; eye irritation, swelling, and pain in rt orbit; proptosis × 1 mo	Eye	30	NHL
28	1977 (42)	42 yo, 13 wk; c/o bilateral breast nodules and marked tenderness	Breast	30	Mastitis
29	1967 (29)	35 yo, 24 wk; c/o breast nodularity × 4 wk; fatigue, jaundice of sclerae, and axillary node enlargement	Breast, lymphatics, liver	42	Lactation and NHL
30	1991 (36)	19 yo, 38 wk; fever, tachypnea, syncopal episodes, mental confusions, and slurred speech; acute onset of a follicular rash	CNS, skin	42	Anxiety, pregnancy
31	1985 (21)	19 yo, 3 mo pp; history of night sweats, fever, wt loss started prior to delivery	Abd mass, bone marrow	97	Abdominal mass
32	1985 (21)	31 yo, 7 wk pp; c/o syncope and fever; suffered from persistent fever and night sweats last 6 wk of pregnancy	Lungs, mediastinum, lymphatics	91	Pregnancy
33	1968 (43)	26 yo, 13 wk; c/o n/v, diarrhea; 27–29 wk epigastric pain, severe heartburn, diarrhea, and vomiting (severe pain different from labor)	Jejunum	112	Pregnancy
34	1967 (29)	20 yo, 4 mo pp; c/o painful breast swelling and nodularity; extremity weakness; incontinence of bowel since third trimester	Breast	114	Lactation
35	1967 (29)	20 yo, 36 wk; nonlactating, breast enlargement; cervical and axillary nodes enlarged	Breast	120	Abnormal breast response to hormones
36	1985 (34)	28 yo, 36 wk; history of neck swelling; stable × 4 mo, then increased	Mediastinum, lymphatics	210	Generalized lymphadenopathy
37	1979 (44)	22 yo; c/o palpable nodularity of lower uterus and cervix, referred for two evaluations (=fibroids); became pregnant, delivered, presented 1 mo pp w/ vaginal bleeding	Uterine cervix	365	Cervicovaginal tumor (fibroids)

abd, abdomen; BM bx, bone marrow biopsy; CNS, central nervous system; c/o, complaints of; CXR, chest x-ray; d, days; Dx, diagnosis; GI, gastrointestinal; lg, large; lt, left; n/v, nausea and vomiting; pp, postpartum; rt, right; SOB, shortness of breath; URI, upper respiratory infection; w/, with; wks, weeks; w/o, without; wt, weight; yo, years old.

Modified from ref. 20, with permission.

TABLE 2. *Stage, histologic subtype, treatment, and maternal and fetal outcome of 96 pregnant women with lymphoma*

					Maternal outcome		Fetal outcome	
Year (ref)	Trimester	Stage at diagnosis	Histologic subtype*	Treatment during pregnancy (1) and after delivery (2)	Status	Date (mo)	Status	Date (mo)
1960 (56)	1	I	—	2: RT	CR	30	Alive	—
1963 (32)	2	—	—	1: Surgery	Death	—	Death	—
1963 (29)	PP	IV	J	—	Death	<1	—	—
1965 (29)	2	IV	J	1: SA	Death	<1	Alive at delivery	—
1965 (29)	3	IV	J	2: SA	Death	9	Death	<1
1965 (29)	PP	IV	J	—	Death	<1	—	—
1964 (43)	2	IV	—	1: Surgery; 2: RT	Death	6	Death	<1
1966 (35)	PP	IV	J	—	Death	<1	—	—
1966 (35)	2	—	—	1: SA	Death	—	Alive	—
1966 (57)	PP	—	I	—	Death	—	—	—
1968 (34)	1	III	—	2: SA	Death	20	Therapeutic abortion	—
1969 (58)	3	IV	G	1: Surgery	Death	1	Alive	30
1970 (41)	3	I	J	1: RT + SA	Death	6	Alive	12
1971 (59)	2	IV	G	1: RT	Death	<1	Alive, premature	—
1972 (60)	3	I	—	1: RT	CR	2	Alive	—
1974 (33)	2	IV	J	2: RT + SA	Death	4	Therapeutic abortion	—
1974 (39)	2	IV	F	1: COP	CR	19	Alive	—
1974 (34)	2	III	I	1: RT; 2: COP	Death	35	Alive	36
1976 (61)	PP	—	J	—	Death	—	—	—
1976 (61)	PP	—	J	—	Death	—	—	—
1976 (30)	2	—	J	1: Surgery	Death	—	Therapeutic abortion	—
1977 (42)	2	IV	J	1: SA	Death	5	Therapeutic abortion	—
1977 (40)	2	IV	I	—	Death	<1	Spontaneous abortion	—
1977 (31)	2	IV	I	1: COP	CR	17	Alive	24
1978 (62)	3	—	G	1: Surgery	CR	—	Alive	—
1979 (61)	3	I	J	1: SA	Death	2	Alive	1
1979 (44)	1	I	—	2: RT + SA	CR	12	Alive, premature	—
1979 (38)	2	IV	J	—	Death	<1	Spontaneous abortion	—
1980 (28)	2	IV	J	2: SA	Death	3	Spontaneous abortion	—
1980 (63)	3	IV	H	2: CHOP	CR	6	Alive, premature	6
1980 (64)	1	IV	E	1: SA	Death	—	Alive, premature	—
1981 (65)	3	IV	—	1: CHOP	CR	40	Alive	26
1981 (34)	3	I	I	2: CHOP	Death	36	Alive	42
1982 (66)	2	IV	J	1: CHOP-like	Death	6	Alive	2
1982 (21)	3	I	I	2: CHOP-like	Death	12	Alive	—
1982 (21)	3	IV	I	2: RT + CHOP	CR	24	Alive	—
1983 (21)	3	IV	E	2: CHOP-like	CR	9	Alive	—
1983 (21)	3	IV	G	2: CHOP-like	Death	6	Alive	—
1983 (27)	3	—	J	2: COP	Death	—	Alive	—
1983 (67)	2	I	I	1: RT; 2: CHOP-like	CR	6	Development failure	72
1984 (67)	3	I	G	2: CHOP-like	CR	12	Alive	12
1984 (67)	2	IV	J	—	Death	<1	Death	<1
1985 (45)	3	IV	G	2: CHOP-like	CR	60	Alive	60
1987 (68)	2	III	G	1: CHOP	CR	36	Alive	—
1989 (26)	3	—	—	2: MR	Death	21	Alive	—
1989 (26)	2	—	—	1: SA	CR	—	Alive	—
1990 (69)	2	IV	G	1: CHOP-like	[a]	—	Alive	—
1990 (69)	1	II	J	1: CHOP-like	[a]	—	Alive	—
1990 (69)	2	IV	G	1: CHOP-like	[a]	—	Alive	—
1990 (69)	1	III	G	1: CHOP-like	[a]	—	Alive	—
1990 (69)	3	IV	H	1: CHOP-like	[a]	—	Alive	—
1990 (69)	1	IV	J	1: CHOP-like	[a]	—	Alive	—
1990 (69)	1	IV	I	1: CHOP-like	[a]	—	Alive	—
1990 (69)	3	III	I	1: CHOP	[a]	—	Alive	—
1990 (69)	1	IV	G	1: CHOP	[a]	—	Alive	—
1990 (69)	2	IV	F	1: CHOP-like	[a]	—	Alive	—
1990 (69)	1	III	G	1: CHOP-like	[a]	—	Alive	—
1990 (69)	2	IV	J	1: CHOP-like	[a]	—	Alive	—
1990 (69)	3	III	G	1: CHOP-like	[a]	—	Alive	—
1990 (69)	1	IV	G	1: CHOP-like	[a]	—	Alive	—
1990 (69)	3	II	F	1: CHOP	[a]	—	Alive	—
1990 (69)	1	IV	G	1: CHOP-like	[a]	—	Alive	—
1990 (52)	3	IV	H	2: CHOP-like	CR	—	Alive	—
1990 (70)	2	—	H	1: CHOP-like	CR	—	Alive, premature	—

TABLE 2. *Continued.*

Year (ref)	Trimester	Stage at diagnosis	Histologic subtype*	Treatment during pregnancy (1) and after delivery (2)	Maternal outcome Status	Maternal outcome Date (mo)	Fetal outcome Status	Fetal outcome Date (mo)
1990 (71)	2	IV	—	1: MR	—	—	Alive	—
1990 (72)	1	—	—	1: RT + SA	CR	—	Alive	5
1990 (24)	1	IV	F	1: No treatment; 2: CHOP-like	Death	—	Alive at delivery	—
1990 (73)	2	II	G	1: CHOP-like	CR	—	Alive	—
1991 (55)	2	—	—	1: CHOP	—	—	Alive	—
1991 (55)	1	—	—	1: COP	—	—	Therapeutic abortion	—
1991 (55)	1	—	—	1: SA	—	—	Alive	20
1991 (55)	1	—	—	1: COP	—	—	Spontaneous abortion	—
1991 (50)	3	IV	H	2: MR	CR	24	Alive	24
1991 (36)	2	II	H	1: MR; 2: RT	Death	6	Alive	11
1991 (74)	PP	IV	H	2: MR	CR	3	Alive	—
1992 (20)	3	IV	G	2: MR	CR	—	Death	<1
1993 (51)	2	IV	G	2: MR	Death	10	Death before term	<1
1993 (75)	—	—	—	No treatment	Death	<1	Death *in utero*	—
1994 (76)	1	IV	F	2: CHOP	Death	4	Therapeutic abortion	
1995 (77)	2	I	—	1: Prednisone + RT	PR	—	Alive at delivery	
1995 (78)	2	II	F	1: MR; 2: MR + RT	CR	48	Alive	48
1995 (79)	2	—	E	1: MR	CR	21	Alive	21
1996 (47)	3	IV	H	2: CHOP + RT	CR	28	Alive, premature	—
1996 (16)	3	IV	G	CT	Alive with disease	5	Alive, premature	—
1996 (16)	—	IV	J	CT	Death	15	Alive, premature	—
1996 (16)	2	III	D	2: CT + RT	CR	—	Therapeutic abortion	—
1996 (16)	—	III	G	2: CT	Death	18	Alive	—
1996 (16)	3	II	G	CT + RT	CR	—	Alive, premature	—
1996 (16)	—	—	G	—	Death	14	Alive	—
1996 (16)	2	I	G	CT	Alive with disease	26	Alive	—
1996 (16)	3	I	J	BMT	CR	—	Alive	—
1996 (16)	3	II	G	CT + RT	CR	—	Alive	—
1996 (16)	2	III	I	CT	CR	—	Alive	—
1996 (16)	3	IV	G	No treatment	Alive with disease	6	Alive	—
1996 (16)	2	IV	H	2: ABMT	Death	10	Alive, premature	—
1997 (49)	3	IV	H	2: CHOP-like	CR	132	Alive, premature	132

ABMT, autologous bone marrow transplantation; BMT,* bone marrow transplantation; CHOP, COP + doxorubicin; COP, cyclophosphamide, vincristine (Oncovin), prednisone; CR, complete remission; CT, chemotherapy; E, diffuse small cleaved; F, diffuse mixed; G, diffuse large cell; H, immunoblastic; I, lymphoblastic; J, small noncleaved cell; MR, multidrug regimen; PP, postpartum; PR, partial recovery; RT, radiation therapy; SA, single-agent chemotherapy.

[a]7 of 16 have expired, 8 of 16 remain in CR 4–9 yr after delivery, and one patient was lost to follow-up.

Adapted from ref. 19, with permission.

42,44,45). The predilection for these organs has been attributed to hormonal influences and/or to increased blood flow to these organs during pregnancy (19,34,38,42). Bilateral breast involvement has been described by many observers, especially in patients with Burkitt's lymphoma, although other histologies have been reported. The breasts may be the only site of involvement or one of many sites (33,38,42,45–47).

In addition to presentations during pregnancy, several observers have reported a characteristic presentation of Burkitt's lymphoma involving the breasts during lactation (22,48). Among 856 patients with Burkitt's lymphoma included in the Cancer Registry at Ibadan, Nigeria, between 1960 and 1975, 26 were Nigerian females older than 15 years. Among these 26 women, five presented with bilateral breast involvement, as well as involvement at other sites. All five women were lactating at the time of presentation (22).

Placental involvement with NHL has been infrequently reported. Only four well documented cases of placental involvement with maternal NHL have been reported: one case of anaplastic large cell lymphoma (49), one case of T-cell immunoblastic lymphoma (50), and two cases of diffuse, large B-cell lymphoma (51,52). In none of these reports was lymphoma ever documented in the infants. In one case, a 33-year-old apparently healthy primigravida delivered a healthy-appearing infant at 41.5 weeks' gestation (52). Examination of the placenta unexpectedly revealed lymphoma. The mother refused further evaluation. Seven months later, the infant was diagnosed with *Pneumocystis carinii* pneumonia. Both mother and infant were then diagnosed with HIV infection. The mother ultimately was diagnosed with high-grade diffuse immunoblastic lymphoma (identical to the histology of the placenta) 9 months after delivery. The child remains free of lymphoma. Dissemination of maternal NHL to the fetus has been reported in only one case (53).

Compared to HD, the effects of NHL on pregnancy and vice versa are less clear, primarily due to a lack of available data. In fact, the first successful pregnancy associated with advanced-stage NHL was not reported until 1977 (39). Some authors have noted relatively stable disease during pregnancy followed by rapid progression after delivery, and suggested that hormonal and immunologic changes occurring during pregnancy may stabilize lymphoma cell proliferation until delivery (18,19,21,34,54). However, other investigators have suggested that pregnancy has no influence on the course of NHL and that response-to-treatment, failure, and progression rates are similar to those in nonpregnant patients (19). Similarly, NHL has been reported by some authors to have an adverse effect on pregnancy due primarily to the mother's death (18). But others have concluded that the incidences of spontaneous abortion, prematurity, and malformations are not influenced by the lymphoma (19,55).

More than 100 cases of NHL associated with pregnancy have been reported. Table 2 details 96 patients in whom sufficient information is available, including trimester at diagnosis, stage at diagnosis, histologic subtype, treatment received during pregnancy and after delivery, and outcome for mother and fetus. Among these 96 women, 23% had small noncleaved-cell lymphoma, 11% had lymphoblastic lymphoma, 36% had diffuse, large-cell or immunoblastic lymphoma, 10% had diffuse small cleaved or diffuse mixed lymphoma, and in 20% the histologic subtype was not available. The majority of patients had advanced-stage disease at diagnosis (stage I, 13%; stage II, 7%; stage III, 10%; stage IV, 50%; and unknown, 20%). Because the ability to adequately stage these pregnant women is limited, the number of patients with advanced-stage disease may actually be underestimated.

Seventy-one of 96 babies are alive, although the follow-up period for the majority was short (less than 1 month) or unknown. Seven percent of pregnancies ended in therapeutic abortion, and 4% ended in spontaneous abortion. Eleven percent of infants were born prematurely and 7% died. Only 31 mothers are known to have achieved a complete remission. Among these 31, one mother had a therapeutic abortion, one infant died less than 1 month after delivery, and 29 infants were alive at last follow-up.

Among the 90 mothers for whom the outcome is known, only 39 are alive and disease-free a median of 21 (range, 2 to 132) months after delivery, four are alive with disease, and 47 died a median of 6 (range, less than 1 to 36) months after delivery (Table 3). Women diagnosed during the third trimester of pregnancy appeared to have a better outcome than those diagnosed in the first or second trimesters. Women with early-stage disease tended to have a better outcome than those with advanced-stage disease. Only 1 of 19 mothers with Burkitt's lymphoma (for whom the outcome is known) is alive and disease-free. She was diagnosed in the third trimester with stage I disease and underwent bone marrow transplantation. Women in whom treatment was initiated during pregnancy did not seem to fare any better than women in whom treatment was delayed until after delivery. Among six women who had therapeutic abortions at the time of diagnosis (two during the first trimester and four during the second trimester), only one is alive. Among the 10

TABLE 3. *Disease outcome in women with non-Hodgkin's lymphoma*

	n	No. (%) alive and disease-free
Gestational period at diagnosis		
First trimester	7	3 (43)
Second trimester	29	11 (38)
Third trimester	27	16 (59)
Stage at diagnosis		
I	12	6 (50)
II	5	4 (80)
III	6	3 (50)
IV	37	13 (35)
Histologic subtype at diagnosis		
Diffuse large cell/immunoblastic	26	15 (58)
Lymphoblastic	9	5 (56)
Small noncleaved cell	19	1 (5)
Any treatment during pregnancy		
Yes	28	13 (46)
No	28	14 (50)
Combination chemotherapy during pregnancy		
Yes	8	6 (75)
No	20	12 (60)

mothers who had spontaneous abortions or whose infants died, only one mother remains alive. All of these observations are retrospective and potentially biased.

In a large review, 13 mothers with NHL received chemotherapy or radiation therapy during the first trimester of pregnancy (19). One patient had a therapeutic abortion, and another had a spontaneous abortion; in 11 of 13 cases, the infants were delivered alive. One infant was premature, but none showed apparent malformations, although cyclophosphamide was administered in 10 cases and methotrexate in two cases. Among the 33 women treated with a multidrug regimen or with radiation therapy during the second or third trimesters, four gave birth to premature infants and 20 to normal infants. One premature infant died, but all the others were alive and in good health.

The outcome for both mother and fetus may have improved in more recent years. Aviles et al. (69) reported on 19 pregnancies in women with NHL between 1975 and 1986. All received doxorubicin-based combination chemotherapy, including eight who received chemotherapy during the first trimester. Three mothers and their fetuses died during induction. The 16 remaining women delivered healthy infants spontaneously (n=12) or by cesarean section (n=4) between 35 and 39 weeks' gestation. Six mothers received their last chemotherapy 1 to 2 weeks prior to delivery; no delivery was complicated by infection or bleeding. Six babies had a subnormal birthweight but no apparent congenital abnormalities. Fifteen children remain alive and well 3 to 11 years after delivery; one died in an automobile accident at age 5 years. Twelve mothers were in complete remission at the time of delivery. Eight remain in complete remission 4 to 9 years after delivery. Seven mothers died from lymphoma, and one was lost to follow-up.

DIAGNOSTIC RADIOLOGY

For nonpregnant patients with lymphoma, the pretreatment radiologic evaluation generally includes chest radiography, computed tomography (CT) of the chest, abdomen, and pelvis, and a gallium scan (in HD). Selected patients may also benefit from specialized tests, such as lymphangiography, bone scan (for patients with suspected bone involvement), and nuclear cardiology (MUGA) studies to establish baseline cardiac function prior to the use of cardiotoxic chemotherapy. The decision to proceed with these studies in a pregnant patient must be individualized, based on the risks and the likelihood that a particular test will affect treatment decisions. Unlike chemotherapy, radiotherapy requires exact anatomic information on target sites to contribute effectively to the care of lymphoma patients (80).

The elective use of ionizing radiation directed at the abdomen and pelvis is almost always contraindicated in pregnant patients during the first 9 to 12 weeks of pregnancy (81). Patients diagnosed with lymphoma during this period should be counseled on the risks that a conventional staging evaluation might pose for the pregnancy and the fetus (82). The diagnostic workup should generally be modified to reflect the known fetal risks observed after even small doses of radiation during this sensitive, early period (83). Table 4 indicates the approximate radiation exposure that one might expect from the studies mentioned above.

According to the National Council on Radiation Protection and Measurements, the maximal permissible elective dose to the embryo and fetus from environmental workplace exposures during the entire gestation period should be 500 mrem (84). This limit is meant as a general environmental guideline and does not directly apply to medically necessary radiation exposure. Nevertheless, it may serve as a rational benchmark for designing a safe and appropriate diagnostic workup for pregnant patients. For most patients, a chest x-ray is safe and appropriate. During the first trimester, an ultrasound evaluation of the abdomen and pelvis (though not nearly as sensitive as CT) may provide an estimate of the extent of gross disease. No data suggest that short-term exposure to magnetic resonance (MR) imaging and electromagnetic fields is harmful to the developing fetus (85,86). The safety of MR imaging contrast material (e.g., gadopentate dimeglumine) has not been fully established, and many radiologists prefer not to perform elective contrast-enhanced MR imaging in pregnant patients in the first trimester (87). Because of the potential and unknown effects of MR imaging, the duration of exposure should be limited and only performed on pregnant women in whom the diagnostic benefit outweighs the theoretic risks. Because of radiation hazard to the fetus, lymphangiography, CT, and isotopic scans should be avoided. Thomas and Peckham (88) indicated that the fetal dose from a single 24-hour abdominal film as part of a lymphangiogram is less than 1 rad (1 cGy) (14). If the results will directly affect management, this test may be performed after the first trimester. However, the usual practice of checking the amount of dye with several films or fluoroscopy makes a complete study hazardous, and a shortened study may be nondiagnostic (10). Certainly, any discretionary radiologic

TABLE 4. *Estimated radiation dose absorbed by the embryo after maternal exposure to selected diagnostic radiology procedures*

Study	Approximate embryo absorbed dose (mrem[a])
Chest x-ray (AP, LAT)	5
Abdomen flat plate (for lymphangiogram)	150–250 per exposure
Lumbosacral spine/pelvis film	400–600
CT abdomen	1000
CT chest	500
CT pelvis	1000
Gallium scan (10 mCi Ga-67)	2500
Bone scan (20 mCi Tc-99m)	300

AP, anteroposterior; CT, computed tomography; Ga-67, gallium Ga 67 citrate; LAT, lateral; Tc-99m, technetium Tc 99m.

[a]Radiation absorbed dose is typically expressed in "rad" (old terminology) or "cGy" (new terminology; 1 cGy = 1 rad). To adjust for the differential biologic effects of some kinds of unusual radiation beams (e.g., neutrons), the unit "rem" is used. For virtually all standard types of medical radiation, including x-rays, gamma rays and electrons, 1 cGy $\cong$ 1 rem.

procedures should be delayed until after week 20 of the pregnancy, if possible, and appropriate shielding (lead apron and so on) should be utilized during all imaging procedures involving ionizing radiation (89).

SURGERY

Although HD and NHL are generally not treated surgically, surgical intervention is occasionally necessary either in the management of the lymphoma (e.g., excisional biopsy for diagnosis) or in cesarean delivery of the infant. Anesthesia during pregnancy is associated with a number of potential risks (e.g., difficult airway and aspiration). The situation may be compounded by the presence of an anterior mediastinal mass, which can obstruct the lower airway or compress the pulmonary artery or right ventricle and alter pulmonary blood flow. Either condition may lead to hypoxia, especially in the supine position. Importantly, the fetus and uteroplacental circulation are exquisitely sensitive to hypoxemia or hypotension. For these and other reasons, anesthesia and airway management in pregnant patients, especially with an anterior mediastinal mass, may be particularly complex, and a discussion is beyond the scope of this text (90–93).

CHEMOTHERAPY

Adverse Chemotherapeutic Effects

The adverse effects of antineoplastic agents on the fetus and neonate can be either immediate or delayed (94). Immediate adverse effects include spontaneous abortion, teratogenesis, organ toxicity, premature birth, and low birthweight. Delayed or long-term complications include carcinogenesis, sterility, retarded physical and/or mental growth and development, mutation, and teratogenesis in the second generation.

Animal studies suggest that almost all chemotherapeutic agents are teratogenic and that the timing of chemotherapy administration is critical (95). Drugs administered during the first 2 weeks of pregnancy probably produce an all-or-nothing phenomenon: either a spontaneous abortion or a normal fetus (94). Weeks 3 to 8 of development are the period of major organogenesis, and chemotherapeutic agents have their greatest teratogenic potential during this time. With the exception of the brain and gonadal tissue, organogenesis is complete by 13 weeks' gestation. Chemotherapy administered during the second and third trimesters (after organogenesis is complete) does not generally result in fetal malformation but is more likely to result in intrauterine growth restriction, impaired functional development, mental retardation, and impaired learning behavior (94–96).

In addition to the gestational time of exposure, adverse chemotherapeutic effects may also be influenced by maternal physiologic changes that may alter pharmacokinetics (94–96). Despite these physiologic changes and their potential effects, standard chemotherapy doses are generally administered during pregnancy. The extent to which individual agents cross the placenta to either enter or exit the fetus, the ability of the fetus to metabolize those drugs, and the concentration obtained within the fetus are variable and poorly understood (94,95). The ability of neonates at birth to metabolize and excrete many drugs is underdeveloped. Consequently, chemotherapy administered shortly before birth may be particularly hazardous to the newborn when placental excretion can no longer occur (94).

Healthy women have a 3% to 5% risk of giving birth to an infant with a serious congenital anomaly (i.e., malformation, mental retardation, or other functional deficits) (91,97,98). The incidence of less serious malformations in the general population may be as high as 9% (94). Approximately 10% to 20% of infants exposed to cytotoxic agents during the first trimester may have major malformations (95). Combination chemotherapy regimens are associated with a higher risk than single agents (94). In one review, Doll et al. (94) identified 7 (16%) of 45 infants with fetal malformations after combination chemotherapy compared to 24 (17%) of 139 infants after single-agent chemotherapy. However, when folate antagonists and concomitant use of radiation were excluded, the incidence associated with single agents was only 6%. Low birthweight has been reported in up to 40% of neonates exposed to chemotherapy during pregnancy (99). Unfortunately, the potential risks associated with individual chemotherapeutic agents or commonly used regimens are difficult to assess because of relatively small numbers of reports and the variation in drug combinations, dosages, routes, and gestational times of administration. Although fetal exposure to chemotherapy in all trimesters of pregnancy has been reported not to induce abnormalities, there is no assurance that deleterious fetal defects will not occur. A Registry of Pregnancies Exposed to Chemotherapeutic Agents has been established at the University of Pittsburgh. Physicians who care for women receiving cancer chemotherapy during pregnancy should contact Dr. John Mulvihill at the University of Pittsburgh for details of the registry or a patient abstract form (phone: 412-624-9951; fax: 412-624-3020; e-mail: jjm@helix.hgen.pitt.edu).

Chemotherapy-induced myelosuppression either in the mother or fetus may pose additional concerns at the time of delivery or cesarean section (95). Nordlund et al. (100) described a patient with HD treated with vinblastine who delivered a normal infant 7 days after receiving the drug. At the time of delivery, the mother's white blood cell count (WBC) was 700/mm^3, but the infant's WBC, absolute neutrophil count, and platelet count were 11,000/mm^3, 5110/mm^3, and 315,000/mm^3, respectively. Neutropenia may increase the risk of maternal infection and require special precautions and treatment. Thrombocytopenia may increase the risk of hemorrhage and require platelet transfusions. As in the mother, chemotherapy may cause transient myelosuppression in the fetus and/or newborn infant (94,101). Some authors have recommended examination of fetal scalp blood and cesarean section if neonatal thrombocytopenia or neutropenia is present, in an attempt to minimize the risk of hemorrhage and/or infection associated with vaginal delivery (102).

Chemotherapeutic Agents

Antineoplastic drugs commonly used in the treatment of HD and NHL include alkylating agents, topoisomerase interactive agents, antimicrotubule agents, antimetabolites, and other miscellaneous agents. The known teratogenic risks of individual agents are described below.

Alkylating Agents

The alkylating agents—for example, chlorambucil (Leukeran), cyclophosphamide, dacarbazine (DTIC-Dome), ifosfamide (IFEX), mechlorethamine hydrochloride (nitrogen mustard) (Mustargen), and procarbazine hydrochloride (Matulane)—are associated with an increased incidence of congenital anomalies if administered during the first trimester. The rate of fetal malformations has been reported to be 14% when these agents are administered during the first trimester but only 4% when administered later in pregnancy (95,103). Women who received cyclophosphamide during pregnancy delivered both normal and malformed infants. Many cases of primarily skeletal and central nervous system (CNS) malformations have been reported. The risk is especially high with exposure during the first trimester and much lower during the second or third trimesters (96,104). Similarly, women who received chlorambucil during pregnancy delivered both normal and deformed infants (96,104). Mechlorethamine has been administered throughout pregnancy. Most reports have not shown an adverse effect, even when it is given during the first trimester (104). Nevertheless, mechlorethamine in combination with procarbazine and vinblastine sulfate (Velban) (i.e., MOPP) has resulted in anomalous infants and spontaneous abortions (96). Anomalies observed have included oligodactyly, cerebral hemorrhage, and malformed kidneys. Administration of procarbazine in combination with other antineoplastic agents has been associated with malformations in infants born to mothers exposed during the first trimester (94,96,104). Abnormalities have included multiple hemangiomas, oligodactyly, malformed kidneys, atrial septal defect, and intrauterine growth restriction. Use of procarbazine as a single agent after the first trimester has not been reported to cause serious teratogenic effects in the fetus (96). Dacarbazine was administered alone or usually in combination with other antineoplastic agents to at least 11 pregnant women—three during the first trimester. No congenital anomalies were observed (17,105,106). No data on ifosfamide use during human pregnancy are available (96,104).

Topoisomerase Interactive Agents

Agents such as doxorubicin, mitoxantrone hydrochloride (Novantrone), and etoposide (VePesid)—topoisomerase interactive drugs—have not been reported to cause birth defects. However, a stillborn fetus with diffuse myocardial necrosis has been reported after *in utero* exposure to daunorubicin hydrochloride (Cerubidine) (94). Turchi and Villasis (107) identified 28 women who received doxorubicin (usually in combination with other drugs) during pregnancy. The pregnancies resulted in 24 normal infants (one set of twins), including four with reversible pathologic findings (marrow hypoplasia, pneumothorax, polycythemia, and neonatal sepsis), two maternal–fetal deaths, two spontaneous abortions, and one therapeutic abortion. Four of these pregnant women were treated with doxorubicin and other antineoplastic agents during the period of embryogenesis. Two infants were normal. One, which was incompletely examined, had a missing digit on one foot. In a series of 31 children born to women who had been treated with doxorubicin and other antineoplastic drugs, no congenital anomalies or developmental abnormalities were observed; 13 had been exposed during the first trimester (106). Mitoxantrone, in association with other chemotherapeutic agents, has been administered to at least two pregnant women. In one case, the pregnant woman received mitoxantrone and cytarabine (Cytosar-U). The fetus developed normally until 28 weeks, when chemotherapy was switched to idarubicin hydrochloride (Idamycin). The woman subsequently delivered a 2200-g stillborn infant with no apparent congenital malformations; however, an autopsy was refused (108). In the other case, a patient received mitoxantrone with a variety of chemotherapeutic agents and delivered a healthy 2960-g infant by cesarean section at 34 weeks (109). At least 13 infants whose mothers were treated with etoposide during gestation have been reported (96,104). None of these babies, including at least two born to mothers treated during the first trimester of pregnancy, had malformations. Transient pancytopenia at the time of delivery was noted in at least two infants.

Antimicrotubule Agents

Antimicrotubule agents, in particular, the vinca alkaloids such as vincristine and vinblastine, appear relatively safe during pregnancy and have only infrequently been associated with malformations in humans (94–96, 104). At least 26 cases of apparently normal infants have been reported whose mothers were treated with vinblastine, often in combination with other antineoplastics, during pregnancy (96). In 17 of these cases, exposure occurred during the first trimester. Three infants with congenital anomalies have been reported whose mothers received vinblastine in combination with other agents during the first trimester of pregnancy. One child had hydrocephalus, the second an atrial septal defect, and the third oligosyndactyly. Similarly, exposure to vincristine in combination with other antineoplastic agents has been described in at least 34 pregnancies, eight during the first trimester. Its use has not been associated with an excessive frequency of congenital anomalies (96).

Antimetabolites

Antimetabolites, such as methotrexate and cytarabine, have been associated with birth defects (94). Methotrexate is an abortifacient and a human teratogen. Among women who received methotrexate early in pregnancy, the rate of miscarriage was high, and infants of these women have had multiple birth defects involving the cranium, extremities, and CNS (95,96,104). Nevertheless, normal children after first-trimester drug exposure have also been reported. The effect on the fetus when exposed during the second and third trimesters is unknown. Cases of severe newborn myelosuppression have also been reported (101,110). Whether the amniotic fluid serves as a third space, a reservoir, where methotrexate accumulates following administration and is then slowly released (similar to a pleural effusion) is unknown. Cytarabine, usually in combination with other antineoplastic agents, has been administered to at least 50 pregnant women. In pregnancies continued to term, most infants appeared normal (96). Although treatment usually commenced during the second or third trimesters, at least 11 normal infants have been born to mothers treated during the first trimester. However, cytarabine was also associated with intrauterine fetal death and congenital and chromosomal abnormalities (95,104,111).

Miscellaneous Antineoplastic Agents

Other miscellaneous antineoplastic agents include cisplatin (Platinol), bleomycin sulfate (Blenoxane), fludarabine phosphate (Fludara), steroids, and interferon alfa.

Cisplatin has been administered to at least seven women during the second and/or third trimesters (96,104). No adverse fetal effects have been confirmed. One infant was exposed 1 week before delivery. At 1-year follow-up, the child was developing normally, except for moderate bilateral hearing loss. The investigators could not determine whether the sensorineural deafness was caused by maternal and neonatal gentamicin therapy or maternal cisplatin chemotherapy (112). Three mothers were treated during the first trimester.

No reports linking the use of bleomycin with congenital defects have been located (17,39,95,104). Twenty-three children with *in utero* exposure to bleomycin (and other antineoplastic agents) had normal growth and development (106). Of note, bleomycin may cause maternal pulmonary toxicity, which may be precipitated or exacerbated by supranormal oxygen levels. Therefore, if general anesthesia is required during pregnancy (e.g., cesarean section) for a woman who received bleomycin before or during pregnancy, the oxygen levels should be administered at room-air concentration (95).

No reports of fludarabine use during human pregnancy have been located (96,104).

Steroids (i.e., prednisone, methylprednisolone, and dexamethasone) are frequently administered in combination with other chemotherapeutic agents. Several large studies have not found any increased incidence of congenital anomalies after maternal treatment (96, 104). Some data suggest that prednisone may retard fetal growth and cause low birthweight; however, this outcome was attributed in some cases to the underlying disease for which the steroids were given (often a collagen-vascular disease or asthma) (96). Pregnant women taking steroids should be closely monitored for the development of gestational diabetes.

Interferon alfa does not appear to pose a significant risk to the developing embryo and fetus (104). Ferrari et al. (113) described a 30-year-old woman with multiply relapsed HD who became pregnant while receiving interferon alfa. The drug was continued until the fourth month of pregnancy. She delivered a healthy, 3200-g male infant. The baby developed normally, and at the time of the report was 2 years old. None of at least 19 infants born to pregnant mothers receiving interferon alfa, often throughout pregnancy, for chronic myelogenous leukemia, essential thrombocythemia, or hairy cell leukemia have had congenital malformations (104).

Several other ancillary drugs are commonly used during the treatment of lymphoma. Prochlorperazine (Compazine) use during pregnancy, including the first trimester, has been studied extensively. Although isolated cases of congenital defects in children exposed to prochlorperazine *in utero* have been reported, the majority of the evidence indicates that this drug is safe if used occasionally in low doses (104). The fetal safety of ondansetron hydrochloride (Zofran) and granisetron hydrochloride (Kytril) is uncertain (104). Three pregnant women (for whom fetal outcome was reported) were treated for hyperemesis gravidarum with ondansetron and other antiemetics at 11 to 13, 30 to 33, and 14 to 33 weeks' gestation. All three mothers delivered healthy infants (114–116). Reports of granisetron use during pregnancy have not been located (104). Allopurinol is often used in patients with lymphoma to minimize the risk of renal failure resulting from tumor lysis syndrome. Eight patients who received allopurinol during pregnancy have been described, six of these in conjunction with antineoplastic agents for malignancy. None of the infants had congenital abnormalities that were attributed to the drug (104). Filgrastim (Neupogen), a hematopoietic growth factor, is normally produced in human placental and decidual tissues and is found in umbilical cord blood at term. No reports of its use or use of sargramostim during pregnancy have been located (96).

RADIATION THERAPY

Available animal data (primarily from rodents) indicate that exposure to ionizing radiation during the preimplantation phase of pregnancy may result in a greatly increased risk of embryonic lethality and resorption. These effects can be seen with doses as low as 5 to 15 cGy. However, if the radiation exposure is limited to the preimplantation phase and the embryo survives, there may be relatively few long-term consequences of the exposure (117). In contrast, radiation exposure during the phase of organogenesis (approximately weeks 2 to 9) produces a high incidence of disastrous and permanent developmental malformations, in addition to increased risk of lethality or intrauterine growth restriction (118). The general sequence of these dose-dependent late effects is in accord with the known high-risk periods for thalidomide and other teratogenic inducers. The accepted threshold for these effects is fairly low, probably in the 10- to 50-cGy range (119). The effects of doses less than 10 cGy are not well documented, even in this critical phase of organogenesis. During the fetal period (roughly week 10 onward in humans), the effects of intrauterine radiation exposure include damage, incomplete formation, or dysregulated function for many organ systems, including the liver, eye, bone marrow, kidneys, and gonads. In general, the exposure threshold at which these effects are commonly observed is significantly higher than the threshold for deleterious effects produced during organogenesis. Low-dose-radiation exposure during the fetal period often produces no demonstrable late effects, although the theoretic risk of carcinogenesis later in life must be assumed (120).

Direct analogies between animal data and available human data are difficult to draw and only partially supported by clinical data. In contrast to the great body of experimental evidence available for fetal radiation exposure in animals, human data come primarily from the detailed observations of Japanese atomic bomb survivors and their medical histories (121). Although a small body of knowledge on medical radiation exposure in pregnant women exists, these data are mostly from the first half of the 20th century, when the effects of ionizing radiation were not yet widely appreciated. Taken together, these human data suggest that the types of effects seen in animal models and the general sequence of the risk periods are largely parallel to the human experience when one corrects for the differing time sequence of pregnancy in humans versus animals. However, the broad spectrum of congenital malformations produced experimentally in rodents is not well documented in atomic bomb survivors (117). Whether this reflects a fundamental difference between rodents and humans or whether it indicates the low likelihood of survival of affected embryos during the postwar era is not clear.

In humans, the principal risk period for birth defects begins at around 15 days' gestational. Very few subjects known to have been exposed at younger gestational ages have survived. Microcephaly and mental retardation are the most commonly observed late effects in atomic bomb survivors (122), and these abnormalities have been observed with exposure doses as low as 10 cGy during weeks 8 to 25 of gestation. Radiation exposure after about 30 weeks' gestation has not generally been associated with major teratogenic consequences, although the risks of organ dysfunction may be significantly increased by high-dose-radiation exposures. Because minor congenital abnormalities are seen in 5% to 10% of the human population, it is extremely difficult to demonstrate small increases in risks after fetal radiation exposure. Thus, even though it is unclear whether radiation exposure in the third trimester involves major risks, the inability to prove that it does not involve risks leads to the current recommendation that all ionizing radiation exposure should be kept to an absolute minimum during all phases of pregnancy.

Whenever possible, radiation therapy should be deferred until the third trimester of pregnancy (123). For patients receiving mantle irradiation, the fetal dose is mainly from internal scatter, with some contribution from machine leakage and collimator scatter (124, 125). Some reports indicate that increasing the energy of the beam can lead to a decrease in internal scatter (126,127). Thus, using the highest energy beam possible without compromising the dose to the areas of disease is encouraged.

The dose to the fetus, as well as the effects of the radiation on the fetus, varies depending on gestational age. Although radiation is more damaging to the fetus at earlier ages of gestation, the fetus is located lower in the pelvis and receives less scatter from a mantle field than a fetus at a more advanced gestational age (128). Reports of patients who became pregnant during radiotherapy for HD have allowed estimation of fetal doses from supradiaphragmatic irradiation. Friedman and Jones (129) estimated the fetal dose received during weeks 8 to 11 of pregnancy for a course of 35 Gy in 20 fractions. The contribution from collimator transmission and source-head leakage was estimated at 0.12%, and the contribution from internal scatter was estimated at 0.29%—for a total dose to the fetus of 0.41% of the total dose or 14.4 cGy. The position of the fetus was taken as the top of the pubic symphysis. Since the authors did not know that the patient was pregnant during the treatment, no attempts at shielding were undertaken. The patient delivered a healthy baby at term, and the child was developing normally at 21 months.

Different authors have proposed a number of shielding techniques to help minimize machine leakage and collimator scatter and thus reduce the dose delivered to the fetus. Cygler et al. (130) proposed a device utilizing a lead shield and an aluminum plate overlying the abdomen. With this device, they estimated that the dose to the fetus accumulated over the course of treatment was 10 cGy and 3 cGy for the fundus and pubis, respectively, for a prescribed dose of 35 Gy in 20 fractions. Because of the physical distance between the skull and the uterus, radiotherapy to the brain (for cranial prophylaxis or for CNS lymphoma) may be delivered safely any time after the first trimester.

At the Cleveland Clinic Foundation, we use an abdominal shielding device to help minimize the dose to the fetus. Thermoluminescent dosimeter measurements taken on a patient who was 4 months pregnant yielded a dose of 24.1 cGy to the fundus and 2.8 cGy to the pubic symphysis. Using this sort of specialized shielding rig, mantle radiotherapy may be delivered safely to a pregnant patient after the first trimester. Shielding techniques are an important component of treatment planning, especially for patients diagnosed with HD in the early part of the second trimester in whom waiting until delivery might compromise the possibility of cure.

With modern shielding techniques and higher energy beams, we can minimize the fetal dose, while still delivering definitive doses of radiation.

MANAGEMENT GUIDELINES

General Considerations

Management of pregnant women with either a history of lymphoma or active disease must be individualized. To provide optimal care, management of these complex patients should involve a multidisciplinary team, which might include a medical oncologist, radiation oncologist, obstetrician, primary care physician, pediatrician, neonatologist, social worker, ethicist, and/or clergy. A member of this management team (usually the medical oncologist) should inform the patient (and her family) of the risks and benefits to both the mother and fetus of the possible diagnostic and therapeutic alternatives.

In pregnant women with a history of lymphoma who are still considered at risk for relapse (which includes most young adults), the usual posttreatment monitoring may not be possible. The physician needs to rely primarily on history and physical examination. The gynecologist must be aware of both the typical and potentially unusual manifestations of lymphoma. Since the presentation of lymphoma during pregnancy may mimic the signs and symptoms of pregnancy, the obstetrician and other involved medical personnel must have a heightened awareness of this possibility and have a low threshold to evaluate changes that are not easily attributable to the pregnancy.

Women diagnosed with HD or NHL should avoid pregnancy. A pregnancy test should be performed prior to the initiation of therapy, and an effective form of birth control should be used from the time of diagnosis, throughout treatment, and even afterward, until the risk of recurrence is relatively low (10). Most studies show that the majority of patients with HD and aggressive NHL who eventually relapse do so within approximately 3 years (131–137). Although no data suggest that pregnancy increases the likelihood of recurrence, this prophylactic measure will hopefully ensure that a developing fetus is not inadvertently exposed to potentially teratogenic therapy, that a patient's posttherapy remission status may be monitored judiciously (e.g., with appropriate radiologic studies), and that in the event of relapse, the patient is not in the difficult position of having to consider a therapeutic abortion and optimal therapy may be initiated in a timely fashion. If the patient does become pregnant and the fetus is inadvertently exposed to potentially teratogenic chemotherapy or radiation in excess of 10 cGy, especially during the first trimester, a therapeutic abortion is recommended (10,14,18,91,138).

For pregnant women with newly diagnosed or relapsed lymphoma, treatment during the first trimester may be necessary. If at all possible, however, treatment should be avoided during the first 8 to 12 weeks of pregnancy (18). If treatment delay is not possible, the most conservative recommendation is a therapeutic abortion (91). Since chemotherapy or radiation therapy during pregnancy may cause spontaneous abortion, congenital malformations, intrauterine growth restriction, or unforeseen delayed effects, patients unwilling to accept any increased risk of adverse fetal outcome potentially attributable to therapy should consider therapeutic abortion (18). Patients who have a therapeutic abortion should be staged and treated as nonpregnant patients (18).

For some patients, a delay in treatment will not adversely affect maternal prognosis, and initiation of treatment may be delayed from the first trimester until the second trimester or from the late second or third trimester until after delivery (91). Patients for whom therapy is delayed should be monitored closely to determine when the fetus may be safely delivered (18). In this situation, early delivery (either by induction or cesarean section) to facilitate the initiation of lymphoma therapy may be considered.

Many patients can be successfully treated while pregnant without apparent adverse effect on the fetus. Some authors have recommended that the least teratogenic chemotherapy regimen be used. However, the majority of these patients have newly diagnosed HD or diffuse, large B-cell lymphoma, and the treatment is currently fairly standardized: ABVD for HD and cyclophosphamide, hydroxydaunomycin (doxorubicin), vincristine (Oncovin), and prednisone (CHOP) for diffuse, large B-cell lymphoma (132,135). Alternative but potentially less teratogenic therapies may not be as efficacious and generally are not an option.

Some authors have suggested that when myelosuppressive chemotherapy is required near term, delivery should be induced or cesarean section be performed at a time when maternal blood counts are not compromised (to minimize the risk of infection and/or bleeding) (91). Since the duration of neutropenia and thrombocytopenia associated with most chemotherapy regimens is predictable and relatively short, and may be shortened even further with hematopoietic growth factors, this approach may not be necessary for most patients. If myelosuppressive therapy has been administered to the mother prior to delivery, a fetal scalp complete blood cell count (CBC) may be checked prior to delivery, and a neonatal CBC should be checked following delivery, even if the mother's CBC is normal, because the mother and the child's CBCs may not correlate (91,102). Patients treated during pregnancy should have staging completed after delivery. Further therapy should consider both the initial and postpartum staging results (realizing that sites of disease present at diagnosis may have already responded completely to therapy).

Hodgkin's Disease

Staging evaluation of pregnant women with newly diagnosed HD should include history, physical examination, routine laboratory tests, chest x-ray with abdominal shielding, and bilateral bone marrow biopsies. An ultrasound may identify gross disease in the abdomen or pelvis. MR imaging (without contrast) of the chest (if more definition of mediastinal adenopathy is required for anticipated radiation therapy), abdomen, and pelvis is safe but should be used sparingly. Echocardiography may be used to assess left ventricular function.

The role of staging laparotomy is diminishing, remains controversial, and is beyond the scope of this text. The interested reader is referred to a recent comprehensive review (139). Generally, staging laparotomy is unnecessary and not indicated. For the exceptional patient in whom a staging laporotomy is considered and will affect management, it should be delayed until after delivery (10).

Based on their own experience and review of the literature, several authors have published treatment recommendations. Jacobs et al. (10) recommended that patients in the first trimester or the first half of the second trimester have a therapeutic abortion, with the possible exception of women with stage IA nonbulky disease in the neck or axilla. If abortion was refused, they recommended approximately 2000 cGy involved-field radiation therapy (with appropriate precautions and shielding) to allow stabilization of the disease, followed by early delivery and then completion of staging and treatment. During the last half of the second trimester and the third trimester, patients with stage I or II supradiaphragmatic disease should have staging and treatment postponed until after a viable infant can be delivered. If the systemic symptoms are so severe that they may be detrimental to the fetus or mother or if the disease is rapidly growing, then treatment with radiation therapy should begin with modification of the field and dose and with appropriate shielding of the abdomen. Patients in the last half of gestation with stage I or II subdiaphragmatic disease and those with stage III or IV disease should have treatment withheld until after delivery. Patients in whom treatment is necessary due to symptoms, rapid progression, or organ compromise should receive low-dose supradiaphragmatic radiation therapy, single-agent vinblastine, or, if necessary, MOPP chemotherapy.

Sutcliffe and Chapman (138) advised either an abortion in early pregnancy or delay of therapy until after the first trimester. They recommended chemotherapy for all patients after the first trimester.

Nisce et al. (14) stated that therapeutic abortion is not justified except in the following circumstances: (a) infradiaphragmatic disease requiring pelvic irradiation, (b) systemic symptoms and/or visceral disease best managed with multiple-agent chemotherapy, (c) diagnosis during the first 10 weeks' gestation when delay of treatment is unacceptable, (d) inadvertent fetal exposure to potentially teratogenic chemotherapy agents or greater than 10 cGy radiation during the first 10 weeks' gestation, or (e) bulky mediastinal disease that requires combined radiation therapy and multiple chemotherapeutic agents.

Ward and Weiss (18) proposed detailed management guidelines. For patients diagnosed during the first half of pregnancy, they recommended therapeutic abortion when any of the following features was present: (a) teratogenic exposure or urgent need for treatment during the first 8 to 12 weeks' gestation, (b) an unwillingness to accept fetal risks of therapy, or (c) bulky mediastinal disease. If abortion is declined, they recommended that therapy be delayed or interrupted, if possible, until after the first trimester. For patients with stable disease not requiring urgent therapy regardless of gestational period, they recommended deferring treatment until disease progression or postpartum. For patients requiring therapy, they recommended single-agent vinblastine during the first trimester and then supradiaphragmatic radiation therapy (with a modified field and dose and abdominal shielding), continued single-agent vinblastine or combination chemotherapy if the patient progresses on vinblastine or possibly has advanced-stage disease. Supradiaphragmatic radiation was not recommended for patients in the third trimester because of the relatively high fetal dose despite abdominal shielding.

Dhedin and Coiffier (19) suggested that a diagnosis of HD during the first trimester is not an indication for a therapeutic abortion, but it may be proposed if a delay in treatment is unacceptable or if bulky disease, visceral involvement, subdiaphragmatic disease, or B symptoms are present or the disease is progressing rapidly. If continuation of pregnancy is elected despite an urgent need to treat a patient, they recommended single-agent vinblastine. For patients presenting in the second half of pregnancy with localized disease, they recommended that treatment be deferred until after delivery. If significant progression occured and delivery was not possible, they recommended a multidrug chemotherapy regimen ABVD (without dacarbazine) or modified CHOP, which they stated are known to be associated with the smallest risk for the fetus.

Most of these recommendations were based on old data and written at a time when the standard treatment for patients with early-stage HD was radiation therapy and the experience with chemotherapy and combined-modality therapy was limited. Among patients with early-stage disease, chemotherapy plus involved-field radiation therapy may be at least as effective as, if not more effective than, traditional extended-field radiation therapy (134,140,141). For patients with advanced-stage disease, combination chemotherapy is standard treatment. In the United States, ABVD is considered the standard combination chemotherapy regimen (132).

Based on this information and our review of the literature, we recommend the following treatment guidelines. Patients diagnosed in the first trimester of pregnancy may be observed until the second trimester unless there is an indication to initiate treatment. Patients who require initiation of treatment during the first trimester because of B symptoms, bulky or advanced-stage disease, or rapid progression should have a therapeutic abortion. If abortion is not an option, the patient should be treated with single-agent vinblastine (which appears safe) until the second trimester or until significant disease progression. If combination chemotherapy is necessary, we recommend ABVD (without dacarbazine) during the first trimester and standard ABVD subsequently. Patients who present in the second or third trimesters should be closely observed, and the fetus should be delivered when it is considered viable. If treatment is necessary, we recommend standard ABVD chemotherapy. In general, postchemotherapy involved-field radiation therapy may be delayed until after delivery but should not be delayed more than 9 weeks following the last cycle of chemotherapy. Mantle radiotherapy with extensive abdominal blocking may be an acceptable alternative if chemotherapy is not effective.

In women with refractory or relapsed HD for whom ABVD and/or radiation therapy are not treatment options, MOPP and MOPP-like regimens have documented efficacy in the treatment of relapsed HD and limited adverse effect on the fetus if administered after the first trimester. The fetal risk of other effective salvage chemotherapy regimens is less well documented. For most patients in whom initial chemotherapy fails, high-dose therapy with autologous blood stem cell transplantation is the treatment of choice. These patients may be treated with salvage chemotherapy until delivery and then proceed with autologous transplantation.

Non-Hodgkin's Lymphoma

The staging evaluation for pregnant women with newly diagnosed NHL should include a history, physical examination, routine laboratory tests, chest x-ray with shielding, abdominal ultrasound, bilateral bone marrow biopsies, and, in some patients, lumbar puncture for cytologic examination of the cerebrospinal fluid. MR imaging (without contrast) of the chest, abdomen, and pelvis is acceptable if the identification of disease in one or more of these sites will significantly alter therapy. Echocardiography may be used to assess left ventricular function.

Young patients with NHL usually present with aggressive and advanced-stage disease. Nevertheless, these patients are potentially curable. Standard treatment depends on the specific histology, stage, and other risk factors. Because of these differences and the timing of diagnosis during pregnancy, management must be individualized. Previous recommendations for patients with NHL during pregnancy are limited.

Ward and Weiss (18) suggested that patients diagnosed during the first half of pregnancy who have had teratogen exposure during the first trimester, have an urgent need to initiate treatment during the first 8 to 12 weeks' gestation, and/or have an unwillingness to accept any fetal risk of therapy should have a therapeutic abortion. For patients who decline an abortion, they recommended delaying or interrupting therapy, if possible, until after the first trimester, although they recognized that this approach is not in the best interests of most patients. If therapy is required, they recommended involved-field radiation therapy, if fetal exposure is acceptable, for some patients with stage I aggressive lymphoma or stage I/II indolent NHL, and chemotherapy for all other patients.

Lishner et al. (142) recommended aggressive chemotherapy, when indicated, after proper counseling of pregnant women and their families. They suggested that rare, localized or low-grade lymphomas might be treated with a more conservative approach.

Dhedin and Coiffier (19) recommended that treatment for pregnant women with a low-grade lymphoma may be delayed until after delivery. Women with an aggressive lymphoma during the first trimester should have a therapeutic abortion and immediate initiation of standard chemotherapy. In a small fraction of these patients with stage I lymphoma, they suggested that localized radiation therapy or no treatment may be acceptable until the second trimester of pregnancy, when a multidrug regimen may be initiated. During the second and third trimesters of pregnancy, they recommended full doses of a multidrug regimen with efficacy in the patient's specific lymphoma subtype. They did not feel that supradiaphragmatic radiation therapy or single-agent chemotherapy to stabilize the disease until after the second trimester is a valid option. However, they recognized that some patients might decline a therapeutic abortion and that a decision regarding treatment must be made that balances the prognosis of the mother and the hazards to the fetus.

Based on our review of the literature, we recommend the following treatment guidelines. Although patients with indolent or low-grade lymphoma and pregnancy have not been reported, these women can theoretically be managed similarly to nonpregnant women. That is, women who are asymptomatic, have a relatively normal CBC, and no impending organ compromise may be safely observed until delivery or significant disease progression. On the other hand, the outcome for pregnant women with aggressive histologic subtypes has been poor. Therefore, their treatment should not be compromised. Women diagnosed during the first trimester and women unwilling to accept any potential therapy-related adverse fetal effect should have a therapeutic abortion. All other women should be treated immediately with standard therapy.

This approach is especially important for pregnant women with Burkitt's lymphoma, a disease for which only one long-term survivor has been reported (16). Whether this poor outcome is due to the aggressive nature of this disease during pregnancy or to suboptimal treatment is uncertain. Recently, Magrath et al. (137) reported outstanding disease-free and overall survival among patients with diffuse, small noncleaved-cell lymphoma (Burkitt's lymphoma and high-grade B-cell lymphoma, Burkitts-like). This approach or a similar approach must be taken if the mother, and potentially the child, are to be saved. Unfortunately, methotrexate is an important component of most regimens shown to be effective in the treatment of this subtype of lymphoma. Consequently, therapeutic abortion for women diagnosed in the first trimester is essential if this therapy is to be initiated.

Lymphoblastic lymphoma in association with pregnancy is exceedingly rare, and specific recommendations are difficult to make. The recently published Revised European–American Lymphoma Classification (REAL) (143) and many large centers do not distinguish between lymphoblastic lymphoma and acute lymphoblastic leukemia. Consequently, patients are often treated using the same protocols. For more information and specific recommendations on the management of these patients, the reader is referred to the chapter on pregnancy and leukemia (see Chapter 9).

The majority of pregnant women with NHL have diffuse, large B-cell or peripheral T-cell lymphoma (i.e., diffuse mixed, diffuse large-cell, or large-cell immunoblastic in the International Working Formulation). The standard treatment is three to eight cycles of CHOP chemotherapy followed by involved-field radiation therapy for women with localized disease, and six to eight cycles of CHOP chemotherapy for women with advanced-stage disease (135,144,145). We recommend that women diagnosed during the first trimester have a therapeutic abortion and that women diagnosed during the second or third trimester proceed with CHOP chemotherapy. For women with localized disease who have completed three to eight cycles of CHOP chemotherapy, radiation therapy may be delayed until after delivery, but no more than 9 weeks after the last cycle of chemotherapy.

For women who relapse during pregnancy, essentially no data are available. Standard therapy consists of several cycles of salvage chemotherapy followed by high-dose therapy and autologous or allogeneic hematopoietic cell transplantation. Since relapsed NHL is often more aggressive than at diagnosis, delayed treatment is generally not an option. For patients for whom a second remission and long-term survival are realistic goals, treatment should not be compromised. Patients who relapse during the first half of pregnancy should probably have a therapeutic abortion. Patients who relapse during the second half of pregnancy may receive salvage chemotherapy. Since the effect on the fetus of standard salvage chemotherapy regimens is unknown, no specific recommendations are available. Following delivery, appropriate patients may receive high-dose therapy with autologous or allogeneic hematopoietic cell transplantation.

OBSTETRIC AND GYNECOLOGIC PROBLEMS AFTER TREATMENT

Antineoplastic therapy may lead to premature ovarian follicle destruction and fibrosis. Affected women subsequently experience symptoms of estrogen deficiency and menopause (e.g., irregular menses and/or amenorrhea, vaginal dryness, dyspareunia, and hot flashes). Laboratory evaluation reveals increased levels of luteinizing hormone and follicle-stimulating hormone, in particular, and decreased levels of estrogen (98,146).

The risk of amenorrhea, premature menopause, and infertility following treatment of women with HD varies. The data are derived from retrospective studies of nonpregnant women who received chemotherapy and/or radiation therapy. Whether the risk for women who received chemotherapy during pregnancy differs from the experience observed among nonpregnant women is unknown. Few, if any, data are available regarding gonadal function following treatment of NHL.

Among the drugs used to treat patients with HD and NHL, the alkylating agents (e.g., cyclophosphamide, mechlorethamine, chlorambucil, and probably procarbazine) are primarily responsible for premature ovarian failure. Other agents that tend not to induce permanent ovarian failure include methotrexate, vincristine, etoposide, cisplatin, doxorubicin, bleomycin, vinblastine, and dacarbazine.

Several studies have reviewed the gonadal function of women following MOPP chemotherapy and reached similar conclusions (147–151). In one of the first reported series, Horning et al. (147) described 34 women who received MOPP chemotherapy without pelvic radiation. Nineteen (56%) had regular menses, 10 (29%) had irregular menses, and five (15%) had amenorrhea following treatment. Menopausal symptoms developed in three (9%) patients. The probability of having regular menses following treatment depended on patient age at the time of treatment, ranging from 80% among 15-year-olds to 20% among 35-year-olds (Fig. 1). Women with amenorrhea and/or postmenopausal symptoms were highly unlikely to become pregnant regardless of age at treatment. Whether menses were regular or irregular had no impact on ability to become pregnant after treatment. Twenty (59%) of 34 women with menses and nonmenopausal symptoms who did not practice birth control subsequently became pregnant. Among women with regular or irregular menses and no menopausal symptoms, the probability of pregnancy decreased with increasing age at the time of treatment, ranging from 60% at age 15 to 5% at age 30. By multivariate analysis, only age at the time of treatment and the presence of menses without menopausal symptoms were statistically significant in identifying women likely to become pregnant (Fig. 2). Forty percent of women became pregnant despite having had temporary amenorrhea with menopausal symptoms lasting several months and up to 3.5 years. A similar experience has been reported in women who received as few as three cycles of MOPP (150,151).

Fertility among women following treatment with ABVD has been less well studied. A randomized study comparing MOPP to ABVD included 61 women younger than 45 years (152). Prolonged amenorrhea (no menses for more than 6 months) developed in 6 of 14 women between ages 30 and 45 years who received MOPP without pelvic radiation therapy, compared to none of eight women in the same age group treated with ABVD.

Data on fertility following treatment with CHOP are not available. However, the effect of cyclophosphamide with or without other agents on subsequent fertility has been reviewed in women treated primarily for breast cancer. The likelihood of permanent amenorrhea depends on both patient age and the cumulative dose of cyclophosphamide (98). Younger women require a significantly higher cumulative dose to induce amenorrhea than older women. Cumulative cyclophosphamide doses of 20 to 50 g, 6 to 8 g, and only 5 g were necessary to cause permanent ovarian failure

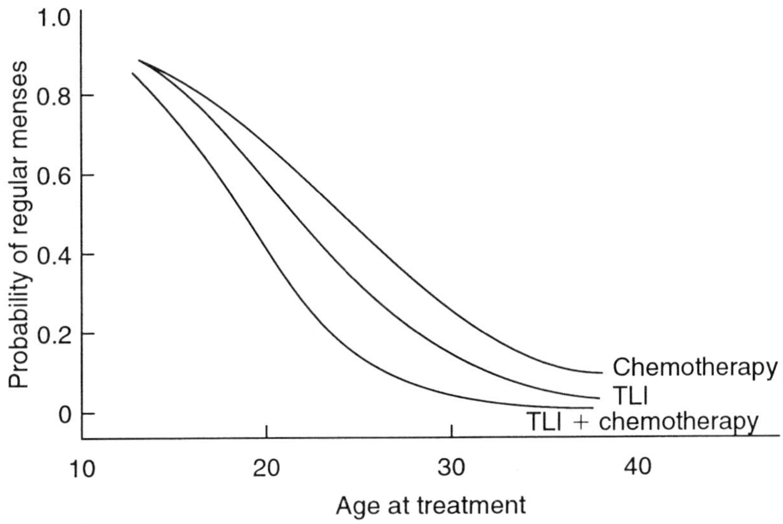

FIG. 1. Probability of regular menses after chemotherapy, total lymphoid irradiation (TLI), or TLI and chemotherapy, according to age at time of treatment.

in women ages 20, 35, and 45, respectively (98). Consequently, eight cycles of CHOP, in which the dose of cyclophosphamide is 0.75 g/m^2 per cycle (and the total dose may be 9 to 12 g for an average-sized woman), will lead to permanent gonadal failure in very few women younger than 20 but in many women older than 35. These data suggest that temporary amenorrhea during chemotherapy is independent of age, while permanent amenorrhea associated with ovarian failure dramatically increases with age. Permanent amenorrhea may

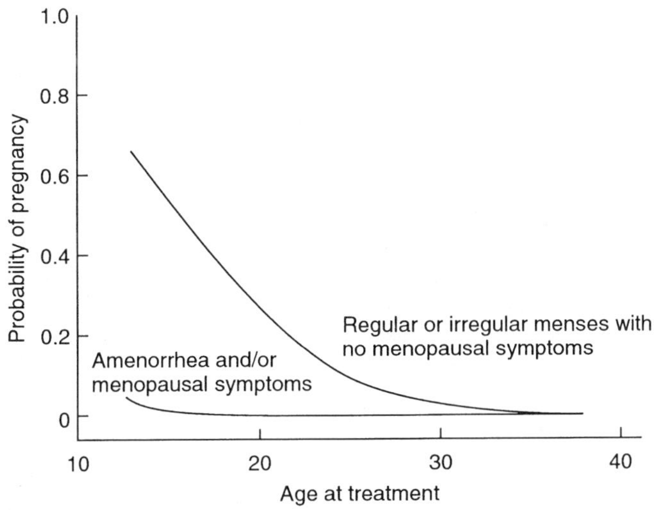

FIG. 2. Probability of pregnancy after treatment with total lymphoid irradiation, chemotherapy, or both, according to menstrual status, menopausal symptoms, and age at treatment. Only women who did not use birth-control measures were considered. (From ref. 147, with permission.)

begin during chemotherapy or several years after the onset of irregular menses. Even if temporary amenorrhea does not occur or if menses resume following temporary amenorrhea, premature menopause may still occur.

Many believe that women who received radiation therapy outside of the pelvis are at increased risk for premature menopause secondary to scatter radiation to the ovaries. Although some women do undergo premature menopause following mantle irradiation for HD, the majority do not do so. A study conducted at the National Cancer Institute reviewed patients treated for childhood cancer who had at least 5 years of follow-up or had reached age 21 years by the time of the analysis (153). All women were younger than 20 and still menstruating at the time of diagnosis. Compared to a control group who did not have cancer, women treated between ages 13 and 19 were significantly more likely to become menopausal during follow-up. The risk was greatest during the first 5 years and varied depending on the treatment regimen. Women treated with surgery alone had no increased risk. However, compared to the control group, the risk increased from fourfold in patients treated with radiation alone, to ninefold for patients treated with alkylating agents, and to 27-fold for patients treated with a combination of alkylating-agent chemotherapy and radiation therapy to areas below the diaphragm.

Madsen et al. (154) reviewed the treatment and follow-up records of 36 patients younger than 50 who were treated for stage I or II supradiaphragmatic HD at Stanford University. All patients underwent mantle, paraaortic, and splenic irradiation. The calculated ovarian dose ranged from 3.2 to 3.5 Gy. Of the 36 women identified, only one (2.7%) experienced premature menopause. This experience is consistent with rates of premature menopause in women who have not undergone radiation therapy (155).

Several relatively recent studies have evaluated outcome of pregnancies in women who have been previously treated for HD. Horning et al. (147) reported 28 pregnancies in 20 women who had previously received chemotherapy (primarily MOPP) and/or radiation therapy for HD. The 28 pregnancies resulted in 21 normal live births (one set of twins), two premature infants, one low-birthweight infant, and five elective therapeutic abortions. No birth defects or developmental abnormalities were reported in the 24 children. The two premature children and the low-birthweight child were developing normally at the time of the report. The median age of the children at the time of the report was 2.3 (range, 1 month to 7.5) years.

Janov et al. (156) reported the outcome of 16 pregnancies of at least 20 weeks' duration that occurred in 109 surviving women who received chemotherapy with or without radiation therapy for HD on any of nine Cancer and Leukemia Group B (CALGB) protocols between 1966 and 1986. Chemotherapy consisted of MOPP, ABVD, MOPP/ABV hybrid, or variations of these regimens that used a nitrosourea, chlorambucil, or streptozocin (Zanosar). Low-birthweight infants (less than 2500 g) were delivered in 2 of 15 pregnancies for which birthweight was available, which was statistically not significantly different from the expected 0.8 based on the National Center for Health Statistics data. No major congenital anomalies or malignancies occurred among these children.

Aisner et al. (157) reviewed the outcome of pregnancies that occurred in women of childbearing age who received treatment for HD between 1965 and 1985. Forty-three of 104 women actively attempted conception after therapy. Thirty-five (81%) of these 43 women had 54 pregnancies. Fourteen of 16 had received radiation therapy alone, and 21 of 27 had received chemotherapy with or without radiation therapy. One woman had stillborn twins but subsequently had three normal, healthy children. Another woman had a stillborn at 32 weeks. Nine women had elective abortions, and one woman had a spontaneous abortion. The median age of the mothers at the birth of the first posttreatment child was 30 (range, 16 to 35) years. The median treatment-free interval at the birth of the child was 5.5 (range, 8 months to 14) years. None of the fetuses was studied. None of the live births was premature. The median birthweight was 2943 g (range, 1896 to 4471 g). Only two children weighed less than 2264 g. The median 5-minute Apgar score was 9 (range, 6 to 10). No major birth defects and no preponderance of minor birth defects were observed. Minor birth defects included pes planus (n=1), congenital hip dislocation (n=1), heart murmur of unknown etiology (n=1), skin hemangioma (n=3), and hepatitis carrier (n=1). Complications during pregnancy included toxemia (n=1), premature placental separation (n=1), postpartum pulmonary embolus (n=1), and cervical laceration with hemorrhage (n=1). Three patients required cesarean deliveries, but two had had a prior cesarean delivery before the treatment of their HD.

Swerdlow et al. (158) studied children of patients treated for HD. They initially mailed a questionnaire to 100 women who had been diagnosed between ages 15 and 40 years from 1970 to 1991. Twenty-six women were identified who had subsequently conceived; 16 were subsequently interviewed. Compared to the general population, they reported no difference in the number of stillbirths, low-birthweight infants, or premature deliveries. Furthermore, no cancers had occurred among these children. By interview, three children had congenital abnormalities (a small cyst on the head, a Mongolian blue spot, and a minor birthmark). Among 10 offspring of women treated with chemotherapy, 10 offspring of women treated with mantle or localized upper-body radiation therapy, and one offspring of a woman treated with combined-modality therapy, no chromosomal abnormalities attributable to the treated parent were identified.

Few data are available on the outcome of pregnancies among women previously treated for NHL. One woman with a history of diffuse lymphoblastic NHL treated with cyclophosphamide, vincristine (Oncovin), procarbazine, and prednisone (COPP) conceived 4 years after completion of therapy and delivered a normal male infant at 38 weeks' gestation (159).

The standard treatment for patients with HD or NHL that has relapsed following chemotherapy usually includes high-dose therapy with autologous or allogeneic blood stem cell or bone marrow transplantation (BMT). Although pregnancy and high-dose therapy are incompatible, an understanding of the effects of high-dose chemotherapy and/or radiation therapy on subsequent gynecologic health may significantly affect the treatment decisions made by some women.

The natural history of gonadal damage following high-dose therapy is variable and depends on the conditioning regimen, underlying disease, and prior chemotherapy (160). Transient recovery with resumption of menses and even pregnancy may occur, but as the number of ova cannot be replenished, premature menopause is probable. Most preparative regimens include high-dose cyclophosphamide. Sanders (161) recently reviewed ovarian function in 65 women between ages 13 and 38 who received cyclophosphamide, 200 mg/kg, with allogeneic BMT for aplastic anemia. All women younger than 26 years at the time of cyclophosphamide administration had evidence of ovarian function recovery between 3 months and 3 years after BMT. Seven of 19 women ages 26 to 38 years never demonstrated evidence of ovarian recovery. No women who received busulfan as part of the preparative regimen had ovarian recovery. Ten women who received total body irradiation as part of the preparative regimen had recovery of ovarian function between 3 and 7 years after BMT. All women who recovered ovarian function were younger than 26 at the time of BMT. Ovarian function recovery following other preparative regimens has not been well studied.

A recent comprehensive review of the English literature identified 142 successful pregnancies in women who received high-dose therapy with allogeneic or autologous blood stem cell and/or BMT for the treatment of aplastic anemia or hematologic malignancies (162). Among women with a history of HD, only seven pregnancies, resulting in eight live births (including two sets of twins), were identified. All eight patients received chemotherapy-based preparative regimens. No successful pregnancies were identified among female survivors of BMT for NHL.

Not surprisingly, HD survivors are at risk for sexual dysfunction. Studies suggest that the prevalence of sexual problems in HD survivors ranges from 22% to 73% and may be particularly high in patients who undergo a treatment-related abortion (163–165). In one study of HD survivors, approximately 25% reported a temporary and 25% a long-term change in their sense of physical attractiveness due either to their cancer diagnosis or to treatment (166). This loss of a sense of physical attractiveness and body image correlated with a loss of energy, decreased frequency of sexual intercourse, and symptoms of depression. These symptoms were greater in patients who had more advanced disease and more treatment. In another study, 73% or more of women questioned had mild or no libido following treatment (163). Often, these young women had not informed anyone of their depressed libido, not even their sexual partners. Among women with documented evidence of chemical castration, hormone replacement therapy led to a return of normal libido. Among participants in the CALGB study, which compared MOPP, ABVD, and MOPP/ABVD, patients who received MOPP were more likely to have sexual problems attributed to the cancer (MOPP, 34%; ABVD, 17%; MOPP/ABVD, 19%), more likely to have decreased interest in sex (MOPP, 23%; ABVD, 9%; MOPP/ABVD, 11%), and more likely to have decreased sexual activity (MOPP, 16%; ABVD, 9%; MOPP/ABVD, 14%), compared to patients in the other two groups, although the differences were not statistically significant (164).

Second malignancies including leukemia, NHL, and solid tumors have been reported among survivors of HD (167,168). Rarely, the solid tumors have included cancer of the cervix, uterus, ovary, and breast. In a recent and detailed study, Hancock et al. (169) identified 885 women with a history of HD who were treated at Stanford University between 1961 and 1986. Breast cancer developed in 25 of these women a mean of 15 (range, 4.5 to 23) years after treatment, for a relative risk (RR) of 4.1. The risk of breast cancer increased over time and was highest (RR, 11 to 15) among women 15 or more years posttreatment. The risk was greatest among children younger than 15 at the time of treatment (RR, 136) and remained elevated until age 30. The majority of the breast cancer observed arose in portions of the breast that received full-dose radiation of approximately 44 Gy. This study showed that women treated with radiation for HD before age 30 years are at markedly increased risk for breast cancer, with risk increasing dramatically more than 15 years after therapy.

SUMMARY

Coincident pregnancy and lymphoma are rare. Yet, as the incidence of lymphoma and the frequency of young lymphoma survivors increase, the likelihood of individual health care providers participating in the management of such patients will also increase. An understanding of the disease presentation during pregnancy, the impact of lymphoma on pregnancy (and vice versa), and the potential immediate and delayed consequences of the available diagnostic and therapeutic options are critical to optimizing the outcome for both the mother and the child. We hope that the information provided in this chapter will provide a rational basis to guide all who are involved in the management of these complex patients.

REFERENCES

1. Haas JF. Pregnancy in association with a newly diagnosed cancer: a population-based epidemiologic assessment. *Int J Cancer* 1984;34:229.
2. Stewart HL, Monto RW. Hodgkin's disease and pregnancy. *Am J Obstet Gynecol* 1952;63:570.
3. Riva HL, Andreson PS, O'Grady JW. Pregnancy and Hodgkin's disease: a report of eight cases. *Am J Obstet Gynecol* 1953;66:866.
4. Landis SH, Murray T, Bolden S, Wingo PA. Cancer statistics, 1998. *CA Cancer J Clin* 1998;48:6.
5. Lin AY, Tucker MA. Epidemiology of Hodgkin's disease and non-Hodgkin's lymphoma. In: Canellos GP, Lister TA, Sklar JL, eds. *The lymphomas.* Philadelphia: WB Saunders, 1998:43.
6. Bachu A. *Fertility of American women: June 1995 (up-*

date). Current population reports. Washington, DC: Census Bureau, U.S. Department of Commerce, 1997: 20–499.
7. Gobbi PG, Attardo-Parrinello A, Danesino M, et al. Hodgkin's disease and pregnancy. *Haematologica* 1984;69:336.
8. Lishner M, Zemlickis P, Degendorfer P, Panzarella T, Sutcliffe SB, Koren G. Maternal and fetal outcome following Hodgkin's disease in pregnancy. *Br J Cancer* 1992;65:114.
9. Lambe M, Ekbom A. Cancers coinciding with childbearing: delayed diagnosis during pregnancy? *BMJ* 1995;311:1607.
10. Jacobs C, Donaldson SS, Rosenberg SA, Kaplan HS. Management of the pregnant patient with Hodgkin's disease. *Ann Intern Med* 1981;95:669.
11. Barry RM, Diamond HD, Graver LF. Influence of pregnancy on the course of Hodgkin's disease. *Am J Obstet Gynecol* 1962;84:445.
12. Hennessy JP, Rottino A. Hodgkin's disease and pregnancy. *Haematologica* 1963;87:851.
13. Tawil E, Mercier JP, Dandavino A. Hodgkin's disease complicating pregnancy. *J Can Assoc Radiol* 1985;36: 133.
14. Nisce LZ, Tome MA, He S, Lee BJ III, Kutcher GJ. Management of coexisting Hodgkin's disease and pregnancy. *Am J Clin Oncol* 1986;9:146.
15. Ebert U, Loffler H, Kirch W. Cytotoxic therapy and pregnancy. *Pharmacol Ther* 1997;74:207.
16. Gelb AB, van de Rign M, Warnke RA, Kamel OW. Pregnancy-associated lymphomas: a clinicopathologic study. *Cancer* 1996;78:304.
17. Sutcliffe SB. ABVD chemotherapy for Hodgkin's disease in pregnancy: a report on three cases and cytogenetic and clinical follow-up at 1, 5 and 7 years. *Ann Oncol* 1996;7(suppl 3):113(abst).
18. Ward FT, Weiss RB. Lymphoma and pregnancy. *Semin Oncol* 1989;16:397.
19. Dhedin N. Coiffier B. Lymphoma and pregnancy. In: Canellos GP, Lister TA, Sklar JL, eds. *The lymphomas*. Philadelphia: WB Saunders, 1998:549.
20. Moore DT, Taslimi MM. Non-Hodgkin's lymphoma in pregnancy: a diagnostic dilemma. Case report and review of the literature. *J Tenn Med Assoc* 1992;85:467.
21. Steiner-Salz D, Yahalom J, Samuelov A, Polliack A. Non-Hodgkin's lymphoma associated with pregnancy: a report of six cases, with a review of the literature. *Cancer* 1985;56:2087.
22. Durodola JI. Burkitt's lymphoma presenting during lactation. *Int J Gynaecol Obstet* 1976;14:225.
23. Benavides Ledezma RR, Barboza Quintana O, Barboza Quintana A, et al. Linfoma indiferenciado tip Burkitt, primario, en ovario y embarazo. *Ginecol Obstet Mex* 1988;56:293.
24. Merimsky O, Reider I, Rahmani R, Chaitchik S. Pregnancy and cavernous sinus involvement in a patient with primary non-Hodgkin's lymphoma of bone. *Isr J Med Sci* 1990;26:520.
25. Spagnoli CU. Primary malignant lymphoma of the uterus. *Diagn Imaging* 1981;50:81.
26. Giovannini M, Saccucci P, Cannone D, Damiani G, Pomini P. Can pregnancy aggravate the course of non-Hodgkin's lymphoma? *Eur J Gynaecol Oncol* 1989; 10:287.
27. Berrebi A, Schattner A, Mogilner BM. Disseminated Burkitt's lymphoma during pregnancy. *Acta Haematol* 1983;70:139.
28. Bornkamm GW, Kaduk B, Kachel G, et al. Epstein-Barr virus-positive Burkitt's lymphoma in a German woman during pregnancy. *Blut* 1980;40:167.
29. Shepherd JJ, Wright DH. Burkitt's tumour presenting as bilateral swelling of the breast in women of childbearing age. *Br J Surg* 1967;54:776.
30. Armon PJ. Burkitt's lymphoma of the ovary in association with pregnancy: two case reports. *Br J Obstet Gynaecol* 1976;83:169.
31. Falkson HC, Simson IW, Falkon G. Non-Hodgkin's lymphoma in pregnancy. *Cancer* 1980;45:1679.
32. Lysyj A, Bergquist JR. Pregnancy complicated by sarcoma: report of two cases. *Obstet Gynecol* 1963;21:506.
33. Finkle HI, Goldman RL. Burkitt's lymphoma: gynecologic considerations. *Obstet Gynecol* 1974;43:281.
34. Iochim HL. Non-Hodgkin's lymphoma in pregnancy: three cases and review of the literature. *Arch Pathol Lab Med* 1985;109:803.
35. Mehta A, Vakil RM. Use of Endoxan in a case of lymphosarcoma with pregnancy during the third trimester. *Indian J Cancer* 1966;3:198.
36. Moore DT, Taslimi MM. Multi-agent chemotherapy in a case of non-Hodgkin's lymphoma in second trimester of pregnancy. *J Tenn Med Assoc* 1991;84:435.
37. Bannerman RHO. Burkitt's tumour in pregnancy. *BMJ* 1966;2:1136.
38. Jones DED, d'Avignon MB, Lawrence R, Latshaw RF. Burkitt's lymphoma: obstetric and gynecologic aspects. *Obstet Gynecol* 1980;56:533.
39. Ortega J. Multiple agent chemotherapy including bleomycin of non-Hodgkin's lymphoma during pregnancy. *Cancer* 1977;40:2829.
40. Case BW, Benaroya S. Dyspnea in a pregnant young woman. *Can Med Assoc J* 1980;122:890.
41. Hardin JA. Cyclophosphamide treatment of lymphoma during third trimester of pregnancy. *Obstet Gynecol* 1972;39:850.
42. Armitage JO, Feagler JR, Skoog DP. Burkitt lymphoma during pregnancy with bilateral breast involvement. *JAMA* 1977;237:151.
43. Henderson M, Paterson WG. Perforation of jejunum by reticulum cell sarcoma in pregnancy. *Am J Surg* 1968;115:385.
44. Tunca JC, Reddi PR, Shah SH, Slack ST. Malignant non-Hodgkin's-type lymphoma of the cervix uteri occurring during pregnancy. *Gynecol Oncol* 1979;7:385.
45. Roumen FJ, de Leeuw JW, van der Linden PJ, Pannebakker MA. Non-Hodgkin lymphoma of the puerperal uterus. *Obstet Gynecol* 1990;75:527.
46. Bucciarelli E, Cavaliere A, Sidoni A, Alberti PF, Sfondalmondo S. Bilateral primary malignant lymphoma of the breast: a case report. *Tumori* 1988;74:587.
47. Kirkpatrick AW, Bailey DJ, Weizel HA. Bilateral primary breast lymphoma in pregnancy: a case report and literature review. *Can J Surg* 1996;39:333.
48. Aghadiuna PU, Akang EE, Ladipo JK. Simultaneous bilateral malignant breast neoplasms in Nigerian women. *J Natl Med Assoc* 1994;86:365.
49. Meguerian-Bedoyan Z, Lamant L, Hopfner C, Pulford K, Chittal S, Delsol G. Anaplastic large cell lymphoma of maternal origin involving the placenta: case report and literature survey. *Am J Surg Pathol* 1997;21:1236.
50. Kurtin PF, Gaffey TA, Habermann TM. Peripheral T-

cell lymphoma involving the placenta. *Cancer* 1992; 70:2963.

51. Tsujimura T, Matsumoto K, Aozasa K. Placental involvement by maternal non-Hodgkin's lymphoma. *Arch Pathol Lab Med* 1993;117:325.
52. Pollack RN, Sklarin NT, Rao S, Divon MY. Metastatic placental lymphoma associated with maternal human immunodeficiency virus infection. *Obstet Gynecol* 1993;81:856.
53. Rothman LA, Cohen CJ, Astarlova J. Placental and fetal involvement by maternal malignancy: a report of rectal carcinoma and review of literature. *Am J Obstet Gynecol* 1973;116:1023.
54. Iochim HL, Moroson H. Lymphoma and pregnancy: clinical observations and experimental investigations. *Leukemia* 1994;8(suppl 1):S198–S201.
55. Zuazu J, Julia A, Sierra J, et al. Pregnancy outcome in hematologic malignancies. *Cancer* 1991;67:703.
56. Vieaux JW, McGuire DE. Reticulum cell sarcoma of the cervix. *Am J Obstet Gynecol* 1964;89:134.
57. Leeks SR. Lymphosarcoma complicating pregnancy. *N Z J Med* 1966;65:465.
58. Ludanyi VI, Donko A. Retikulosarkom in der Gravidität. *Zentralbl Gynakol* 1969;49:1609.
59. Bergamaschi P, Magni M, Recevuti G. Reticulosarcoma in gravidanza: studio anatomoclinico. *Ann Obstet Ginecol Med Perin* 1973;94:255.
60. Inoue Y, Masuda H, Shiojima Y. Pregnancy complicated by sarcoma. *Acta Obstet Gynaecol Jpn* 1972;19:222.
61. Durodola JI. Administration of cyclophosphamide during late pregnancy and early lactation: a case report. *J Natl Med Assoc* 1979;71:165.
62. Villasanta U, Attar S, Jiji R. Malignant histiocytic lymphoma (reticulum cell sarcoma) in pregancy. *Gynecol Oncol* 1978;6:383.
63. Cheson BD, Johnston JL, Junco DD, Kjeldsberg CR. Cytologic evidence for disseminated immunoblastic lymphoma. *Am J Clin Pathol* 1981;75:621.
64. Schapira DV, Chudley AE. Successful pregnancy following continuous treatment with combination chemotherapy before conception and throughout pregnancy. *Cancer* 1984;54:800.
65. Garg A, Kochupillai V. Non-Hodgkin's lymphoma in pregnancy. *South Med J* 1985;78:1263.
66. Lowenthal RM, Funnell CF, Hope DM, Stewart IG, Humphrey DC. Normal infant after combination chemotherapy including teniposide for Burkitt's lymphoma in pregnancy. *Med Pediatr Oncol* 1982;10:165.
67. Spitzer M, Citron M, Ilardi CF, Saxe B. Non-Hodgkin's lymphoma during pregnancy. *Gynecol Oncol* 1991;43:309.
68. Toki H, Okabe K, Kamei H, et al. Successful chemotherapy on a pregnant non-Hodgkin's lymphoma patient. *Acta Med Okayama* 1990;44:321.
69. Aviles A, Diaz-Maqueo JC, Torras V, Garcia EL, Guzman R. Non-Hodgkin's lymphomas and pregnancy: presentation of 16 cases. *Gynecol Oncol* 1990;37:335.
70. Nantel S, Parboosingh J, Poon MC. Treatment of an aggressive non-Hodgkin's lymphoma during pregnancy with MACOP-B chemotherapy. *Med Pediatr Oncol* 1990;18:143.
71. du Bois A, Runge M, Schmid J, Hillemanns HG. Disseminiertes, hochmalignes Non-Hodgkin-Lymphom und Schwangerschaft: Polychemotherapie im 2. und 3. Trimester. *Geburtshilfe Frauenheilkd* 1990;50:405.
72. Ba-Thike K, Oo N. Non-Hodgkin's lymphoma in pregnancy. *Asia Oceania J Obstet Gynecol* 1990;16:229.
73. Lambert J, Wijermans PW, Dekker GA, Ossenkoppele GJ. Chemotherapy in non-Hodgkin's lymphoma during pregnancy. *Neth J Med* 1991;38:80.
74. Sheil O, Redman CW, Pugh C. Renal failure in pregnancy due to primary renal lymphoma: case report. *Br J Obstet Gynaecol* 1991;98:216.
75. Morice P, Cristalli B, Heid M, Briere J, Levardon M. Grossesse et lymphome non-hodgkinien: un cas. *J Gynecol Obstet Biol Reprod* 1993;22:68.
76. Lees CC, Tsirigotis M, Carr JV, Richards MA. T-cell non-Hodgkin's lymphoma presenting in the first trimester of pregnancy. *Postgrad Med J* 1994;70:371.
77. Imai A, Kawabata I, Tamaya T. Primary brain malignant lymphoma newly diagnosed during pregnancy. *J Med* 1995;26:333.
78. Goldwasser F, Pico JL, Cerrina J, et al. Successful chemotherapy including epirubicin in a pregnant non-Hodgkin's lymphoma patient. *Leuk Lymphoma* 1995; 20:173.
79. Rodriguez JM, Haggag M. VACOP-B chemotherapy for high-grade non-Hodgkin's lymphoma in pregnancy. *Clin Oncol (R Coll Radiol)* 1995;75:319.
80. Shulman LN, Mauch PM. Current role of radiotherapy in Hodgkin's and non-Hodgkin's lymphoma. *Curr Opin Oncol* 1995;7:421.
81. Carmichael JHE. Management of radiation hazard: radiology in late pregnancy and the neonate. In: Preger L, ed. *Induced disease:* drug, *irradiation, occupation.* New York: Grune & Stratton, 1980:137.
82. Mossman KL. Medical radiodiagnosis and pregnancy: evaluation of options when pregnancy status is uncertain. *Health Phys* 1985;48:297.
83. Hart GC. Diagnostic medical exposures to ionizing radiation during pregnancy (editorial). *Nucl Med Commun* 1994;15:403.
84. Jankowski CB. Radiation and pregnancy: putting the risks in proportion. *Amer J Nurs* 1986:261.
85. Mayo-Smith WW, Lee MJ. MR imaging of the female pelvis. *Clin Radiol* 1995;50:557.
86. Levine D, Edelman RR. Fast MRI and its application in obstetrics. *Abdom Imaging* 1997;22:589.
87. Elster AD. Questions and answers: does MR imaging have any known effects on the developing fetus? *Am J Roentgenol* 1994;162:1493.
88. Thomas PR, Biochem D, Peckham MJ. The investigation and management of Hodgkin's disease in the pregnant patient. *Cancer* 1976;38:1443.
89. Swartz HM, Reichling BA. Hazards of radiation exposure for pregnant women. *JAMA* 1978;239:1907.
90. Orr JW Jr, Shingleton HM. Cancer in pregnancy. *Curr Probl Cancer* 1983;8:1.
91. Doll DC, Ringenberg QS, Yarbo JW. Management of cancer during pregnancy. *Arch Intern Med* 1988;148: 2058.
92. Ferrari LR, Bedford RF. Anterior mediastinal mass in a pregnant patient: anesthetic management and considerations. *J Clin Anesth* 1989;1:460.
93. Martin JW. Cesarean section in a pregnant patient with an anterior mediastinal mass and failed supradiaphragmatic irradiation. *J Clinc Anesth* 1995;7:312.
94. Doll DC, Ringenberg QS, Yarbro JW. Antineoplastic agents and pregnancy. *Semin Oncol* 1989;16:337.
95. Sorosky JI, Sood AK, Buekers TE. The use of chemo-

therapeutic agents during pregnancy. *Obstet Gynecol Clin North Am* 1997;24:591.
96. Brier KL, Tornow JJ, Ries AJ, Weber MP, Downs JR. Forecasting patient outcomes in the management of hyperlipidemia. *Arch Intern Med* 1999;159:569.
97. Kalter H, Warkany J. Congenital malformations. *N Engl J Med* 1983;308:424.
98. Meistrich ML, Vassilopoulou-Sellin R, Lipshultz LI. Gonadal dysfunction. In: DeVita VT Jr, Hellman S, Rosenberg SA, eds. *Cancer: principles and practice of oncology*, 5th ed. Philadelphia: Lippincott–Raven Publishers, 1997:2758.
99. Nicholson HO. Cytotoxic drugs in pregnancy. *J Obstet Gynaecol Br Commonwlth* 1968;75:307.
100. Nordlund JJ, DeVita VT, Cabbone PP. Severe vinblastine-induced leukopenia during late pregnancy with delivery of a normal infant. *Ann Intern Med* 1968;69:581.
101. Okun DB, Groncy P, Sieger L, Tanaka KR. Acute leukemia in pregnancy: transient neonatal myelosuppression after combination chemotherapy in the mother. *Med Pediatr Oncol* 1979;7:315.
102. Meader JM, Armentrout SA, Slater LM. Third trimester chemotherapy and neontal hematopoiesis. *Cancer Chemother Pharmacol* 1987;19:177.
103. Glantz JC. Reproductive toxicology of alkylating agents. *Obstet Gynecol Surv* 1994;49:709.
104. Briggs GG, Freeman RK, Yaffe SJ. *Drugs in pregnancy and lactation*, 5th ed. Baltimore: Williams & Wilkins, 1998.
105. Toussi T, Blais M, Langevin P, et al. Metastatic melanoma treated in a pregnant woman: pre- and postnatal implications. *Union Med Can* 1974;103:1968.
106. Aviles A, Diaz-Maqueo JC, Talavera A, Guzman R, Garcia EL. Growth and development of children of mothers treated with chemotherapy during pregnancy: current status of 43 children. *Am J Hematol* 1991;36:243.
107. Turchi JJ, Villasis C. Anthracyclines in the treatment of malignancy in pregnancy. *Cancer* 1988;61:435.
108. Reynoso EE, Huerta F. Acute leukemia and pregnancy: fatal outcome after exposure to idarubicin during the second trimester. *Acta Oncol* 1994;33:703.
109. Azuno Y, Kaku K, Funjita N. Mitoxantrone and etoposide in breast milk. *Am J Hematol* 1995;48:131.
110. Pizzuto J, Aviles A, Noriega L, Niz J, Morales M, Romero F. Treatment of acute leukemia during pregnacy: presentation of nine cases. *Cancer Treat Rep* 1980;64:679.
111. Caligiura MA, Mayer RJ. Pregnancy and leukemia. *Semin Oncol* 1989;16:388.
112. Raffles A, Williams J, Costeloe K, Clark P. Transplacental effects of maternal cancer chemotherapy: case report. *Br J Obstet Gynaecol* 1989;96:1099.
113. Ferrari VD, Jirillo A, Lonardi F, Pavanato G, Bonciarelli G. Pregnancy during alpha-interferon therapy in patients with advanced Hodgkin's disease [Letter]. *Eur J Cancer* 1995;31A:2121.
114. Guikontes E, Spantideas A, Diakakis J. Ondansetron and hyperemesis gravidarum. *Lancet* 1992;340:1223.
115. World MJ. Ondansetron and hyperemesis gravidarum. *Lancet* 1993;341:185.
116. Tincello DG, Johnstone JM. Treatment of hyperemesis gravidarum with the 5-HT_3 antagonist ondansetron (Zofran). *Postgrad Med J* 1996;72:688.
117. Hall EJ. *Radiobiology for the radiologist*, 4th ed. Philadelphia: JB Lippincott Co, 1994.
118. Rugh R. Low levels of x-irradiation and the early mammalian embryo. *Am J Roentgenol* 1962;87:559.
119. Russell LG, Russell WL. An analysis of the changing radiation response of the developing mouse embryo. *J Cell Physiol* 1954;43:1030.
120. Miller RW. Effects of prenatal exposure to ionizing radiation. *Health Phys* 1990;59:57.
121. Otake M, Schull WJ. *In utero* exposure to A-bomb radiation and mental retardation: a reassessment. *Br J Radiol* 1984;57:409.
122. Miller RW, Blot WJ. Small head size after *in utero* exposure to atomic radiation. *Lancet* 1972;2:784.
123. Byram D. Mantle irradiation for Hodgkin's disease during pregnancy: safe and practical? *Australas Radiol* 1996;40:101.
124. Leung JT, Kuan R, Patel V. Radiotherapy for Hodgkin's disease in pregnancy. *Australas Radiol* 1996; 40:146.
125. Brent R. The effect of embryogenic and fetal exposure to x-ray, microwaves, and ultrasound: counseling the pregnant and nonpregnant patient about risks. *Semin Oncol* 1989;16:347.
126. Becker MH, Hyman GA. Management of Hodgkin's disease coexistent with pregnancy. *Radiology* 1965;85: 725.
127. Becker MH. Hodgkin's disease and pregnancy. *Radiol Clin North Am* 1968;6:111.
128. D'Angio GJ, Nisce LZ. Problems with the irradiation of children and pregnant patients. *JAMA* 1973;223: 171.
129. Friedman E, Jones GW. Fetal outcome after maternal radiation treatment of supradiaphragmatic Hodgkin's disease. *Can Med Assoc J* 1993;149:1281.
130. Cygler J, Ding GX, Kendal W, Cross P. Fetal dose for a patient undergoing mantle-field irradiation for Hodgkin's disease. *Med Dosim* 1997;22:135.
131. Rosenberg SA, Kaplan HS. The evolution and summary results of the Stanford randomized clinical trials of the management of Hodgkin's disease: 1962–1984. *Int J Radiat Oncol Biol Phys* 1985;11:5.
132. Canellos GP, Anders JR, Propert KJ, et al. Chemotherapy of advanced Hodgkin's disease with MOPP, ABVD, or MOPP alternating with ABVD. *N Engl J Med* 1992;327:1478.
133. Morel P, Lepage E, Brice P, et al. Prognosis and treatment of lymphoblastic lymphoma in adults: a report on 80 patients. *J Clin Oncol* 1992;10:1078.
134. Carde P, Hagenbeek A, Hayat M, et al. Clinical staging versus laparotomy and combined modality with MOPP versus ABVD in early-stage Hodgkin's disease: the H6 twin randomized trial from the European Organization for Research and Treatment of Cancer Lymphoma Cooperative Group. *J Clin Oncol* 1993;11: 2258.
135. Fisher RI, Gaynor KR, Dahlberg S, et al. Comparison of a standard regimen (CHOP) with three intensive chemotherapy regimens for advanced non-Hodgkin's lymphoma. *N Engl J Med* 1993;328:1002.
136. Shipp MA, Harrington DP, Anderson JR, et al. A predictive model for aggressive non-Hodgkin's lymphoma. *N Engl J Med* 1993;329:987.
137. Magrath IT, Adde M, Shad A, et al. Adults and children with small non-cleaved-cell lymphoma have a similar excellent outcome when treated with the same chemotherapy regimen. *J Clin Oncol* 1996;14:925.

138. Sutcliffe SB, Chapman RM. Lymphomnas and leukemias. In: Allen HH, Nisker JA, eds. *Cancer in pregnancy.* Mt Kisco, NY: Futura Publishing, 1986:135.
139. Mauch PM. Controversies in the management of early stage Hodgkin's disease. *Blood* 1994;83:318.
140. Radford JA, Cowan RA, Ryder WDJ, et al. Four weeks of neoadjuvant chemotherapy significantly reduces the progression rate in patients treated with limited-field radiotherapy for clinical stage IA/IIA Hodgkin's disease: results of a randomized pilot study. *Ann Oncol* 1996;7:66(abst).
141. Carde P, Noordijk EM, Hagenbeek A, et al. Superiority of EBVP chemotherapy in combination with involved-field irradiation (EBVP/IF) over subtotal nodal irradiation (STNI) in favorable clinical stage (CS) I-II Hodgkin's disease: the EORTC GPMC H7F randomized trial. *Proc Am Soc Clin Oncol* 1997;16:13a(abst).
142. Lishner M, Zemlickis D, Sutcliffe SB, Koren G. Non-Hodgkin's lymphoma and pregnancy. *Leuk Lymphoma* 1994;14:411.
143. Harris NL, Jaffe ES, Stein H, et al. A revised European-American classification of lymphoma neoplasms: a proposal from the International Lymphoma Study Group. *Blood* 1994;84:1361.
144. Glick JH, Kim K, Earle JD, O'Connell MJ. An ECOG randomized phase III trial of CHOP vs. CHOP + radiotherapy (XRT) for intermediate-grade early-stage non-Hodgkin's lymphoma (NHL). *Proc Am Soc Clin Oncol* 1995;14;391a(abst).
145. Miller TP, Dahlberg S, Cassady R, et al. Chemotherapy alone compared with chemotherapy plus radiotherapy for localized intermediate- and high-grade non-Hodgkin's lymphoma. *N Engl J Med* 1998;339;21.
146. Goldman S, Johnson FL. Effects of chemotherapy and irradiation on the gonads. *Endocrinol Metab Clin North Am* 1993;22:617.
147. Horning SJ, Hoppe RT, Kaplan HS, Rosenberg SA. Female reproductive potential after treatment for Hodgkin's disease. *N Engl J Med* 1981;304:1377.
148. Schilsky RL, Sherins RJ, Hubbard SM, Wesley MN, Young RC, DeVita VT. Long-term follow-up of ovarian function in women treated with MOPP chemotherapy for Hodgkin's disease. *Am J Med* 1981;71:552.
149. Cunningham J, Mauch P, Rosenthal DS, Canellos GP. Long-term complications of MOPP chemotherapy in patients with Hodgkin's disease. *Cancer Treat Rep* 1982;66:1015.
150. Andrieu JM, Ochoa-Molina ME. Menstrual cycle, pregnancies and offspring before and after MOPP therapy for Hodgkin's disease. *Cancer* 1983;52:435.
151. Koziner B, Myers J, Cirrincione C, et al. Treatment of stages I and II Hodgkin's disease with three different therapeutic modalities. *Am J Med* 1986;80:1067.
152. Viviani S, Santoro A, Ragni G, Bonfante V, Bestetti O, Bonadonna G. Gonadal toxicity after combination chemotherapy for Hodgkin's disease: comparative results of MOPP vs. ABVD. *Eur J Cancer Clin Oncol* 1985;21:601.
153. Byrne J. Fertility and pregnancy after malignancy. *Semin Perinatol* 1990;14:423.
154. Madsen BL, Giudice L, Donaldson SS. Radiation-induced premature menopause: misconception. *Int J Radiat Oncol Biol Phys* 1995;32:1461.
155. Cohen I, Speroff L. Premature ovarian failure update. *Obstet Gynecol Update* 1991;46:156.
156. Janov AJ, Anderson J, Cella DF, et al. Pregnancy outcome in survivors of advanced Hodgkin's disease. *Cancer* 1992;70:688.
157. Aisner J, Wiernik PH, Pearl P. Pregnancy outcome in patients treated for Hodgkin's disease. *J Clin Oncol* 1993;11:507.
158. Swerdlow AJ, Jacobs PA, Marks A, et al. Fertility, reproductive outcomes, and health of offspring of patients treated for Hodgkin's disease: an investigation including chromosome examinations. *Br J Cancer* 1996;74:291.
159. Pajor A, Zimonyi I, Koos R, Lehoczy D, Ambrus C. Pregnancies and offspring in survivors of acute lymphoid leukemia and lymphoma. *Eur J Obstet Gynecol Reprod Biol* 1991;40:1.
160. Chatterjee R, Goldsone AH. Gonadal damage and effects on fertility in adult patients with haematological malignancy undergoing stem cell transplantation. *Bone Marrow Transplant* 1996;17:5.
161. Sanders JE. Growth and development after bone marrow transplantation. In: Forman SJ, Blume KG, Thomas ED, eds. *Bone marrow transplantation.* Oxford: Blackwell Science, 1994:527.
162. Gulati SC, Paznak CV. Pregnancy after bone marrow transplantation. *J Clin Oncol* 1998;16:1978.
163. Chapman RM, Sutcliffe SB, Malpas JS. Cytotoxic-induced ovarian failure in Hodgkin's disease. II. Effects on sexual function. *JAMA* 1979;242:1882.
164. Kornblith AB, Anderson J, Cella DF, et al. Comparison of psychosocial adaptation and sexual function of survivors of advanced Hodgkin disease treated by MOPP, ABVD, or MOPP alternating with ABVD. *Cancer* 1992;70:2508.
165. Yellen SB, Cella DF, Bonomi A. Quality of life in people with Hodgkin's disease. *Oncology* 1993;7:41.
166. Fobair P, Hoppe RT, Bloom J, Cox R, Varghese A, Spiegel D. Psychosocial problems among survivors of Hodgkin's disease. *J Clin Oncol* 1986;4:805.
167. Tucker MA, Coleman CN, Cox RS, Varghese A, Rosenberg SA. Risk of second cancers after treatment for Hodgkin's disease. *N Engl J Med* 1988;318:76.
168. Van Leeuwen FE, Klokman WJ, Hagenbeek A, et al. Second cancer risk following Hodgkin's disease: a 20-year follow-up study. *J Clin Oncol* 1994;12:312.
169. Hancock SL, Tucker MA, Hoppe RT. Breast cancer after treatment of Hodgkin's disease. *J Natl Cancer Inst* 1993;85:25.

11

Adnexal Masses and Ovarian Cancer in Pregnancy

J. Rebecca Liu, James F. Lilja, and Carolyn Johnston

Department of Obstetrics and Gynecology, University of Michigan and University of Michigan Medical Center, Ann Arbor, Michigan 48109

INCIDENCE OF PELVIC MASSES IN PREGNANCY

The incidence of adnexal masses in pregnancy has been reported to range from 1 in 81 to 1 in 2500 live births (1). Since ultrasound examination has become a routine component of current obstetric management, nearly 1% of women have an adnexal mass diagnosed during pregnancy (2,3). Prior to the widespread use of ultrasound, most adnexal masses remained undetected until cesarean section or postpartum evaluation. The management of sonographically identified adnexal masses in the gravid patient has remained controversial. Some investigators advocate surgical excision of all adnexal masses persisting into the second trimester, quoting a malignancy rate of up to 6% (1,4). Other investigators have found that with advances in sonographic technology, ultrasound characterization can determine which patients are at risk for malignancy and which may be followed expectantly (5). Most investigators define an adnexal mass in pregnancy as a simple or complex mass 4 to 6 cm or greater in diameter found to be persistent on ultrasound beyond the first trimester (2,5).

The majority of adnexal masses detected during pregnancy are benign. Differential diagnoses of ovarian pathology can often be made on the basis of sonographic findings. The histologic diagnosis and relative frequency of ovarian neoplasms diagnosed during pregnancy from several studies is summarized in Table 1. Functional ovarian cysts, from follicles or corpora lutea, are the most common adnexal masses detected during pregnancy. These usually resolve by the second trimester. Among persistent adnexal masses diagnosed during pregnancy, dermoids are the most common, followed by benign serous or mucinous cystadenomas. Malignant ovarian neoplasms account for 2% to 6% of all persistent adnexal masses diagnosed during pregnancy. Epithelial ovarian carcinoma usually occurs in elderly women and is relatively rare among reproductive-age women. Ovarian cancer in pregnancy

TABLE 1. *Relative frequency of adnexal masses diagnosed during pregnancy*

Diagnosis	n	Percent
Dermoid	109	43
Endometrioma	18	7.1
Serous or mucinous cystadenoma	47	18.6
Fibroids	16	6.3
Follicular cyst	23	9
Corpus luteum	30	12
Malignancy	6	2.4
Other	4	1.6

Data from refs. 1, 5–7, with permission.

TABLE 2. *Relative frequency of malignant ovarian tumors diagnosed during pregnancy*

Histologic diagnosis	n	Percent
Serous cystadenoma	4	17.4
Borderline serous tumor	6	26.2
Mucinous cystadenoma	3	13.0
Borderline mucinous tumor	2	8.7
Dysgerminoma	4	17.4
Granulosa cell tumor	3	13.0
Undifferentiated	1	4.3

From ref. 10, with permission.

has been reported to occur with a frequency ranging from 1 in 18,000 to 1 in 25,000 pregnancies (8,9).

Most of the literature regarding invasive ovarian carcinoma during pregnancy comprises only case reports. In 1989, Dgani et al. (10) reported a series of 23 patients with ovarian carcinoma diagnosed during pregnancy in Israel over 25 years, representing an incidence of 0.12 per 100,000 women older than 14 years. In this series, the most common malignant ovarian neoplasms diagnosed during pregnancy included serous or mucinous tumors of low malignant potential, invasive serous or mucinous cystadenocarcinoma, dysgerminoma, and granulosa cell tumors. The relative frequency of malignant ovarian neoplasms diagnosed during pregnancy is described in Table 2.

DIAGNOSIS

Because most adnexal masses are asymptomatic, an adnexal mass discovered in pregnancy is often detected on routine pelvic examination at a prenatal visit or on prenatal ultrasound examination. Prior to the widespread use of ultrasound, adnexal masses were most commonly diagnosed as an incidental finding at the time of cesarean section or as a result of acute complications, such as abdominal pain from cyst torsion, rupture, hemorrhage, or infection. Several investigators have reported successful diagnosis of ovarian pathologic conditions on the basis of sonographic appearance, especially for dermoids, endometriomas, and simple cysts (11,12). Bromley and Benacerraf (5) classified persistent adnexal masses (4 cm or greater in diameter) as benign in sonographic appearance in 89.3% of 125 patients diagnosed during pregnancy; 10.7% of lesions were classified as suggestive of malignancy. In their study, the malignancy rate was only 0.8% overall. Only 1 (7%) of 14 suspicious masses detected by ultrasound was diagnosed as true malignancy. Suspicious characteristics included complex masses consisting of both solid and cystic components with nodularity, irregular borders, thick septations, or solid masses containing irregular echoes. These data confirm the work of Hogston and Lilford (13) who reported that only complex cysts or multilocular, thick-walled, or semisolid cysts should be removed during pregnancy. They investigated 137 adnexal masses diagnosed during pregnancy; 10% were surgically excised electively early in pregnancy, and 2% were removed when patients presented with acute pain later in pregnancy. One case of malignancy resulted in a malignancy rate of 0.5%.

In addition to routine ultrasonography, Wheeler and Fleischer (14) described using color Doppler sonography to establish specific criteria to help distinguish between benign and malignant adnexal masses in pregnancy. In their study, only patients with persistent complex adnexal masses were investigated. Thirty-four women were analyzed, all of whom had persistent complex masses with ultrasound, including irregular septa, papillary excrescences, or solid components. Low pulsatility index of less than 1.0 and low impedance were associated with malignant ovarian masses detected during pregnancy. However, a considerable overlap in blood flow patterns resulted in a high false-positive rate. Overall, the sensitivity of high-resolution ultrasound to distinguish benign from malignant disease is 96.6% and specificity 77%. The negative predictive value is as high as 99%.

In addition to ultrasonography, other investigators have described using magnetic resonance (MR) imaging in pregnancy to examine women with abnormal pregnancy or persistent adnexal mass. Lowe et al. (15) described using

MR imaging in addition to ultrasound and showed that the procedure provided detailed imaging of normal and abnormal maternal or fetal anatomy without putting the patient or the fetus at risk with exposure to x-rays. MR imaging produces high-resolution cross-sectional body images that can be used to characterize adnexal masses in detail. Curtis et al. (16) described using MR imaging in the differential diagnosis of adnexal masses in five pregnant women. Based on MR imaging findings suggesting a benign-appearing process, all women avoided laparotomy during pregnancy. MR imaging characteristics of adnexal masses are not well defined in nongravid women, and thus a standard of comparison is lacking.

Tumor markers in the setting of a gravid patient are generally not helpful in distinguishing between a benign or malignant process, as most tumor markers used in the management of ovarian carcinoma can be elevated in a normal pregnancy. Niloff et al. (17) reported elevated CA125 antigen levels in the serum of 15 (16%) of 94 women in the first trimester of pregnancy. Maternal serum CA125 levels declined as gestational age progressed. CA125 was found in high concentrations in amniotic fluid samples from 26 gestations, and concentrations appeared to be greater in the second than in the third trimester. Other tumor markers such as the β chain of human chorionic gonadotropin, alpha-fetoprotein, or lactate dehydrogenase are all constitutively high in the serum of gravid patients. In addition, germ cell tumors such as dysgerminoma and sex cord–stromal tumors rarely present during pregnancy with clinically significant hormonal manifestations.

Pathologic diagnosis may be affected by pregnancy. In particular, serous tumors of low malignant potential have been reported to have microscopic features suggestive of aggressive behavior. However, these features appear to regress postpartum (18).

MANAGEMENT

Management of an adnexal mass discovered during pregnancy remains controversial. As mentioned above, nearly 1% of pregnant women have an adnexal mass diagnosed on ultrasound (19). Because the majority of adnexal masses diagnosed in pregnancy are related to pregnancy, such as corpus luteum or theca-lutein cysts, most will resolve during the second trimester. Therefore, if a mass is diagnosed early in pregnancy, most physicians will follow it conservatively with serial pelvic and ultrasound examinations.

In the past, all pregnant women with persistent adnexal masses were managed by surgical intervention, optimally during the second trimester. The rationale for operative intervention was to rule out ovarian malignancy and avoid acute complications such as torsion, rupture, infection, obstructed labor, or pregnancy loss. Several investigators now advocate the use of sonographic characterization of adnexal masses in pregnancy to determine which patients are at high risk for malignancy versus which can be followed expectantly (2,5,14). As mentioned above, Bromley and Benacerraf (5) noted a malignancy rate of 0.8% in 125 pregnant patients with persistent nonsuspicious adnexal masses followed expectantly. Doppler sonography was not used routinely to evaluate blood flow.

Persistent simple cysts may be managed with ultrasound-guided percutaneous or transvaginal drainage to potentially reduce the incidence of rupture, torsion, pain, hemorrhage, or obstruction of labor. Ultrasound-guided cyst drainage is associated with a low risk of infection, hemorrhage, or other complications related to the pregnancy such as preterm labor or infection. Selected patients may benefit from these procedures to reduce the need for surgical intervention during pregnancy. Platek et al. (2) reported on five patients who underwent ultrasound-guided percutaneous or transvaginal drainage of a simple cyst. Three patients had the procedure because of symptoms of early torsion and two to prevent dystocia in labor. Khaw and Walker (20) reported on four pregnant patients who underwent transabdominal (n=2) and transvaginal (n=2) ultrasound-guided fine-needle aspiration of benign adnexal cysts during pregnancy. Three patients had recurrent cysts later in pregnancy, and two required repeat aspiration. Furthermore, in a retrospective review of women with ovarian torsion treated by laparoscopic intervention, Morice et al. (21) described six pregnant patients who were successfully treated between 6 and 13 weeks' gestation, four undergoing detorsion followed by cyst puncture. There were no adverse operative or obstetric sequelae.

When surgical intervention is required for management of a persistent adnexal mass in pregnancy, several factors require careful consideration. Hess et al. (1) reported on 15 of 54 pregnant women with adnexal masses who required emergent exploratory laparotomy. These investigators discovered that of pregnant women requiring laparotomy during pregnancy for definitive diagnosis and treatment of a persistent adnexal mass, those women who underwent emergent laparotomy were more likely to develop complications related to their pregnancy. Indications for emergent surgery in these 15 pregnant women included cyst rupture (n=6), adnexal torsion (n=7), and acute infarction (n=1). Six patients underwent emergent laparotomy in the first trimester, resulting in a 50% spontaneous abortion rate within 7 days of laparotomy. Five patients underwent laparotomy in the second trimester, resulting in one spontaneous abortion 4 weeks following surgery. Four women underwent emergent laparotomy in the late second (n=2) or third (n=2) trimesters. Both patients operated on in the third trimester developed preterm labor and delivered soon after surgery despite tocolytic therapy. Of the two women who underwent laparotomy in the second trimester, one developed preterm labor 12 weeks later and delivered at 35 weeks.

Of the 54 patients in this study by Hess et al. (1), all who underwent emergent laparotomy had a worse outcome than those who underwent elective surgery. Consequently, this group of investigators recommended elective removal of any mass 6 cm or greater in diameter, regardless of sonographic appearance (1). Likewise, Struyk and Treffers (22) reported a high rate of complications in 90 pregnancies with adnexal masses. Complications included severe pain (26%), adnexal torsion (12%), cyst rupture (9%), and obstruction of labor (17%). We concur with the more conservative management plan of Platek et al. (2), which takes into account sonographic characterization of adnexal masses (Fig. 1).

If surgical intervention is deemed necessary for patients without acute symptoms, the ideal time for laparotomy is between 16 and 22 weeks' gestation. Physiologic cysts will have resolved by this time. If oophorectomy is required, the placenta has replaced the hormonal function of the corpus luteum after 12 weeks' gestation. The prophylactic use of tocolytic agents remains controversial (23). If surgical intervention is deemed necessary, indomethacin (Indocin), 100 mg per rectum, may be used once, followed by oral indomethacin, 25 mg every 6 hours for 24 hours, postoperatively. Intraoperative obstetric monitoring is indicated for operative intervention at 24 weeks' gestation to term. This would include fetal heart rate monitoring, as well as monitoring for uterine contractions. Both anesthesia-induced hypotension and hypoxia can alter uterine perfusion and fetal oxygenation. In the event that laparotomy is performed after 24 weeks' gestation, administration of steroids to enhance lung maturity should be considered several days prior to surgery in case preterm labor or preterm delivery occurs (24). If an adnexal mass is discovered in the third trimester, surgery can often be delayed until postpartum or at the time of cesarean section.

The incision chosen should optimize exposure and minimize both uterine manipulation and operative time. Surgical intervention may range from diagnostic laparoscopy, to laparotomy with ovarian cystectomy, to full staging laparotomy. Guerrieri and Thomas (25) reported performing open laparoscopy on a patient at 15 weeks' gestation for a persistent 7-cm complex adnexal mass. On exploratory laparoscopy, the mass was noted to be a pedunculated 7-cm fibroid arising from the left posterior aspect of the uterus, and further sur-

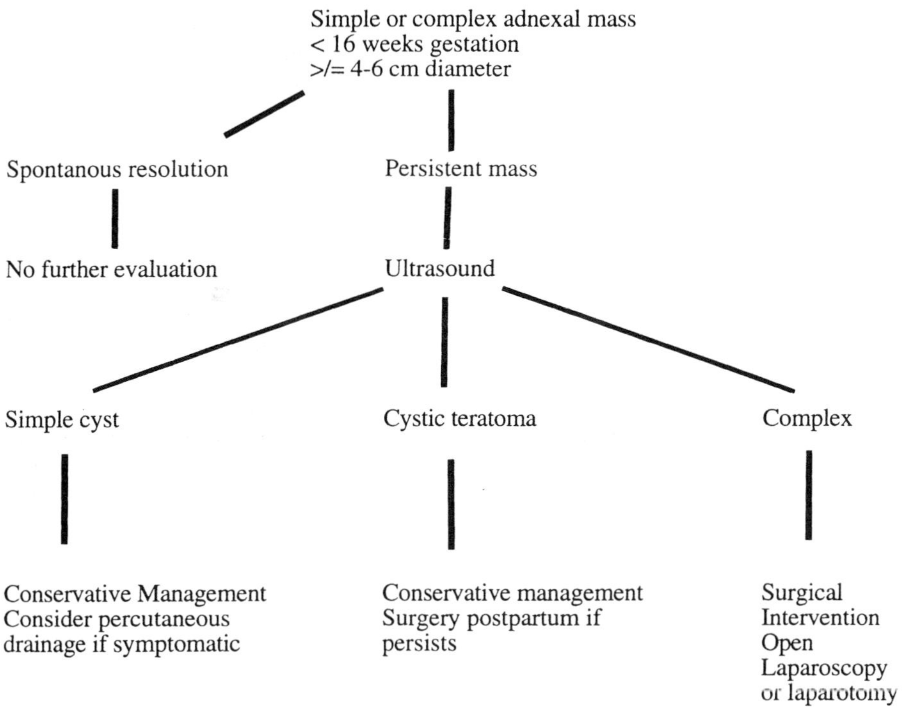

FIG. 1. Recommended management of adnexal masses in pregnancy. (From ref. 2, with permission.)

gical intervention was avoided. Other surgeons have performed laparoscopic oophorectomies and cystectomies with low morbidity in patients ranging from 9 to 18 weeks' gestation (26–28). The first report to address complications and safety in laparoscopy during pregnancy specifically noted five intraoperative and 10 postoperative complications in 413 patients. Of note, this was a retrospective survey of surgical experience within the Society of Laparoscopic Surgeons with a reply from 192 surgeons (29). Recommendations have been made for the monitoring of fetal heart rate with transvaginal ultrasound, maternal end-tidal carbon dioxide, and oxygen saturation during laparoscopy. These recommendations are not necessarily uniformly accepted (30). Most published reports do not document monitoring techniques, making definitive conclusions difficult. Although most of the experience with laparoscopy in pregnancy is with nongynecologic disease, particularly cholecystectomy, laparoscopy appears to be a safe technique that can be performed in the first, second, and early third trimester, with the potential for reduction of hospital stay and narcotic use (26,31).

Full staging laparotomy during pregnancy is rare (32). The surgical management of ovarian cancer diagnosed during pregnancy should be the same as in a nonpregnant patient. Because most tumors in pregnant women present as stage I disease, unilateral oophorectomy or unilateral salpingo-oophorectomy with omentectomy and possible pelvic and paraaortic lymph node sampling is the procedure of choice. Rarely will a hysterectomy be indicated. For more advanced-stage disease, the extent of surgery and tumor debulking will depend on the stage of disease, fetal viability, and patient choice.

EMERGENT COMPLICATIONS

The incidence of pregnant women requiring emergent laparotomy for acute complications involving adnexal masses is unknown. As mentioned, Hess et al. (1) reported on 54 patients with persistent adnexal masses during pregnancy who required laparotomy, 15 (28%) of whom underwent emergent laparotomy for acute complications. In contrast, Dgani et al. (10) reported a series of 23 patients with malignant ovarian carcinoma diagnosed during pregnancy, 17 (74%) of whom were symptomatic. Although most pregnant patients diagnosed with ovarian carcinoma present with early-stage disease, these patients may tend to present with emergent complications because of rapid tumor growth more frequently than nonpregnant patients with early-stage disease. Pregnant women with a large adnexal mass may present with abdominal pain due to torsion, acute abdomen due to rupture of the mass and subsequent hemorrhage, pelvic impaction, obstructed labor, or infection. Sophisticated ultrasound or MR imaging techniques can be helpful in clarifying the diagnosis.

CHEMOTHERAPY DURING PREGNANCY

Administration of chemotherapy during pregnancy raises concerns about transplacental passage of cytotoxic agents to a maturing fetus. Unfortunately, the gynecologic literature consists primarily of case reports and case series. The paucity of data concerning the treatment of pregnant patients with ovarian malignancy makes it difficult to determine the risks of administering modern combination chemotherapy. The literature concerning pregnant patients treated for nongynecologic cancers provides additional information, but not enough on which to base solid conclusions. It is difficult to compare data from case reports and case series because of variations in treatment combinations and doses of chemotherapy administered. Moreover, other factors, including gestational age, disease status, and medications, make it even more difficult to interpret cause and effect.

In the past, first-line chemotherapeutic agents for epithelial ovarian carcinoma included doxorubicin hydrochloride (Adriamycin) and cyclophosphamide. Currently, chemotherapy based on cisplatin (Platinol) and paclitaxel (Taxol) is the treatment of choice (33). More recently, carboplatin (Paraplatin) and paclitaxel have been used as first-line combination therapy for epithelial ovarian cancer (34–36).

Reports concerning the effects of cisplatin with cyclophosphamide for the treatment of epithelial ovarian cancer during pregnancy are summarized in Table 3. Carboplatin has been reported once in the literature as being used during pregnancy, supplanting cisplatin initiated at 20 weeks' gestation (38). Carboplatin was administered at 30 weeks, and the patient delivered at 36 weeks. No adverse effect on the fetus was reported. Paclitaxel has not been reported to be used in a pregnant patient. Animal studies on paclitaxel, however, indicate embryotoxicity in rats (41,42).

Germ cell tumors are commonly treated with triple-agent chemotherapy. The Gynecologic Oncology Group recommended vincristine, dactinomycin (actinomycin D), and cyclophosphamide (VAC) to treat these tumors in the past (43). Current recommendations for

TABLE 3. *Effect of cisplatin and cyclophosphamide on fetal outcome*

Histology	Reference	Initiation of treatment (gestational age, wk)	Fetal outcome
Recurrent Sertoli-Leydig cell	37	24	34-wk elective induction; normal development at 12 mo
Primary papillary serous	38	20 (cisplatin) 30 (carboplatin)	36-wk premature delivery
Primary papillary serous	39	16	36.5-wk premature delivery; <24 h ventilatory support
Primary papillary serous	40	16	Term delivery

treatment of germ cell tumors includes cisplatin, etoposide, and bleomycin (PEB) are also used to treate germ cell tumors (44,45). Cisplatin, vincristine, and bleomycin (PVB) have been used as well (46,47). Table 4 summarizes the relevant gynecologic literature with regard to chemotherapy for germ cell tumors during pregnancy.

The data regarding chemotherapy in pregnant patients with gynecologic tumors and chemotherapy are limited. However, outcome data from studies of pregnant patients with other malignancies are available. Ebert et al. (54) summarized 217 cases of pregnant patients treated for leukemias, lymphomas, rheumatic disorders, and gynecologic neoplasms between 1983 and 1995. Although this review is clearly limited by the fact that multiple diseases are represented and various combinations of agents were utilized, some conclusions can be drawn. Toxicity was considered to be the presence of fetal morphologic and chromosomal alterations. The rates of preterm delivery, stillbirth, hematologic anomalies, and spontaneous abortion were also tabulated. The study noted that 83.3% of malformed live-born children involved the use of chemotherapy in the first trimester. Twelve of 15 infants with anomalies were treated with antimetabolites of deoxyribonucleic acid, ribonucleic acid, or proteins: methotrexate, mercaptopurine (Purinethol), thioguanine, 5-fluorouracil, or cytarabine (Cytosar-U). Low-dose methotrexate used to treat rheumatic disorders in this survey did not result in any abnormal congenital development. The fact that the majority of infants with birth defects had exposure to chemotherapy in the first trimester is not surprising because this is the period of organogenesis (55).

The four cases of stillbirth all involved antimetabolites; 4 of 15 patients who had spontaneous abortions received methotrexate. Only one case of third-trimester delivery of chemotherapy had an adverse outcome, with an infant with a normal karyotype and physical gaps in the chromosomes. Overall, 50% of all infants born were prematurely delivered. Overall, 77 (35%) of 217 children were delivered at term without complications. Table 5 collates study data with respect to drug and fetal outcome for all diseases and all gestational ages.

Breast-feeding during chemotherapy treatment is generally contraindicated. The effects of most agents on infants are unknown, and bottle-feeding is a reasonable alternative. There are scant data for the effects of cyclophosphamide, cisplatin, or doxorubicin on breast-fed infants. The published case reports are summarized in Table 6.

Summarizing the data for the various combination chemotherapy regimens is the only method of gathering significant numbers of cases to analyze to determine the fetotoxic effects of chemotherapy. A Registry of Pregnan-

TABLE 4. *Chemotherapy for germ cell tumors during pregnancy*

Histology	Reference	Chemotherapy regimen	Initiation of treatment (gestational age, wk)	Fetal outcome
Endodermal sinus tumor/ immature teratoma	48	PEB	20.5	Term delivery
Immature teratoma	49	PVB	19 (one course)	Term delivery
Endodermal sinus tumor	50	PVB	26.5	32-wk elective cesarean section; transient tachypnea
Endodermal sinus tumor	51	VAC	16	Term delivery; normal development at 33 mo
Endodermal sinus tumor	52	VAC	17	Induction at term
Endodermal sinus tumor	53	VAC	23	Premature delivery 33 wk

PEB, cisplatin (Platinol), etoposide, and bleomycin; PVB, cisplatin, vincristine, and bleomycin; VAC, vincristine, doxorubicin (Adriamycin), and cyclophosphamide.

TABLE 5. *Adverse fetal outcomes with chemotherapy*

Disease	Drug	No. of infants
Leukemias (n=96)	Cyclophosphamide	2 with ACD 1 with CA 4 with HA
	Cytarabine (Cytosar-U)	5 with ACD 1 with CA 6 with HA 3 stillborn
	Anthracycline antibiotics: daunorubicin HCl (Cerubidine), doxorubicin HCl (Adriamycin), idarubicin HCl (Idamycin)	3 with ACD 1 with CA 5 with HA
	Thiolated purines: 6-mercaptopurine (Purinethol), 6-thioguanine	4 with ACD 1 with CA 7 with HA
Malignant lymphomas (n=57)	Anthracycline antibiotics: daunorubicin, doxorubicin, idarubicin	1 spontaneous abortion 1 stillborn
	Thiolated purines: 6-mercaptopurine, 6-thioguanine	1 spontaneous abortion
	Vincristine sulfate	2 with ACD 2 spontaneous abortions 1 stillborn
	Vinblastine sulfate (Velban)	2 with ACD
	Procarbazine HCl (Matulane)	3 with ACD 2 spontaneous abortions
Rheumatic disorders (n=16)	Methotrexate	6 spontaneous abortions 2 immature
Gynecologic and breast neoplasms (n=26)	Methotrexate	2 with ACD 3 immature
	Cyclophosphamide	1 with ACD 1 spontaneous abortion
	Anthracycline antibiotics: daunorubicin, doxorubicin, idarubicin	4 immature
Severe miscellaneous disorders (n=22)	Methotrexate	2 with ACD 1 spontaneous abortion
	Interferon alfa	2 immature

ACD, abnormal congenital development; CA, chromosomal anomaly; HA, hematologic anomalies.
From ref. 54, with permission.

cies Exposed to Chemotherapeutic Agents has been established at the University of Pittsburgh. All clinicians who care for women receiving cancer chemotherapy during pregnancy should report their experiences to this database. For details or a patient abstract form, clinicians should contact Dr. John Mulvihill at the University of Pittsburgh (phone: 412-624-9951; fax: 412-624-3020; e-mail: jjm@helix.hgen.pitt.edu). Current first-line agents for the treatment of epithelial ovarian and germ cell tumors have unknown effects on the unborn fetus. Based on collated case report data, chemotherapy should be avoided in the first trimester, if at all possible. Treatment must be individualized for pregnant patients. The range of known toxicities must be discussed, along with the impact of delay of treatment for the

TABLE 6. *Adverse fetal effects of chemotherapeutic agents*

Age	Adverse fetal effect	Reference
Cyclophosphamide	Neutropenia	56, 57
Cisplatin	Unknown—present in milk	58
Doxorubicin	Unknown—present in milk	59

particular malignancy. Thus, the decision to delay or modify treatment plans can be made in conjunction with the wishes of the patient.

PROGNOSIS

Ovarian carcinoma diagnosed during pregnancy is rare, with an incidence of 1 in 18,000 to 1 in 25,000 pregnancies (8,9). Because of its rarity, there are no well designed studies outlining optimal treatment of ovarian cancer associated with pregnancy. Likewise, because the literature regarding ovarian cancer in pregnancy consists only of case reports and case series, it is difficult to estimate accurate survival rates. The largest reported series by Novak et al. (60) described 60 cases of malignant ovarian carcinoma during pregnancy, and the second largest series by Dgani et al. (10) described 23 cases. In all of these cases, multiple operations were performed, ranging from conservative to radical, and various regimens of radiotherapy and/or chemotherapy were used. Therapy was administered over a 25-year period, and many different modalities were used. Both series reported a high rate of 5-year survival: 76% (60) and 61% (10), including all stages. The high survival rates described in these studies are related to the early stage at which the disease was detected and the fact that the majority of neoplasms were not carcinomas, but tumors of low malignant potential. In general, survival rates for pregnant patients with ovarian malignancy parallel those for age-matched nonpregnant patients. As with ovarian cancers in general, the main prognostic parameters are tumor stage and histology.

REFERENCES

1. Hess, LW, Peaceman A, O'Brien WF, Winkel CA, Cruikshank DP, Morrison JC. Adnexal mass occurring with intrauterine pregnancy: report of fifty-four patients requiring laparotomy for definitive management. *Am J Obstet Gynecol* 1988;158:1029.
2. Platek DN, Henderson CE, Goldberg GL. The management of a persistent adnexal mass in pregnancy. *Am J Obstet Gynecol* 1995;173:1236.
3. Thornton C, Wells M. Ovarian cysts in pregnancy: does ultrasound make traditional management inappropriate? *Obstet Gynecol* 1987;69:717.
4. Roberts JA. Management of gynecologic tumors during pregnancy. *Clin Perinatol* 1983;10:369.
5. Bromley B, Benacerraf B. Adnexal masses during pregnancy: accuracy of sonographic diagnosis and outcome. *J Ultrasound Med* 1997;16:447.
6. Kort B, Kurtz VL, Watson WJ. The effect of nonobstetric operation during pregnancy. *Surg Gynecol Obstet* 1993;177:371.
7. Ballard CA. Ovarian tumor associated with pregnancy termination patients. *Am J Obstet Gynecol* 1984;149:384.
8. Jubb EB. Primary ovarian carcinoma in pregnancy. *Am J Obstet Gynecol* 1963;85:345.
9. Creasman WT, Rutledge F, Smith JP. Carcinoma of the ovary associated with pregnancy. *Obstet Gynecol* 1971;38:111.
10. Dgani R, Schwartz Z, Atar E, Zosmer A, Lancet M. Ovarian cancer during pregnancy: a study of 23 cases in Israel between the years 1960 and 1984. *Gynecol Oncol* 1989;33:326.
11. Benacerraf BR, Finkler NJ, Wolciechowski C, et al. Sonographic accuracy in the diagnosis of ovarian masses. *J Reprod Med* 1990;35:491.
12. Timor-Tritsch IE, Lerner JP, Monteagudo A, et al. Transvaginal ultrasonographic characterization of ovarian masses by means of color flow-directed Doppler measurements and a morphologic scoring system. *Am J Obstet Gynecol* 1993;168:909.
13. Hogston P, Lilford RJ. Ultrasound study of ovarian cysts in pregnancy: prevalence and significance. *Br J Obstet Gynaecol* 1986;83:625.
14. Wheeler TC, Fleischer AC. Complex adnexal mass in pregnancy: predictive value of color Doppler sonography. *J Ultrasound Med* 1997;16:425.
15. Lowe TW, Weinreb J, Santos-Ramos R, Cunningham FG. Magnetic resonance imaging in human pregnancy. *Obstet Gynecol* 1985;66:629.
16. Curtis M, Hopkins MP, Zarlingo T, Martino C, Graciansky-Lengyl M, Jenison EL. Magnetic resonance imaging to avoid laparotomy in pregnancy. *Obstet Gynecol* 1993;82:833.
17. Niloff JM, Knapp RC, Schaetzl E, Reynolds C, Bast RC. CA125 antigen levels in obstetric and gynecology patients. *Obstet Gynecol* 1984;64:703.
18. Mooney J, Silva E, Tomas C, Gershenson D. Unusual features of serous neoplasms of low malignant potential during pregnancy. *Gynecol Oncol* 1997;65:30.
19. Nelson MJ, Cavalieri R, Graham D, et al. Cysts in Pregnancy discovered by sonography. *J Clin Ultrasound* 1986;14:509.
20. Khaw T, Walker WJ. Ultrasound-guided fine needle aspiration of ovarian cysts: diagnosis and treatment in pregnant and non-pregnant women. *Clin Radiol* 1990;41:105.
21. Morice P, Louis-Sylvestre C, Chapron C, Dubuisson JB. Laparoscopy for adnexal torsion in pregnant women. *J Reprod Med* 1997;42:435.
22. Struyk AP, Treffers PE. Ovarian tumors in pregnancy. *Acta Obstet Gynecol Scand* 1984;63:421.
23. Fergusson JE II, Albright GA, Ueland K. Prevention of preterm labor following surgery. In: Baden JM, Brodsky JB, eds. *The pregnant surgical patient.* Mt Kisco, NY: Futura Publishing, 1985:223.
24. Effect of corticosteroids for fetal maturation on perinatal outcomes. NIH Consensus Development Conference Feb 28–Mar 2, 1994. *JAMA* 1995;273:413.

25. Guerrieri JP, Thomas RL. Open laparoscopy for an adnexal mass in pregnancy. *J Reprod Med* 1994;39:129.
26. Yuen PM, Chang A. Laparoscopic management of adnexal masses during pregnancy. *Acta Obstet Gynecol Scand* 1997;76:173.
27. Parker WH, Childers JM, Canis M, Phillips DR, Topel H. Laparoscopic management of benign cystic teratomas during pregnancy. *Am J Obstet Gynecol* 1996;174:1499.
28. Neiswander LL, Toub D. Laparoscopic excision of pelvic mass during pregnancy. *J Am Assoc Gynecol Laparosc* 1997;4:269.
29. Ready MB, Galan HL, Richards WE, et al. Laparoscopy during pregnancy: a survey of laparo-endoscopic surgeons. *J Reprod Med* 1997;42:33.
30. Curet MJ, Vogt DA, Schob O, Qualls C, Izquierdo LA, Zucker KA. Effects of CO_2 pneumoperitoneum in pregnant ewes. *J Surg Res* 1996;63:339.
31. Curet MJ, Allen D, Josloff RK, et al. Laparoscopy during pregnancy. *Arch Surg* 1996;131:546.
32. Beicher NA, Battery BW, Fortune DW, Macafee CA. Growth and malignancy of ovarian tumors in pregnancy. *Am J Obstet Gynecol* 1971;11:208.
33. Thigpen JT, Blessing JA, Ball H, Hummel SJ, Barrett RJ. Phase II trial of paclitaxel in patients with progressive ovarian carcinoma after platinum-based chemotherapy: a Gynecologic Oncology Group study. *J Clin Oncol* 1994;12:1748.
34. Ozols RF. Gynecologic Oncology Group trials in ovarian carcinoma. *Semin Oncol* 1997;24(1 suppl 2):S2–S10.
35. du Bois A, Luck HJ, Meier W, et al. Carboplatin plus paclitaxel as first-line chemotherapy in previously untreated advanced ovarian cancer. German AGO Study Group Ovarian Cancer. Arbeitsgemeinschaft Gynäkologische Onkologie. *Semin Oncol* 1997;24(4 suppl 11):S11.
36. Meerpohl HG, du Bois A, Luck HJ, et al. Paclitaxel combined with carboplatin in the first-line treatment of advanced ovarian cancer: a phase I trial. *Semin Oncol* 1997;24(1 suppl 2):S2–S17.
37. Tomlinson MW, Treadwell MC, Deppe G. Platinum-based chemotherapy to treat recurrent Sertoli-Leydig cell ovarian carcinoma during pregnancy. *Eur J Gynaecol Oncol* 1997;18:44.
38. Henderson CE, Giovanni E, Garfinkel D, Poirier MC, Shamkhani H, Runowicz CD. Platinum chemotherapy during pregnancy for serous cystadenocarcinoma of the ovary. *Gynecol Oncol* 1993;49:92.
39. King LA, Nevin PC, Williams PP, Carson LF. Treatment of advanced epithelial ovarian carcinoma in pregnancy with cisplatin-based chemotherapy. *Gynecol Oncol* 1991;41:78.
40. Malfetano JH, Goldkrand JW. Cis-platinum combination chemotherapy during pregnancy for advanced epithelial ovarian carcinoma. *Obstet Gynecol* 1990;75: 545.
41. Scialli AR, Waterhouse TB, Desesso JM, Rahman A, Goeringer GC. Protective effect of liposome encapsulation on paclitaxel developmental toxicity in the rat. *Teratology* 1997;56:305.
42. Kai S, Kohmura H, Hiraiwa E, et al. Reproductive and developmental toxicity studies of paclitaxel. III. Intravenous administration to rats during the perinatal and lactation periods. *J Toxicol Sci* 1994;19(suppl 1):9.
43. Slayton RE, Park RC, Silverberg SG, Shingleton H, Creasman WT, Blessing JA. Vincristine, dactinomycin, and cyclophosphamide in the treatment of malignant germ cell tumors of the ovary: a Gynecologic Oncology Group study (a final report). *Cancer* 1985;56:243.
44. Wong LC, Collins RJ, Ngan HY, Ma HK. Etoposide combination chemotherapy in refractory ovarian malignant germ cell tumor. *Gynecol Oncol* 1990;39:123.
45. Hansen SW, Daugaard G, Rorth M. Treatment of persistent or relapsing advanced germ cell neoplasms with cisplatin, etoposide and bleomycin. *Eur J Cancer Clin Oncol* 1986;22:595.
46. Motzer RJ, Sheinfeld J, Mazumdar M, et al. Etoposide and cisplatin adjuvant therapy for patients with pathologic stage II germ cell tumors. *J Clin Oncol* 1995;13: 2700.
47. De Palo G, Zambetti M, Pilotti S, et al. Nondysgerminomatous tumors of the ovary treated with cisplatin, vinblastine, and bleomycin: long-term results. *Gynecol Oncol* 1992;47:239.
48. Horbelt D, Delmore J, Meisel R, Cho S, Roberts D, Logan D. Mixed germ cell malignancy of the ovary concurrent with pregnancy. *Obstet Gynecol* 1994;84:662.
49. Christman JE, Teng NNH, Lebovic GS, Sikic BI. Delivery of a normal infant following cisplatin, vinblastine, and bleomycin (PVB) chemotherapy for malignant teratoma of the ovary during pregnancy. *Gynecol Oncol* 1990;37:292.
50. Malone JM, Gershenson DM, Creasy RK, Kavanagh JJ, Silva EG, Stringer CA. Endodermal sinus tumor of the ovary associated with pregnancy. *Obstet Gynecol* 1986; 68(suppl):86S.
51. Kim DS, Moon IP. Maternal and fetal survival following surgery and chemotherapy of endodermal sinus tumor of the ovary during pregnancy: a case report. *Obstet Gynecol* 1989;73:503.
52. Metz SA, Day TG, Pursell SH. Adjuvant chemotherapy in a pregnant patient with endodermal sinus tumor of the ovary. *Gynecol Oncol* 1988;32:371.
53. Weed JC, Roh RA, Mendenhall HW. Recurrent endodermal sinus tumor during pregnancy. *Obstet Gynecol* 1979;55(suppl):90S.
54. Ebert U, Loffler H, Kirch W. Cytotoxic therapy and pregnancy. *Pharmacol Ther* 1997;74:207.
55. Barber HR. Fetal and neonatal effects of cytotoxic agents. *Obstet Gynecol* 1981;58(suppl):41S.
56. Wiernik PH, Duncan JH. Cyclophosphamide in human milk. *Lancet* 1971;1:912.
57. Amato D, Niblett JS. Neutropenia from cyclophosphamide in breast milk. *Med J Aust* 1977;1:383.
58. De Vries EGE, Van Der Zee AGJ, Uges DRA, Sleijfer D. Excretion of platinum into breast milk. *Lancet* 1989; 1:497.
59. Egan PC, Costanza ME, Dodion P, Egorin MJ, Baccur NR. Doxorubicin and cisplatin excretion into human milk. *Cancer Treat Rep* 1985;69:1387.
60. Novak ER, Lambrou CO, Woodruff JO. Ovarian tumors in pregnancy. *Obstet Gynecol* 1975;46:401.

12

Other Cancers in Pregnancy

Seamus O'Reilly and *Anuradha Chakravarthy

Department of Oncology, Waterford Regional Hospital, Waterford, Ireland;
Johns Hopkins University School of Medicine, Baltimore, Maryland 21287;
**Department of Radiation Oncology, Vanderbilt University, Nashville, Tennessee 37232*

The American College of Obstetricians and Gynecologists estimates that approximately 3500 cases of cancer occur in pregnant women annually in the United States (1). No situation in oncology evokes more fear and anxiety in patients and physicians than the discovery of malignancy in pregnancy. Cancer complicates pregnancy even more frequently than appendicitis, thyrotoxicosis, nephrolithiasis, or deep vein thrombosis (2). It has been estimated that 1 in 1000 pregnant women will be affected by some malignancy, with 1 in 118 malignancies being associated with pregnancy (3,4). Although most neoplasms have their peak incidences beyond the reproductive years, 13% of all cancers occur between ages 15 and 34 years. With the trend toward delaying pregnancy until the fourth decade, the incidence of cancer in pregnancy is likely to increase. Pregnancy neither predisposes women to nor protects them from the development of cancer; therefore the most frequently encountered malignancies during pregnancy are similar to those observed in nonpregnant women of similar ages (2) (Table 1). Management of these malignancies involves the care of two patients, the mother and the fetus, and should involve a multidisciplinary team including medical, surgical, gynecologic, and radiation oncologists, neonatologists, obstetricians, midwives and social workers. Treatment decisions must be individualized, based on the nature and location of the tumor, the period of gestation, and the desire to continue with the pregnancy.

As illustrated in Table 1, the most common malignancies affecting pregnancy are the hematologic malignancies and breast, cervical, and ovarian cancers. The purpose of this chapter is to discuss the management of the other, less common solid tumor malignancies during pregnancy. Symptoms of pregnancy may confound the presentation of malignancies, and delays in diagnosis in this population are therefore common. Once a malignancy is diagnosed, concerns exist because of the toxicity of therapies and diagnostic procedures for the mother and fetus, as well as the effect of the timing of these diagnostic and therapeutic procedures on the birth of the in-

TABLE 1. *Incidence of cancer during pregnancy*

Type	Estimated frequency
Cervix	1/1200 to 1/2200
Breast	1/3000 to 1/10,000
Melanoma	1/360 to 1/7100
Hodgkin's lymphoma	1/6100
Ovary	1/12,000 to 1/25,000
Colorectal	up to 1/10,000
Leukemia	1/75,000
Non-Hodgkin's lymphoma	Rare
Thyroid	Rare

From ref. 1, with permission.

TABLE 2. *Pharmacokinetic factors affected during pregnancy*

Pharmacokinetic factor	Effect
Volume of distribution	Increased
Peak drug concentration	Decreased
Half-life	Increased or decreased
Concentration over time (AUC)	Increased or decreased
Drug absorption	Increased or decreased
Enterohepatic recirculation	Increased or decreased
Protein binding	Increased
Renal clearance	Increased
Hepatic clearance	Increased or decreased

AUC, area under the plasma concentration versus time curve.
Modified from ref. 5, with permission.

fant. As in nonpregnant patients, the management of such patients may require surgery, chemotherapy, or radiotherapy. Of these modalities, chemotherapy use in pregnancy is the most complex in terms of risks both to the mother and to the fetus. Use of these agents, which have a narrow therapeutic index, is compounded by physiologic changes in pregnant patients that alter drug exposure (5) (Table 2) and by the relative dearth of information concerning the use of anticancer drugs during pregnancy.

Chemotherapeutic agents act on rapidly proliferating cells and are therefore teratogenic. The effects of chemotherapy on the fetus are influenced by the agent, timing of exposure, duration and frequency of exposure, and ability of the agent to cross the placenta. Fetal drug metabolism may be immature, allowing certain drugs to accumulate, particularly in newborn infants who lack a placental route of excretion. The risks of chemotherapy are generally greatest in the first trimester, when organogenesis occurs and is completed for all organs except the central nervous system (CNS) and the gonads (6). After the first trimester, the risk of birth defects is decreased, and intrauterine growth retardation (IUGR) becomes the dominant effect (7). Chemotherapy may also induce myelosuppression in the fetus and newborn infant. The Toronto Leukemia Study Group reported that one-third of all infants exposed *in utero* had pancytopenia at birth (8).

While standardized treatment regimens exist for many solid tumor malignancies, available data on the use of chemotherapy in pregnancy are limited. Treatment decisions should be individualized for each patient (9). There is evidence that synergistic teratogenic interactions may occur with combination chemotherapy (10) or combinations of chemotherapy and radiotherapy (11). In a comprehensive review of chemotherapy use in pregnancy, Wiebe and Sipila (5) suggested several strategies by which fetal risk from cancer chemotherapy could be reduced (Table 3). These strategies should be incorporated into the development of individualized treatment regimens for pregnant patients receiving chemotherapy. A Registry of Pregnancies Exposed to Chemotherapeutic Agents has been established by the National Cancer Institute to in-

TABLE 3. *Pharmacologic variables that increase fetal risk during pregnancy*

Pharmacologic variable	Avoidance of risk
Stage of fetal development during drug exposure	Avoid exposure during the first trimester, particularly weeks 3–12
High concentration over time (AUC)	Avoid high-dose, long-term therapy
Extent of placental drug penetration	Avoid high-dose, long-term therapy
Mechanism of action of drug	Avoid agents known to cause birth defects: folic acid antagonists, purine and pyrimidine antagonists, and alkylating agents
Timing of delivery to last dose of chemotherapy	Allow sufficient time between delivery and last dose of chemotherapy Provide enough time for both fetal and maternal counts to recover
Route of drug administration	Avoid using peritoneal and orally administered agents whose absorption may be altered in late pregnancy
Pharmacologic third spacing of drugs	Avoid drugs known to accumulate in fluid-filled compartments, such as methotrexate, particularly in late pregnancy

AUC, area under the plasma concentration versus time curve.

crease knowledge in this area (12). All clinicians who care for women receiving cancer chemotherapy during pregnancy should report their experiences to this database. For details or a patient abstract form, clinicians should contact Dr. John Mulvihill at the University of Pittsburgh (phone: 412-624-9951, fax: 412-624-3020, email: jjm@helix.hgen.pitt.edu).

Several factors need to be considered in the evaluation of the role of radiation in pregnancy. First and foremost, the well-being of the pregnant cancer patient must be taken into account. Whether the fetus can be saved with a reasonable chance for normal fetal development is a secondary consideration. To better understand the effects of radiation in pregnancy, it is necessary to review some of the fundamentals of radiobiology.

BASICS OF RADIOBIOLOGY

Radiation during pregnancy can cause somatic effects such as the induction of cancer (carcinogenesis) or developmental effects on the fetus (teratogenesis). Lethal effects can occur before birth (prenatal death) or at or about the time of birth (neonatal death). Malformations or gross abnormalities of body structures or IUGR without gross malformations may also occur (13).

The important factors are (a) dose and (b) stage of gestation. Dose rate is also an important variable. Many congenital anomalies are present without any radiation. Any conclusions regarding the role of radiation in causing fetal damage must be compared to this natural level of birth defects. Approximately, 15% of developing embryos spontaneously abort, 3% have major malformations, 4% have IUGR, and 10% have genetic diseases (14). Therefore, one needs to study enormous numbers of patients to reliably determine changes from this natural baseline.

The linear accelerator is currently the most common method of delivering external-beam radiation for the treatment of cancer. It is a device that uses high-frequency electromagnetic waves to accelerate charged particles such as electrons to high energies through a linear tube. The high-energy electron beam can be used to treat superficial tumors or to strike a target to produce photons to treat deep tumors. To shape the treatment beam, it is collimated by pairs of tungsten blocks. To further shape the beam, special blocks are molded for each patient. At times, specially shaped blocks called wedges are needed to ensure dose homogeneity and compensate for varying body shapes.

The dose to the fetus is the sum total of both the primary and scattered components. The primary dose is that contributed by the original photons emitted from the linear accelerator. In cases in which the fetus can be entirely excluded from the radiation field, this primary dose can be eliminated. There are two forms of scattered dose. This includes the dose that results from scatter caused by the patient's body (internal scatter) and that from external sources such as the collimator, blocks, and wedges.

The fetal dose varies with the energy of radiation used, field size, and distance from the site requiring treatment to the fetus. Although internal scatter occurring from radiation to the mother cannot be reduced, secondary scatter can be reduced by a variety of methods. Methods to decrease secondary scatter include avoiding the use of wedges and blocks. In this case, use of small, collimated fields would be more effective.

Since radiation dose falls in proportion to the square of the distance, the single most important factor to decrease fetal dose is distance from the field edge to the fetus (15). The larger the field size is, the greater is the ratio of the dose to the fetus to the central-axis dose. As a general guide, at 10 cm from the field edge, the dose is 1% of the mother's exposure dose (16).

The effects of radiation on the fetus vary with gestational age (13). Gestation can be divided into the following periods:

- Preimplantation: 0 to 9 days
- Early organogenesis: 2 to 8 weeks
- Late organogenesis: 8 to 15 weeks
- Fetal period: 15 weeks onward

The preimplantation period is the most sensitive to the lethal effects of radiation. This leads to spontaneous abortions that are often not even recognized as pregnancies. It is therefore impossible to study this in humans. Experiments in rats show that 10 cGy in this period results in embryonic resorption in 11.9% versus 4.7% in unirradiated controls. Embryos that survive are normal with no congenital anomalies or abnormalities of growth (16).

During early organogenesis, the risk of structural malformations, as well as IUGR, is highest. Neonates of mothers who underwent abdominal diagnostic x-rays with doses of 0.5 Gy or greater were found to have malformations such as microcephaly (17). The risk of microcephaly was increased in Hiroshima and Nagasaki atomic bombing survivors who received 0.06 to 0.31 Gy of radiation.

During late organogenesis, mental retardation was observed in survivors of the atomic bombings. The frequency of mental retardation appears to vary linearly with dose. The dose–response relationship is consistent with a threshold dose of 0.25 to 0.28 Gy (18). The Committee on the Biological Effects of Ionizing Radiations (BEIR III) concluded that readily measurable damage could be observed at doses less than 10 cGy delivered during sensitive stages of development (19).

A retrospective case–control study initially suggested that *in utero* exposure to radiation from diagnostic x-rays increased the risk of cancer (20). Although initial follow-up of prenatally exposed atomic bombing survivors did not support this study (21), a more recent review found that patients exposed *in utero* have an excess absolute risk coefficient of approximately 6% per gray (22). As these patients are now approaching the age when the cancer incidence begins to rise, it will be important to continue close follow-up to determine whether *in utero* exposure increases adult cancer risk. Several studies have demonstrated no increase in abortion, IUGR, or congenital malformations from diagnostic exposures less than 0.05 Gy delivered at any time during gestation (14). Nevertheless, no proven safe threshold dose of radiation exposure to the fetus has been established (23). Therefore, diagnostic studies using ionizing radiation should be limited to those that are absolutely essential.

BLADDER CANCER

Cancer of the urinary bladder is rarely observed during pregnancy. By 1995, 13 cases of nonbilharzial tumors had been reported in the literature (24). The histology in nine of these cases was transitional cell carcinoma, with the majority of patients presenting with hematuria. Initial evaluation of patients presenting with hematuria should include urine culture and subsequently cytologic examination and ultrasonography. Cystoscopy can be performed safely under local anesthesia during pregnancy, as can subsequent transurethral resection of a bladder tumor. If an invasive tumor is found, then formal staging for metastatic disease is required. Magnetic resonance (MR) imaging is safe during pregnancy (25). In cases diagnosed late in the second or in the third trimester, a cesarean section can be performed at the time of radical cystectomy and urinary diversion. In invasive disease at earlier stages of pregnancy, management is dictated by parental wishes about termination of pregnancy.

CENTRAL NERVOUS SYSTEM MALIGNANCIES

Intracranial and spinal tumors are rare in the general population, and the presentation of such tumors during pregnancy is even more uncommon. In the former East Germany, where all CNS malignancies were recorded, 17 pregnant patients were diagnosed with malignant brain tumors between 1961 and 1979, yielding a frequency of 3.6 per 1 million live births (26). It has been estimated that in the United States 90 women per year would be pregnant and have a brain tumor (27). The types of brain tumors seen in such patients are identical to those observed in nonpregnant women of the same age (28,29) (Table 4).

TABLE 4. *Brain tumors in pregnancy*

Tumor	n
Glioma	62
Meningioma	57
Acoustic neuroma	30
Cerebellar astrocytoma	12
Medulloblastoma	6
Plexus papilloma	5
Ependymoma	3
Pinealoma	1
Other	19
Total	195

Modified from refs. 28, 29, with permission.

These tumors present with a combination of nonspecific and specific symptoms and signs. Nonspecific symptoms include headache in about 50% of patients and nausea and vomiting in 25% (29). The latter can be confused with morning sickness. However, unlike morning sickness, it does not resolve after the first trimester and does not improve with time. Constant, daily headache should not be attributed to pregnancy, particularly in patients without a prior history of headache. Development of seizures during pregnancy is more likely to suggest eclampsia, particularly if it occurs in the second half of pregnancy. However, focal seizures are rare with eclampsia, and associated signs of edema, proteinuria, hypertension, and generalized hyperreflexia are absent in patients with brain tumors. The presence of lateralizing neurologic symptoms or signs necessitates neurodiagnostic evaluation with a gadolinium-enhanced MR imaging.

Of diagnosed tumors, glial neoplasms are the most common. Some of these tumors are categorized into low-grade tumors consisting of astrocytomas and oligodendrogliomas. Treatment for these low-grade tumors involves surgical resection. While surgery can be safely performed during pregnancy, urgent treatment of a low-grade glioma is almost never necessary, as often it has been present for several years before diagnosis and may persist for many more without causing disability. The role of adjuvant radiation in these low-grade lesions is controversial. As they are slow-growing tumors, adjuvant radiation for incompletely resected lesions could be deferred until after delivery. There is no established role for chemotherapy in this disease.

In contrast to low-grade gliomas, anaplastic astrocytoma, anaplastic oligodendroglioma, and glioblastoma multiforme are highly malignant and aggressive neoplasms that require prompt diagnosis and treatment. Patients with these lesions should undergo surgical debulking of the tumor. Surgery may not be feasible if the tumor is bilateral, involves the midline, or is restricted to deep structures. In patients with such tumors, surgery should not be delayed until after the completion of pregnancy. Following surgery, adjuvant radiotherapy and in some cases chemotherapy are recommended (30). The timing of these procedures is dictated by the stage of pregnancy, as these modalities pose considerable risk to the fetus and should be tailored to the individual patient. Cranial radiotherapy (using abdominal shielding and small collimated beams to reduce external scatter, and carefully designed fields and ports to reduce internal scatter) may have to be administered to some pregnant patients for whom it is unsafe to wait until after delivery (e.g., those with unresectable tumors in the second trimester). Phantom studies, as well as clinical measurements, in patients using thermoluminescent dosimeters show that brain tumors can be irradiated to a high-dose resulting in fetal exposures of less than 0.1 Gy.

Additional considerations in the management of these patients during pregnancy include the use of anticonvulsants and corticosteroids (31). Because of the teratogenic potential of these agents, women treated for CNS malignancies should be jointly managed with a neurologist. Prednisone is the preferred corticosteroid because it is metabolized before crossing the placenta. Systemic corticosteroids may serve a dual purpose in pregnant women being considered for early delivery to facilitate treatment of a brain tumor, as agents such as dexamethasone hasten pulmonary maturation *in utero*. Labor and delivery can result in significant increases in intracranial pressure that are normally well tolerated but can lead to brain stem herniation in patients with intracranial tumors (32). Consequently, most patients with significant space-occupying lesions will require cesarean section. For discussion of benign intracranial neoplasms in pregnancy, the reader is referred to several recent reviews (29,33).

Brain metastases are rarely diagnosed during pregnancy. However, their management follows similar lines to those for nonpregnant patients. Surgical resection is usually reserved for patients who have a single metastatic lesion or require urgent decompression (e.g., those with a tumor obstructing the fourth ventricle). Chemotherapy and radiotherapy are usually avoided because of the risks to the fetus. If the clinical situation does not permit delaying treatment until after delivery, radiation with appropriate shielding can be utilized to help palliate symptoms.

COLORECTAL CANCER

The incidence of colon cancer during pregnancy has been variously estimated at 0.1% to 0.001% (34,35). The coexistence of these conditions is rare, with only 205 cases in the medical literature between 1842 and 1991 (36). Review of these cases and a postal survey of the membership of the American Society of Colon and Rectal Surgeons indicate a predominance of rectal lesions in this population and a tendency for patients to have more advanced stages of disease, with more than 60% of patients presenting with Dukes' stage C or D disease (36). The basis for the predominance of these tumors in the rectum is unclear and may reflect a detection bias based on performing rectal examinations during pregnancy, or straining during labor and delivery that makes these lesions more detectable. Delay in diagnosis, reflected by the advanced stage of most patients, is common because the initial symptoms may be attributable to normal pregnancy.

Management of pregnant patients with colorectal cancer depends on gestational age. If the tumor is diagnosed before week 20 of pregnancy, treatment of the cancer should take precedence, and a definitive cancer operation should be performed (37). Abdominoperineal resection for low-lying tumors is feasible up to 20 weeks' gestation (38). A colostomy may be performed if the tumor is obstructing or unresectable. However, the majority of these tumors are diagnosed in late pregnancy. In this regard, surgical treatment, particularly for low-lying tumors, should wait until after uterine involution, as there is an increased risk of bleeding due to engorgement of the pelvic veins (37).

Following surgery, adjuvant chemotherapy with 5-fluorouracil (5-FU) and radiotherapy should be considered for patients with Dukes' stages B2 or C lesions (39). Use of 5-FU during pregnancy has been associated with complications: multiple anomalies when used in the first trimester, and reversible bone marrow suppression in the neonatal period when used in the second trimester (40). Therapeutic doses of radiation administered to the fetus are lethal, and therefore patients requiring such treatment would need to undergo a therapeutic abortion. Consequently, adjuvant therapy or chemotherapy for palliative treatment of metastatic disease should not be used during pregnancy.

LUNG CANCER

Lung cancer is now the most common fatal malignancy in women (41). Despite recent advances in treatment, the overall long-term survival of patients with lung cancer remains poor with 5-year survival rates of 10% to 15%. In a recent epidemiologic study from Detroit, Michigan, the majority of cases of lung cancer were found to occur in the sixth, seventh, and eighth decades of life, with only 9% of cases occurring in patients younger than 50 years and 1.2% occurring in patients younger than 40 (42). Consequently, the occurrence of lung cancer during pregnancy is rare but is likely to increase as the prevalence of smoking in young women continues to rise. In addition, this study demonstrated that younger patients were less likely to present with localized, and therefore potentially curable, disease.

The occurrence of lung cancer in pregnancy has been reported in 12 cases in the literature (43). In all cases, the outcome was poor, with maternal death occurring in 9 of 10 cases within 9 months of diagnosis. Such poor outcomes were related in part to delays in diagnosis. Symptoms of hemoptysis and dyspnea are often assumed to be due to infection, while pain from bone metastasis may often be assumed to be pregnancy-related. This issue is further compounded because of concerns regarding the effects of using imaging studies during pregnancy.

Once lung cancer is diagnosed, management is guided by the histologic subtype and stage of the malignancy, gestational age, and whether or not the patient wishes to continue the pregnancy. Patients with resectable (stages I and II and selected patients with stage IIIA) non–small cell lung cancer should be treated with surgical resection (44). In these patients, surgery can be delayed until the second trimester when organogenesis is complete and the risk of spontaneous abortion is lower. For patients with more advanced stages of disease or with unresectable tumor, treatment is palliative and may involve radiotherapy to symptomatic sites (e.g., painful bone lesions, superior vena cava obstruction) with appropriate abdominal shielding. In nonpregnant patients with localized unresectable intrathoracic disease, the addition of cisplatin-based chemotherapy to radiotherapy may improve survival (44). However, use of such radiosensitizing treatment in pregnancy is compounded by the dearth of information about the safety of cisplatin in pregnancy. Preclinical studies indicate that this agent can cross the placenta and accumulate in fetal tissue (45). Three case reports of its use in pregnancy have not documented any fetal side effects when it was administered in the second or third trimester (5).

For small cell lung cancer, a combination of chemotherapy and thoracic radiotherapy is used when the disease has a limited stage, whereas patients with extensive-stage disease are managed with chemotherapy alone. Management of pregnant patients with this condition is particularly complex because of concerns regarding the safety of chemotherapy. Because of the risks during organogenesis, it is best to avoid treatment in the first trimester, if possible. However, if the situation arises where chemotherapy must be used, then doxorubicin hydrochloride (Adriamycin) and vinca alkaloids appear to be less teratogenic than other agents (5). In the second or third trimester, single-agent cisplatin (Platinol) or combination cisplatin and doxorubicin would be reasonable. However, treatment decisions need to be individualized, and the benefits of combination therapy must outweigh the risks of higher toxicity to the mother and greater risk to the fetus.

MELANOMA

Melanoma complicating pregnancy has a reported incidence of 2.8 per 1000 deliveries (46). Since 1951 when Pack and Scharnagel (47) reported an unfavorable outcome for patients diagnosed with melanoma during pregnancy, the biologic behavior of this disease during pregnancy has been controversial. However, more recent studies have demonstrated no difference in survival between pregnant patients and stage-matched, nonpregnant controls (48–50).

A majority of melanomas arise in a preexisting nevus, usually located on the lower extremities in women. Melanoma can be diagnosed very early in its development. Grin et al. (51) reported the clinical diagnosis of melanoma was correct in almost 85% of a series of 265 histologically confirmed melanomas. Physical examination and biopsy of suspicious lesions is essential. Pigmented lesions that change rapidly (over weeks to months) in color, shape, or size or that bleed, become inflamed, itch, or are more than 7 mm in diameter should be assessed (52). Treatment of these lesions is surgical excision with adequate margins depending on lesion size. Recent studies have demonstrated a survival advantage for patients with high-risk melanoma who received interferon alfa-2b (Intron A) for 1 year after surgical excision (53). However, data on the use of this biologic-response modifier in pregnancy is limited. For patients who present with metastatic disease or in whom metastatic disease develops, treatment options are limited regardless of pregnancy. Single-agent dacarbazine (DTIC-Dome) has a response rate of 20% in this disease (54) and has been used successfully in the second and third trimesters of pregnancy (55).

PHEOCHROMOCYTOMA

In 1982, Schenker and Granat (56) reported that maternal and fetal mortality from pheochromocytoma occurring during pregnancy were 40% and 56%, respectively, if the condition was undiagnosed during pregnancy. With correct diagnosis and management, these rates can decline to 0 and 15%, respectively (57). The diagnosis of pheochromocytoma during pregnancy is often missed, as the tumor has no pathognomonic signs or symptoms. Hypertension, though the most common sign of this tumor, may often be attributable to essential hypertension, preeclampsia, or eclampsia. Supine hypertension is an important sign in pregnant patients (58). Additional symptoms and signs include sweating, palpitations, headache, and tachycardia.

Diagnosis of pheochromocytoma is made by analysis of a 24-hour urine collection sample for epinephrine, norepinephrine, metanephrine, and vanillylmandelic acid (59). Plasma catecholamine levels can also be used (60). Pregnancy does not elevate urinary catecholamine values into the diagnostic range for pheochromocytoma. Once the tumor is diagnosed, localization involves ultrasonography or MR imaging. Ultrasonography has a sensitivity of 89% to 97% for adrenal masses; however, extramedullary tumor can occur, limiting ultrasound's role. Iodine-131 metaiodobenzylguanidine, used in scintigraphy, has never been tested in pregnancy (61–64).

For all patients, preoperative α-adrenergic blockade is necessary (65–67). Phenoxybenzamine hydrochloride (Dibenzyline) or prazosin hydrochloride (Minipress) is started 1 to 2 weeks before surgery. Once adequate α-adrenergic blockade has been established, β-adrenergic blockade with propranolol hydrochloride (Inderal) can be initiated. Once blood pressure is controlled, surgery can be performed usually through a midline incision, allowing visualization of adrenal glands and periaortic tissues and permitting delivery by cesarean section. While successful vaginal delivery has been performed in patients with pheochromocytoma (68), it should be avoided, as labor and delivery may cause significant autonomic stress. Despite adequate adrenergic blockade, hypertensive crisis can occur during surgery, particularly during tumor palpation. Sodium nitroprusside (Nitropress) is the agent of choice to control these events because of its fast onset of action; intraoperative cardiac arrhythmias can be managed by lidocaine hydrochloride (Xylocaine HCl) or β-aderenergic blocking agents (69,70).

THYROID CANCER

The exact incidence of thyroid cancer in pregnancy is unknown (71). However, certain types, such as papillary adenocarcinoma, have a peak incidence in the reproductive years (72). The majority of these tumors present as a thyroid nodule that is evaluable by clinical examination, ultrasonography, and thyroid function testing. Use of radioisotopes during pregnancy is contraindicated (73). Management involves surgery and radioiodine use and depends on tumor stage, degree of differentiation, histologic subtype, and gestational age at diagnosis. Radioactive iodine is used to ablate remaining thyroid tissue following thyroidectomy for thyroid cancer. Unfortunately, once the fetal thyroid begins to function and accumulate radioiodine (10 to 12 weeks' gestation), fetal absorbed doses of 5000 cGy per 1 mCi of I 131 administered to the mother can occur. Therefore, pregnancy is an absolute contraindication to the use of radioactive iodine; the risk of cretinism is too high. As thyroid cancer is often a slow-growing disease, treatment can often be delayed until after delivery.

Patients previously treated with high doses of I 131 for thyroid cancer safely undergo pregnancy. In a study of 70 women treated with I 131, the estimated gonadal dose was 10 to 63 cGy. Seventy-three children were followed: One child had tetralogy of Fallot, and three had low birthweight. Two spontaneous abortions occurred (74). We advise patients to wait at least 1 year following administration of I 131 to become pregnant.

SUMMARY

The diagnosis of cancer rarely complicates pregnancy. For patients with malignancies during pregnancy, management is predominantly surgical, with radiotherapy and chemotherapy having relatively limited roles. Occasionally, the latter two modalities offer the only reasonable hope for palliation or cure in patients with cancer. Their use is complicated by risks to the mother, as well as to the fetus. Ionizing radiation should be avoided during pregnancy whenever possible. If it cannot be avoided, it must be delivered with as little dose to the fetus as possible, utilizing the lowest energy, smallest field, and maximal blocking. With respect to chemotherapy, the timing of its use is probably the single most important variable in terms of its effects on the fetus, because there are no reports of an increase in the incidence of congenital malformations in infants exposed after the first trimester. Exposure to chemotherapy during this crucial stage of organogenesis has been reported to result in malformations in 17% to 25% of infants (75). However, when folic acid antagonists were excluded, the incidence of congenital malformations among exposed infants fell to 6%. Use of chemotherapy in the second and third trimesters can result in IUGR and pancytopenia. Further studies are needed to document the effects of chemotherapy administration on neurologic function, as brain development continues during the second and third trimesters (76). It is hoped that with the development of a National Cancer Institute database, information about the long-term effects of cancer chemotherapy can improve. In the interim, management of pregnant patients needs to be individualized and multidisciplinary, with careful consideration of the risks and benefits involved at each stage of pregnancy.

REFERENCES

1. Waalen J. Pregnancy poses tough questions for cancer treatment. *J Natl Cancer Inst* 1991;83:900.
2. Shivvers SA, Miller DS. Preinvasive and invasive breast and cervical cancer prior to or during pregnancy. *Clin Perinatol* 1997;24:369.
3. Donegan WL. Cancer and pregnancy. *CA Cancer J Clin* 1993;33:194.
4. Allan HH, Nisker JA. Cancer in pregnancy: an overview. In: Allen HH, Nisker JA, eds. *Cancer in pregnancy:* therapeutic guidelines. Mt Kisco, NY: Futura Publishing, 1986:3.
5. Wiebe VJ, Sipila PEH. Pharmacology of antineoplastic agents in pregnancy. *Crit Rev Oncol Hematol* 1994;16:75.
6. Sorosky JI, Sood AK, Buekers TE. The use of chemotherapeutic agents during pregnancy. *Obstet Gynecol Clin North Am* 1997;24:591.
7. Nettleton J, Long H, Kuban D, et al. Breast cancer during pregnancy: quantifying the risk of treatment delay. *Obstet Gynecol* 1996;87:414.
8. Reynoso EE, Shepherd FA, Messner HA, et al. Acute leukemia during pregnancy: The Toronto Leukemia Study Group experience with long-term follow-up of children exposed *in utero* to chemotherapeutic agents. *J Clin Oncol* 1987;5:1098.
9. Ebert U, Loffler H, Kirch W. Cytotoxic therapy and pregnancy. *Pharmacol Ther* 1997;74:207.
10. Mulvihill JJ, McKeen EA, Rosner F. Pregnancy outcome in cancer patients: experience in a large co-operative group. *Cancer* 1987;60:1143.
11. Toledo TM, Harper RC, Moser RH. Fetal effects during cyclophosphamide and irradiation therapy. *Ann Intern Med* 1971;74:87.
12. Randall T. National registry seeks scarce data on pregnancy outcomes during chemotherapy. *JAMA* 1993;269: 323.
13. Hall EJ, Effects of radiation on the embryo and fetus. In: Hall ED, ed. *Radiobiology for the radiologist*, 4th ed. Philadelphia: JB Lippincott Co, 1994:363–378.
14. Brent RL. The effects of embryonic and fetal exposure to x-ray, microwaves, and ultrasound: counseling the pregnant and non-pregnant patient about these risks. *Semin Oncol* 1989;16:347.
15. Nakagawa K, Aoki Y, Kusama T, Ban N, Nakagawa S, Sasaki Y. Radiotherapy during pregnancy: effects on fetuses and neonates. *Clin Ther* 1997;19:770.
16. Brent RL, Ghorson RO. Radiation exposure in pregnancy. *Curr Probl Radiol* 1972;2:2.
17. Debaken AS. Abnormalities in children exposed to x-radiation during various stages of gestation: tentative timetable of radiation injury to the human fetus. *J Nucl Med* 1968;9:471.
18. Otake M, Schull WJ, Lee S. Threshold for radiation-related severe mental retardation in prenatally exposed A-bomb survivors: a re-analysis. *Int J Radiat Biol* 1996; 70:755.

19. Committee on the Biological Effects of Ionizing Radiations BEIR III. *The effects on populations of exposure to low levels of ionizing radiation*. Washington, DC: National Academy of Sciences, 1980.
20. Stewart A, Kneale GW. Radiation dose effects in relation to obstetric x-rays and childhood cancers. *Lancet* 1970;1:1185.
21. Jablon S, Kato H. Childhood cancer in relation to prenatal exposure to atomic-bomb radiation. *Lancet* 1970;2:1000.
22. Doll R, Wakeford R. Risk of childhood cancer from fetal irradiation. *Br J Radiol* 1997;70:130.
23. Mole RH. Childhood cancer after prenatal exposure to diagnostic x-ray examinations in Britain. *Br J Cancer* 1990;62:152.
24. Loughlin KR. The management of urologic malignancies during pregnancy. *Br J Urol* 1995;76:639.
25. Weinreb JC, Brown CE, Lowe TW, Cohen JM, Erdman WA. Pelvic masses in pregnant patients: MR and US imaging. *Radiol* 1986;159:717.
26. Hass JF, Janisch W, Staneczek W. Newly diagnosed primary intracranial neoplasms in pregnant women: a population-based assessment. *J Neurol* 1986;49:874.
27. Simon RH. Brain tumors in pregnancy. *Semin Neurol* 1988;8:214.
28. Roelvink NCA, Kamphorst W, van Alphen HAM, Rao R. Pregnancy-related primary brain and spinal tumors. *Arch Neurol* 1987;44:209.
29. DeAngelis LM. Central nervous system neoplasms in pregnancy. In: Devinsky O, Feldmann E, Hainline B, eds. *Neurologic complications of pregnancy*. New York: Raven Press, 1994:139.
30. Glass J, Hochberg FH, Gruber ML, Louis DN, Smith D, Rattner B. The treatment of oligodendrogliomas and mixed oligodendroglioma-astrocytomas after PCV chemotherapy. *J Neurosurg* 1992;76:741.
31. Weissman DE. Glucocorticoid treatment for brain metastases and epidural spinal cord compression: a review. *J Clin Oncol* 1988;5:543.
32. Finfer SR. Management of labor and delivery in patients with intracranial neoplasms. *Br J Anaesth* 1991;67:784.
33. Fox MW, Harms RW, Davis DH. Selected neurologic complications of pregnancy. *Mayo Clin Proc* 1990;65: 1595.
34. Potter JF, Schoeneman M. Metastasis of maternal cancer to the placenta and fetus. *Cancer* 1970;25:380.
35. Hendleman L, Mestel AC. Multiple carcinomatosis of the colon complicating pregnancy. *Obstet Gynecol* 1958;11:119.
36. Bernstein MA, Madoff RD, Caushaj PF. Colon and rectal cancer in pregnancy. *Dis Colon Rectum* 1993;36: 172.
37. Nesbitt JC, Moise KJ, Sawyers JL. Colorectal carcinoma in pregnancy. *Arch Surg* 1985;120:636.
38. McLean DW, Arminski TW, Bradley GT. Management of primary carcinoma of the rectum diagnosed during pregnancy. *Am J Surg* 1955;90:816.
39. Heise RH, Van Winter JT, Wilson TO, Ogburn PL. Colonic cancer during pregnancy: case report and review of the literature. *Mayo Clin Proc* 1992;67:1180.
40. Stephens JD, Golbus MS, Miller TR, Wilber RR, Epstein CJ. Multiple congenital anomalies in a fetus exposed to 5-fluorouracil during the first trimester. *Am J Obstet Gynecol* 1980;137:747.
41. Parker SL, Tong T, Bolden S, et al. Cancer statistics. *Ca Cancer J Clin* 1996;65:5.
42. Ramalingam S, Pawlish K, Gadgeel S, Demers R, Kalamkerian GP. Lung cancer in young patients: analysis of a surveillance, epidemiology and end-results database. *J Clin Oncol* 1998;16:651.
43. Van Winter JT, Wilkowske MA, Shaw EG, Ogburn PL, Pritchard DJ. Lung cancer complicating pregnancy: case report and review of literature. *Mayo Clin Proc* 1995;70:384.
44. American Society of Clinical Oncology. Clinical practice guidelines for the treatment of unresectable non-small cell lung cancer. *J Clin Oncol* 1997;15:2996.
45. Kopf-Maier P. Stage of pregnancy dependent transplacental passage of 195m Pt after cisplatinum treatment. *Eur J Cancer Clin Oncol* 1983;19:533.
46. Smith RS, Randall P. Melanoma during pregnancy. *Obstet Gynecol* 1969;34:825.
47. Pack JT, Schnargel IM. Prognosis for malignant melanoma in the pregnant woman. *Cancer* 1951;4:324.
48. Slingluff CL, Reintgen DS, Vollmer RT, Seigler HF. Malignant melanoma arising during pregnancy. *Ann Surg* 1990;211:552.
49. MacKie RM, Bufalino R, Morabito A, et al. Lack of effect of pregnancy on outcome of melanoma. *Lancet* 1991;337:653.
50. McManamny DS, Moss ALH, Pocock PV, et al. Melanoma and pregnancy: long-term follow-up. *Br J Obstet Gynaecol* 1989;96:1419.
51. Grin CM, Kopf AW, Welkovich B, Bart RS, Levenstein MJ. Accuracy in the clinical diagnosis of malignant melanoma. *Arch Dermatol* 1990;126:763.
52. Rivers JK. Melanoma. *Lancet* 1996;347:803.
53. Kirkwood JM, Strawderman MH, Ernstoff MS, Smith TJ, Borden EC, Blum RH. Interferon alfa-2b adjuvant therapy of high-risk resected cutaneous melanoma: the Eastern Co-operative Oncology Group trial EST 1684. *J Clin Oncol* 1996;14:7.
54. Ho RCS. Medical management of stage IV malignant melanoma. *Cancer* 1995;75:735.
55. Harkin KP, Drumm JE, O'Brien P, Daly A. Metastatic malignant melanoma in pregnancy. *Ir Med J* 1990; 83:116.
56. Schenker JG, Granat M. Phaeochromocytoma and pregnancy—an updated appraisal. *Aust N Z J Obstet Gynaecol* 1982;22:1.
57. Harper MA, Murnaghan GA, Kennedy L, Hadden DR, Atkinson AB. Phaeochromocytoma in pregnancy: five cases and review of the literature. *Br J Obstet Gynaecol* 1989;96:594.
58. Ellison GT, Mansberger JA, Mansberger AR. Malignant recurrent pheochromocytoma during pregnancy: case report and review of the literature. *Surgery* 1988; 103:484.
59. Smith AM. Phaeochromocytoma and pregnancy. *J Obstet Gynaecol Br Commonwlth* 1973;80:848.
60. McCullough DL. Pheochromocytoma. In: Resnick MI, Kursh E, eds. *Current therapy in genitourinary surgery.* Philadelphia: CV Mosby, 1987:4.
61. Freier DT, Thompson NW. Pheochromocytoma and pregnancy: the epitome of high risk. *Surgery* 1993;114: 1148.
62. Bowerman RA, Silver TM, Jaffee MH, Struck KJ, Hinerman DC. Sonography of adrenal pheochromocytomas. *Am J Roentgenol* 1981;137:1227.

63. Greenberg M, Mowad A, Weities B. Extraadrenal pheochromocytoma: detection during pregnancy using MR imaging. *Radiology* 1986;161:475.
64. Sisson JC, Frazer MS, Valk TW. Scintigraphic localization of pheochromocytoma. *N Engl J Med* 1981;305:12.
65. Griffith MI, Felts JH, James FM, Meyers RT, Shealy GM, Woodruff LF. Successful control of pheochromocytoma in pregnancy. *JAMA* 1974;229:427.
66. Burgess GE. Alpha blockade and surgical intervention of pheochromocytoma in pregnancy. *Obstet Gynecol* 1979;53:266.
67. Wheeler MH, Chare MJB, Austin TR, Lazarus JH. The management of the patient with catecholamine excess. *World J Surg* 1982;6:735.
68. Davies AE, Navaratnarajah M. Vaginal delivery in a patient with a phaeochromocytoma. *Br J Anaesth* 1984;56:913.
69. Desmonts JM, Marty J. Anaesthetic management of patients with phaeochromocytoma. *Br J Anaesth* 1984;56:781.
70. Mitchell ZS, Frelich JD, Brant D, Flynn M. Anesthetic management of pheochromocytoma resection during pregnancy. *Anesth Analg* 1987;66:478.
71. Stuart GCE, Temple WJ. Thyroid cancer in pregnancy. In: Allen HH, Nisker JA. eds. *Cancer in pregnancy: therapeutic guidelines.* Mt Kisco, NY: Futura Publishing, 1986:191.
72. Moore JL, Martin JN. Cancer and pregnancy. *Obstet Gynecol Clin North Am* 1992;19:815.
73. Zanzonico PB. Radiation dose to patients and relatives incident to 131-I therapy. *Thyroid* 1997;7:199.
74. Casara D, Rubello D, Saladini G, et al. Pregnancy after high therapeutic doses of iodine-131 in differentiated thyroid cancer: potential risks and recommendations. *Eur J Nucl Med* 1993;20:192.
75. Doll DC, Ringenburg QS, Yarbro JW. Management of cancer during pregnancy. *Arch Intern Med* 1988;148:2058.
76. Aviles A, Diaz-Maqueo JC, Talavera A, Guzman R, Garcia EL. Growth and development of children of mothers treated with chemotherapy during pregnancy: current status of 43 children. *Am J Hematol* 1991;36:243.

Subject Index

Notes: Page numbers followed by f indicate figures; those followed by t indicate tables.

M

Q

R

S